ADVANCE PRAISE FOR

Intercultural Health Communication

"This edited volume provides a rich intersectional compilation from different expert scholars on how race, gender, sexuality, and even religion interplay with and inform culture and health. It underlines how each of these constructs are intrinsically essential to the inquiry of human communication, identity, and health behaviors.

I always encourage students to interrogate the required readings; to ask of it if their lived experiences are accurately and thoroughly depicted. I want them to become critical thinkers who push the boundaries of our heteronormative, patriarchal, typically binary scholarship and research. This book offers the groundwork for what inclusive, robust scholarship should look like. Each chapters of this text provides dynamic, transparent, even healing confirmation of how the multi-layered realities of the individual interplay with health.

I am appreciative to be able to add this text to my canonical of highly-regarded books."

—Angela Cooke-Jackson, Associate Professor, Health Communication and Behavioral Science, California State University, Los Angeles

"Spieldenner and Toyosaki's *Intercultural Health Communication* is a much needed and ground-breaking resource that disrupts the whiteness of health communication through compelling and intersectional case studies that center Other bodies and experiences by bringing to bear theories and methods of intercultural communication. This book brings together senior and up-and-coming scholars to address emerging issues in intercultural health communication."

—Bernadette Marie Calafell, Professor and Chair, Critical Race and Ethnic Studies, Gonzaga University

"*Intercultural Health Communication* is perhaps the most forward-thinking book within health communication I have seen in many years! This volume offers a brilliant set of essays on identities, body politics, health, and agency, finally giving us a rich resource for understanding the complexities of marginalized bodies."

—Ronald L. Jackson II, Author of *Scripting Black Masculine Bodies in Popular Media* and Past President of the National Communication Association

"*Intercultural Health Communication* adopts a critical perspective and connects health communication scholarship with intercultural communication. Rooted in lived experiences and cultural identities, the essays in this collection examine and interrogate the different aspects of health in the context of culture. Moreover, this collection employs global perspectives and is committed to social justice issues in the context of health communication. While this book fills a void in the literature and offers a much-needed outlook by connecting intercultural and health communication discourses, it also encourages a more expansive dialogue between these two areas in the field of communication. The essays in this collection employ critical, qualitative, and interpretive approaches to illuminate different areas and issues of intercultural health communication. Hence, they are bold, personal, provocative, critical, and thoughtful."

—Ahmet Atay, Associate Professor,
Department of Communication, College of Wooster

Intercultural Health Communication

Health Communication

Gary L. Kreps, Series Editor

Vol. 16

The Health Communication series is part of
the Peter Lang Media and Communication list.
Every volume is peer reviewed and meets
the highest quality standards for content and production.

PETER LANG
New York • Bern • Berlin
Brussels • Vienna • Oxford • Warsaw

Intercultural Health Communication

Edited by
Andrew R. Spieldenner
and Satoshi Toyosaki

PETER LANG
New York • Bern • Berlin
Brussels • Vienna • Oxford • Warsaw

Library of Congress Cataloging-in-Publication Data

Names: Spieldenner, Andrew R., editor. | Toyosaki, Satoshi, editor.
Title: Intercultural health communication / edited by Andrew R. Spieldenner and Satoshi Toyosaki.
Description: New York: Peter Lang, 2020.
Series: Health communication; vol. 16 | ISSN 2153-1277
Includes bibliographical references and index.
Identifiers: LCCN 2019057284 (print) | LCCN 2019057285 (ebook)
ISBN 978-1-4331-5652-6 (hardback) | ISBN 978-1-4331-5653-3 (paperback)
ISBN 978-1-4331-5654-0 (ebook pdf) | ISBN 978-1-4331-5655-7 (epub)
ISBN 978-1-4331-5656-4 (mobi)
Subjects: LCSH: Communication in public health. | Communication in medicine. | Intercultural communication. | Medical policy. | Health education. | Health promotion.
Classification: LCC RA423.2 .I55 2020 (print) | LCC RA423.2 (ebook) | DDC 362.101/4—dc23
LC record available at https://lccn.loc.gov/2019057284
LC ebook record available at https://lccn.loc.gov/2019057285
DOI 10.3726/b13517

Bibliographic information published by **Die Deutsche Nationalbibliothek.**
Die Deutsche Nationalbibliothek lists this publication in the "Deutsche Nationalbibliografie"; detailed bibliographic data are available on the Internet at http://dnb.d-nb.de/.

80 Broad Street, 5th floor, New York, NY 10004
www.peterlang.com

Table of Contents

Introduction: Intercultural Health Communication Studies

BY ANDREW R. SPIELDENNER, GLORIA N. PINDI, AND SATOSHI TOYOSAKI

Drawing a map is a matter of delineating boundaries between two (or more) spaces, tracing the contours of its declared territory. Within any academic discipline, these maps are meant to focus attention rather than contain knowledge. When they do contain and restrict knowledge, it becomes easier to overlook the connective tissues in the field's body. In the relatively new and often interdisciplinary field of communication, these rifts have grown such that students, faculty, and researchers in one area may not necessarily know how to engage another even though they overlap and are synergistic to collaborate and approach questions that defy our artificially constructed disciplinary demarcations. Health communication and intercultural communication are two such areas; interdisciplinary collaborations between them have already begun, and its potentiality for further interdisciplinary growth is grand.

Health communication scholarship looks at health in every conceivable way, yet often leaves issues related to culture—or even intercultural communication—untouched or operationalized in such a way that a particular discourse of identity politics is advanced. While much of the health communication scholarship examines or intervenes in people of color or international communities, intercultural communication is not involved in conceptualizing the exchange or information sharing that should occur. For instance, health communication scholars can play in a role in translational science for low health literacy or low health access communities, but how does this information become legible and important to those same groups?

Similarly, international and intercultural communication scholarship, generally speaking, does not pay explicit attention to human health and the ways in which cultural identity politics may complicate and/or situate the politics of human health. Human health threats, such as communicable diseases and pollution, do not know national boundaries and cause international and regional conflicts. In today's globalizing world, the intersection between health communication and international/intercultural communication is an imperative scholarly bridge for both to become meaningfully more complex, particular, and nuanced in our understandings of human health and culture simultaneously.

Health in/and Cultures

Health is not a neutral concept: it is historically, socially, and culturally constructed and situated. Changing notions of healthy behaviors (or ill health) are not just a matter of knowledge; they live inside discourses about the body, aesthetics, science, and the world. While health research may reveal more about a certain health condition, individuals act within particular narratives. Tanning, for instance, has been understood as healthy and beautiful in some places where a bronze glow is revered. In other regions, darker skin is considered "less desirable." Some of those regions may have skin whitening agents in body lotions that are commercially available. Based on data emerging over decades of research on skin conditions, health agencies and some organizations have begun to actively promote increased sun protection in order to prevent skin cancers. The three narratives about tanning each form a discourse that is all-encompassing and mutually exclusive.

Communities and individuals who participate in one narrative may not believe in the others—or at least enough to alter actions or lifestyles. This example is derived from a single health behavior and a single health concern. Within the broader realms of health and disease, the behaviors are a multitude, and individuals make choices based on what is communicated to them, what they know, what they value, and what they can do. The concept of health is constantly moving at various locations in the world. Capturing such a concept as it moves and evolves is important for today's globalizing and increasingly diversifying world, cultures, and communities.

Health is often understood and practiced through the biomedical and Western cultural technologies (Dutta, 2008), rendering an image of health as fixed, neutral, and objective. However, as argued earlier, health is not a neutral concept; it is performed and constrained in various ways at various locations throughout the world. In the current context, health and healthcare are embedded in neoliberalism, "emphasiz[ing] individual responsibility for health [and] minimizing the role of the state" (Cross, Davis & O'Neil, 2017, p. 7). The concept of health is developed, performed, managed, and politicized through communal and cultural practices. The issue of culture is integral to health communication studies.

Intercultural Communication and Health

Within the US context, health concerns and disparities are firmly embedded in socioeconomic status as well as identity. Race, gender, sexuality and geographic region play key factors in which illnesses and conditions enter people's lives. Police violence, for instance, is disproportionately experienced by African Americans and poor people in the US. Some of this is due to the racist history of policing in the US, and some of it has to do with increased police presence in low-income areas (thus increasing the likelihood of interaction with law enforcement). While health communication may be adept at understanding how law enforcement communicates these acts or how communities organize against this, intercultural communication provides the additional context to better understand how these forces come into play.

Within the category of people of color, health outcomes differ widely. Within the HIV epidemic, African Americans bear the largest brunt of the disease burden. According to the federal Centers for Disease Control and Prevention (CDC), African Americans are 13% of the US population, but accounted for 43% of new HIV diagnoses in 2017 (CDC, 2019a). While White HIV diagnoses have decreased since 2010, the number of Native American and Alaska Native HIV diagnoses increased by 46% (CDC, 2019c). Even within these racial categories, differences of gender and sexuality alter the picture of the epidemic. African American gay and bisexual men are more affected by HIV than any other group in the country, accounting for 26% of all new HIV diagnoses in 2017 (CDC, 2019b). Each of these identities have their own cultural values, community structures and languages around HIV risk, sex, substance use, trauma, social support and healing. In addition, each identity has specific structural challenges based on socioeconomic, education, housing and regional opportunities.

We argue that health at the individual, community and institutional levels is firmly entrenched within culture, and that interventions that reduce people to bodies without culture will remain ineffective. Latinos in the US are also more likely than White counterparts to be diagnosed with HIV and less likely to benefit from treatment due to access (CDC, 2018b). Latino gay and bisexual men have been the only population category whose HIV rate has increased since 2015 in the US, which requires an intercultural lens to respond (CDC, 2018a). HIV prevention and treatment messages cannot be just Spanish-translations of English-language social marketing; Latino gay and bisexual men have different concerns that are influenced by culture and community connections. Without understanding the intercultural aspects of this communication, then HIV prevention and services will be poorly prepared to accommodate communities of color.

The International in Intercultural Health Communication Studies

We acknowledge that intercultural health communication studies must also be inclusive of the global. Therefore intercultural health communication studies connects several interrelated areas, such as global public health, international and intercultural communication, transnationalism, and global studies. As we look at systems of communication—and how beliefs, values and understandings of the body/health/illness are embedded within it—we begin to understand how borders are structured. These borders can be regional, domestic, governmental, political, physical, cultural, ideological, and linguistic or determined by dimensions of identity such as nationality, socioeconomic class, gender, and/or sexuality. Intercultural health communication studies examines more closely how these borders are constructed and politicized and problematizes their enforcement individually, interpersonally, communally, and institutionally.

Migration is one of the defining issues of our current moment. Whether people migrate by choice or are forced into it, this movement disrupts everything in migrants' lives. As people on the move, migrants must manage new community norms, institutions, opportunities, and challenges in employment, education, and healthcare. Indeed, as migration has increased over the past decade, the profile of migrants has also changed. From the figure of the lone person going in order to send money "back home," the new migrants are families or people fleeing violence associated with their identity (e.g., religion, ethnicity, sexuality, gender identity, and health status). As these migrants create communities in their new homes, the existing populations may begin to feel threatened and respond with propaganda, policies or violence to discourage public displays of difference. When dealing with health and well-being, these discriminatory acts further exacerbate disparities.

Understanding health as a transnational issue is vital in developing appropriate solutions to critical health concerns globally such as tuberculosis, malaria,

HIV, and sexual and reproductive rights. When we allow borders to determine how we examine these health concerns, we run the risk of ignoring ongoing challenges in various regions or amongst certain groups. In the US, for instance, "End the Epidemic" initiatives have erupted across the country about HIV, which often involves increased focus on surveillance, HIV testing, access to HIV treatment, and access to HIV Pre-Exposure Prophylaxis (PrEP). While the "End the Epidemic" advocates use this as a means to focus on expansion of specific services, it also sends a message to philanthropy and government that the HIV epidemic is manageable and that it is close to being over. This is not true globally—or even in much of the US amongst key populations, such as people of trans experience, African Americans, women who experience violence, gay and bisexual men of color, immigrants, and people who engage in sex work. While US HIV advocates and organizations advance "End the Epidemic" initiatives, they need to be cautious about the potential deleterious impact this rhetoric can have in developing resourcing and policies that make sense to all communities (Spieldenner, Robinson & Woodruffe, 2019).

In this way, intercultural health communication studies begins conversations between and among parts of the field. Communication studies programs often do not connect health and intercultural communication, yet health inequities, domestically in the US and globally, are often along lines of race, ethnicity, nationality, region, religion, and socioeconomic background. We see rich possibilities in using intercultural communication as a framework to better understand the ways that communities and individuals understand health. Health communication scholars engage communities of health through research and advocacy. Intercultural health communication studies involves a range of communication scholars/activists who utilize health communication studies and intercultural communication studies. Such labor in communication studies has already begun. In the following section, we examine more closely Dutta's (2008) culture-centered approach to health communication studies.

Culture-Centered Approach

The Culture-Centered Approach (CCA) emerged as an alternative way of looking at health issues that is "value-centered and built on the notion that the ways of understanding and negotiating the meanings of health are embedded within cultural contexts and the values deeply connected with them" (Dutta, 2008, pp. 2–3). Such meaning-making process is both structural and contextual. Whereas structure "refers to the ways the healthcare system is organized and its services are delivered, and to the organization of healthcare organizations" (Dutta, 2008, p. 6), context is understood as "the rich web of intertwined local environments within which health meanings are constantly negotiated [as well as] the local setting within which life is lived" (Dutta, 2007, p. 320). As such, cultural meanings result from this structure-context dialectic as "contexts connect local cultural systems with broader social structures and provide a culturally nuanced basis for the co-construction of meanings" (Dutta, 2007, p. 320).

Central to the CCA is deconstructing "the taken-for-granted value of Western knowledge as the only way of looking at health, illness, and treatment" (Dutta, 2008, p. 88). CCA stipulates that such knowledge is "rooted in European value systems and European ways of knowing the world [as] connected to the Enlightenment project, which used the universal rationality of science to dominate over other ways of knowing" (Dutta, 2008, p. x). CCA questions how these assumptions are used in the health system "to retain the privileged position of the dominant paradigm and the power of those who practice it" (Dutta, 2008, p. 87). For example, CCA decries how the colonial legacy of Western knowledge serves as ideological tool in the medical field to reproduce "the cultural exotic other" (Dutta, 2008, 2015; Sastry & Dutta, 2012). In this othering process, state rationality and modernization of the "Western expert" is pitted against the backwardness/primitiveness of the "Third-world other." Ultimately, "central to the conceptualization of the "other" is the creation of a system of categorization, [which] serves as the basis for the intervention" (Dutta, 2007, p. 316) of Western medical approaches on the Third World body marked as "a passive body" (Sastry & Dutta, 2012, p. 524).

As a postcolonial health communication theory, CCA "seeks to critically examine the continual construction of the world into bifurcations of the 'modern' versus the 'primitive' and the discursive processes that constitute such bifurcations" (Sastry & Dutta, 2012, p. 521). In doing so, this theory interrogates the historical, political, economic, cultural, and social conditions of Western imperialism that reproduce hegemonic/colonial interventions of health in the Third World often resulting into systemic oppressions/inequities (Dutta & Basu, 2009; Sastry & Dutta, 2012). CCA challenges the universal Western medicalization of the colonized Third World body as site of disease and intervention because it often fails to take into consideration the historical context of power dynamics characterizing the West positioned as the "developed" First World in opposition to the "underdeveloped" Third World (Lupton, 1995; Sastry & Dutta, 2012). In contrast to this view, claims Dutta (2008), any medical process remains deeply contextual "such that the meaning of health is both continuous and transformative, shifting through interactions with these [historical] contexts" (p. 320).

Scholars have used the CCA to explore the health experiences of immigrant communities living in the U.S. (Dutta, 2008; Dutta & Jamil, 2013; Gao, Dutta, & Okoror, 2016; Koenig, Dutta, Kandula, & Palaniappian, 2012). Within this body of scholarship, research has mainly focused on the experiences of Asian migrants including Bangladeshi (Dutta & Jamil, 2013), Chinese (Gao et al., 2016), and Indians (Koening, Dutta, Kandula, & Palaniappan, 2012). These studies have decried health care providers' ignorance about the important role that various layers of migrants' identity–such as birthplace, immigration status, occupational status, socioeconomic status, religious background, linguistic background, and more –play in health settings (Dutta & Jamil, 2013; Gao et al., 2016; Koenig et al., 2012). In contrast, health scholars emphasize that factors such as language, cultural beliefs/ expectations, cultural understanding, and communication style should necessarily be taken into consideration because they significantly impact immigrants' access to health and the process of providing them with culturally appropriate health services (Bollini, 1993; Bollini & Siem, 1995; Dutta & Jamil, 2013; Kandula, Kersey, & Lurie, 2004).

Additionally, this body of literature has pointed that "immigrant communities are often constructed as monoliths and the voices of immigrant communities are traditionally absent from mainstream health policy and program discourses" (Dutta & Jamil, 2013, p. 170). Because the immigrant's culture is framed as an "obstacle" rather than an "asset" in the communication process, immigrants' cultural background is generally dismissed "based on the assumption that the immigrant needs to be educated in order to acculturate adequately into the [host] culture" (Dutta & Jamil, 2013, p. 172). Bollini's (1993) study on health policies for immigrant populations demonstrated that the U.S. has a "passive attitude" (p. 110) towards immigrants' health issues, "that is, which expect[s] immigrants to adapt to the health system designed for the native population" (p. 110). Additionally, Bollini and Siem (1995) decried that immigrants are faced with racism and discrimination in health settings due to their culture often perceived as alien and inappropriate. Ultimately, immigrants are monolithically interpreted as "pathologies in need of intervention" (as cited by Dutta & Jamil, 213, p. 172) within a narrow ideal of Eurocentric Western lens of what is considered as healthy or "sick"/"ill" (Dutta, 2008; Koening et.al., 2012).

Intercultural Health Communication

We editors hope that this book follows the efforts made by those who are interested in the intersection between health and cultures, such as Dutta (2008) and others. This book grew out of conversations between the editors. I (Andy) specialize in health communication, and I (Satoshi) in intercultural communication. We have developed a great professional relationship and friendship over the last few years after we met. Through our many conversations and collaborations, our approaches to our own research have increasingly complemented each other's. We also discussed that we would need to be teaching the rich intersection of health communication and intercultural communication studies. While our teaching assignments and curricula expected us to keep health communication and intercultural communication somehow "separate," we were reminded of the difficulty and near-impossibility of doing so. While frustrated, we saw an opportunity for developing a course with an interdisciplinary twist. We developed classes at our separate institutions that spoke more directly to the interdisciplinary intersection. We found a range of material to support these courses from the field of Communication but also from Anthropology, History, Sociology, and the Humanities. We wanted to have central resources to inform this approach both for research and pedagogy that would look at health and cultures as interrelated phenomena.

We hope this book functions as one of the primary sources for those who see a value in researching and teaching from the intersection between health communication studies and intercultural communication studies. In doing so, we were lucky to run into scholars from both health communication and international/intercultural communication who are interested in the interdisciplinary intersection, such as Gloria Pindi, our co-author of this introduction chapter. We are, indeed, lucky and privileged to work with the authors featured in this book.

This book is based on a premise: neither health nor culture is a neutral concept. The authors of this collection employ critical, qualitative, and interpretive research methodologies in order to engage the transnational, political, and intersectional nature of health and cultures simultaneously. We see this book as an important step towards developing a more transnational view of health communication. *Intercultural Health Communication* ties together critical public health with critical intercultural communication. Through these connections, the authors engage the health research in, amongst others: HIV, cancer, trauma, celiac disease, radioactive pollution, food politics, and prenatal care. The authors in this collection engage both health communication and international/intercultural communication studies to enrich their research. Some authors are interested in translating the rich intersection between these fields into their pedagogy.

Intercultural Health Communication is comprised of four sections. Each of these serve to advance knowledge and approaches to what we understand as health communication and intercultural communication with an international scope. At these intersections, the authors each explore a particular area that deepens what we know about how bodies, communities, health and illness are understood and communicated. These book chapters, together, continue the work started in interdisciplinary approaches to communication and health.

We entitle the first section "Engaging Interdisciplinary Approaches: Analysis, Interpretation, Critique, and Action." This section gathers researchers and thinkers that engage in emerging methodological approaches that help us research complex intersections among health and cultures. These chapters engage Dutta's (2007, 2008) culture-centered approach to health communication studies and give textual and performative means to materialize the culture-centered approach. As a result, their works help readers conceive of, envision, and engage interdisciplinary analyses, interpretations, critiques, and actions in doing intercultural health communication research.

Chen and Parsloe, in their chapter "Health Narratives and Body Politics on the Margins: Proposing Six Principles of 'EMBODY' with Cultural Others," work with Dutta's (2007, 2008) culture-centered approach to health communication research with crucial attention paid to the body politics of/from/within cultural margins. Engaging tenets of critical and interpretive intercultural communication studies, their EMBODY approach—Exposing, Mobilizing, Bearing, Othering, Disrupting, and Yin and Yang—help advance how we use the culture-centered approach to analyze, interpret, critique, and transform ourselves as narrative beings and social/cultural makings of health politics. Eguchi offers their chapter whose title is "Queer(ing) Spaces: Sexualities as Critical Intersections among Health and Intercultural Communication." In their chapter, Eguchi uses an interdisciplinary approach that queers the artificial demarcation of health communication and intercultural communication studies in order to labor toward meaningfully complex interpretations of sexuality as an always already intersectional construct, identity, and performativity. They discuss the importance of queering our research space and calls for our reflexivity to examine our own academic training of how we research. The next chapter is written by Scott and Harris. In their chapter, "The Construction of Women and their Health Across Cultures," they offer detailed analyses of how women's health, such as menstruation, has been historically and culturally constructed. Their metaresearch reviews the extensive amount of literature and shows the importance of analyzing cultures and histories in order to understand health as a temporally emerging and culturally various construct. Madlock Gatison writes the final chapter in this section. Her chapter is entitled "Moving beyond Awareness Social Media in Health and Policy Communication: The Case of the Black Women's Health Imperative's Black Women Vote 2018 National Health Policy Agenda." Her chapter begins with a claim that social, cultural, and political aspects have significant influences on health outcomes and various health disparities. Focusing on media messaging,

Madlock Gatison contemplates ways to move beyond awareness and to practice health advocacy.

The second section of this book is entitled "Engaging Selfhoods: Contextual Complexity between Biomedical and Cultural Narratives." The authors in this section bravely interrogate their own selfhood emerging from a complex context where biomedical narratives and cultural narratives interact, collide, and/or crushes. Navigating our selfhood in such a complex context is not an easy task. The researchers in this section use their own lived experiences bravely, layer them with existent research, and/or construct their personal narratives and autoethnographic essays evocatively while inviting readers to engage back their writing.

Pindi brings to us her autoethnographic piece, which reminds us how culturally complex and contested one interaction between a patient and a doctor may be, predicated upon multiple layers of biomedical narratives, (inter)cultural narratives, and personal lived experiences. In her "'I am Not Sick, I'm Hairy': Cultural Constructions of Women's Bodies in the Ob/Gyn Exam," she explores her lived experiences with her body at medical contexts both in the Democratic Republic of Congo and the United States. Robinson continues on to demonstrate how complex doctor-patient interactions can be, layered with biomedical and cultural narratives. In her "People of Color Don't Get That: An Analytic Autoethnography of Living with Celiac Disease," she describes how her identity and cultural heritage have been phenotypically reduced by her doctor, preventing her from receiving a test she needed to be diagnosed. Biomedical narratives simplify and reduce cultures to phenotypical demarcations, judged by doctors' observations, such as "people of color," while cultures are indeed more complex than such demarcations.

The third section is "Engaging Communities: Communal Complexity, Identity Politics, and Advocacy." The authors in this section rigorously research the complex interconnectedness of health and identity politics within particular communities. Further, these authors make us think of what it means to engage in health advocacy when health is constructed in various ways in various communities. These researchers employ qualitative methodologies to get at communal complexity among health, identity politics, and advocacy.

For example, Basu, Dillon, and Sastry write a chapter entitled "HIV Drugs [Are] Like My Birth Control Pill: Lived Narratives of Black and Latino MSM in an Urban American Context." Employing various qualitative interview approaches, they investigate how men of color who have sex with men, particularly Black and Latino men, understand and communicate about health and HIV/AIDS. They delve into the collected interview data and unpack how health and culture/identity politics intersect in the participants' lived experiences. Cooper and Palmedo look at how communities emerge digitally in "Social Media as a Transformative Force in

Intercultural Health Communications: A Case Study of The BADASS Army." The BADASS Army is an online group of cyber sexual assault (CSA) survivors. With the increase in revenge porn circulating online, the BADASS Army presents a way for communities to come together, educate and support each other, as well as advocate in real life and online. Hernandez offers a chapter whose title is "Mexican-American Women, Prenatal Testing, and Definitions of Fetal Health: Challenging Social Perceptions of What Is 'Healthy.'" Hernandez approaches "health" as a socially and culturally constructed concept. Particularly attending to gender, relational status, and ethnic identity, she investigates prenatal testing. In her chapter, she employs an intersectional qualitative Chicana feminist analysis to understand how two communities of Mexican-American women culturally construct "fetal health" through their lived experiences of prenatal testing.

The fourth section gathers researchers who are interested in investigating how "health" and "health practices" become complicated and contested around international, intercultural, and intercommunal borders and while border-crossing. This section is called "Engaging Borders: Intercultural Complexity, Identity Politics, and Advocacy." The researchers in this section use various qualitative and critical methodologies to investigate how "health" gets messy and politicized at the cultural borders, often implicating the marginalized.

In their "Health in the Margins: Cultural Borders in Contestation," Dutta and Kaur-Gill employ culture-centered interrogations and unearth the often hidden and erased voices of those who live in the margins of state borders. They attend to culture-centered readings of health politics that migrant laborers in Singapore experience up against the state's construction of "health" as "disease free body." They share their ethnographic and narrative research of low-skilled migrant workers in Singapore. Lengel, Smidi and Abdul-Aziz share their chapter entitled "Transcending In/Visibility, Isolation, and Stigma: Trauma-Inforced and Culture-Centric Mental Health." They locate their research at the intersection among critical intercultural communication, health, and organizational communication research. Using qualitative methodologies, they study and analyze Muslim faith-based health organizations and discuss complex marginalizing effects of mental illnesses, xenophobia, and anti-Muslim Othering and trauma associated with islamophobia. The last chapter in this section is Tullis' "Searching for a Good Death." This chapter outlines the historical and communicative origins of a good death, and considers how communities of color, people with disabilities, poor and working class, and evangelical values challenge mainstream conceptions of what it means to die well. The author aims for a more inclusive and varied definition of a good death that will open avenues for more goal-focused communication among people who are terminally ill, their families, and healthcare practitioners.

The final content section before our conclusion chapter is entitled "Engaging Classrooms: Meaningful Complexity of Teaching and Learning." The pedagogues in this section try to implement and experiment various innovative pedagogical techniques to teach and learn (from) the complex intersections among health and cultures. Capturing the complexity in teaching and learning is not easy as it requires educators to juggle theoretical, contextual, experiential, instructional, and performative complexities. These chapters engage these complexities.

Toyosaki, Seick, Swafford, Valenta, and Wagner, for example, offer each other their autoethnographic unpacking of their own lived experiences where intercultural and health politics collided. In their "Critical Intercultural Health Communication Pedagogy: An Autoethnographic Approach," they use autoethnography as a pedagogical and collaborative learning method to explore how their lived experiences are complex and particular, materializing the intersection of intercultural and health politics. Wagner, in his "Photovoice and Photobodies: Public Pedagogies of Health and Corporeality," engages his students to use technologies to productively challenge the wall between education and communities, aiming at public pedagogies. Wagner documents the uses of Photovoice technologies in the communication classroom, with particular emphasis on how embodiment, perception and identity can be brought out through Photovoice and class discussions. Finally, Wright offers her chapter entitled "When Cultural Identity Impacts Health Decisions: Using *Grey's Anatomy* to Teach Communication Theory of Identity and Agency-Identity Model." She builds a teaching plan whose goal is to complicate her health communication students' learning meaningfully. Layering Communication Theory of Identity and Agency-Identity Model, she aims at developing the students' theoretical and analytical skills to unpack their observations of doctor-patient communication and decision-making processes.

After these content sections, Toyosaki and Spieldenner, the editors of this edited collection, write a conclusion chapter. In "Intercultural Health Communication Studies: Looking Forward," we reflect upon their journey of editing this collection. We reaffirm that health communication and intercultural communication can benefit from each other. The interdisciplinary approach of intercultural health communication helps us investigate and interrogate how health and cultures are historically, socially, economically, politically, and ideologically co-constructed and situated within our everyday lives. It may be advantageous for Intercultural health communication studies to model Martin and Nakayama's (1999) dialectic approach. Such complex interparadigmatic approaches help researchers explore the complexity and messiness of health and cultural politics. They further offer several discussion points on which health communication and intercultural communication scholars can come together to continue collaborating for the future.

Concluding Thoughts

Intercultural Health Communication emerges from a broad need to address connections and challenges to incorporating health communication with intercultural communication approaches. After compiling this book, we see ready connections to public health, global studies, gender and sexuality studies and ethnic studies. In this day and age, nation-states have to be considered within the broader frameworks of globalization, transnationalism and global health. To ignore these connections is to pretend that we are still living 20th century lives, where borders are structured as matter-of-fact or already-established lines. We recognize that the contemporary health issues require an understanding of culture as integral towards eliminating health disparities.

References

Bollini, P. (1993). Health for immigrants and refugees in the 1990s. A comparative study in seven receiving countries. *Innovation: The European Journal of Social Science Research, 6*, 101–110.

Bollini, P., & Siem, H. (1995). No real progress towards equity: Health of migrants and ethnic minorities on the eve of the year 2000. *Social Science & Medicine, 41*, 819–828.

CDC. (2018a). *HIV and Hispanic/Latino gay and bisexual men.* Washington, DC: Department of Health and Human Services. Accessed May 5, 2019 at: https://www.cdc.gov/hiv/pdf/group/msm/cdc-hiv-factsheet-msm-hispanic-latino.pdf

CDC. (2018b). *HIV and Hispanics/Latinos.* Washington, DC: Department of Health and Human Services. Accessed May 5, 2019 at: https://www.cdc.gov/hiv/pdf/group/racialethnic/hispaniclatinos/cdc-hiv-latinos.pdf

CDC. (2019a). *HIV and African Americans.* Washington, DC: Department of Health and Human Services. Accessed May 5, 2019 at: https://www.cdc.gov/hiv/pdf/group/racialethnic/africanamericans/cdc-hiv-africanamericans.pdf

CDC. (2019b). *HIV and African American gay and bisexual men.* Washington, DC: Department of Health and Human Services. Accessed May 5, 2019 at: https://www.cdc.gov/hiv/pdf/group/msm/cdc-hiv-bmsm.pdf

CDC. (2019c). *HIV and American Indians and Alaska Natives.* Washington, DC: Department of Health and Human Services. Accessed May 5, 2019 at: https://www.cdc.gov/hiv/pdf/group/racialethnic/aian/cdc-hiv-aian-fact-sheet.pdf

Cross, R., Davis, S., & O'Neil, I. (2017). *Health communication: Theoretical and critical perspectives.* Cambridge, UK and Malden, MA: Polity Press.

Dutta, M. J. (2007). Communicating about culture and health: Theorizing culture-centered and cultural sensitivity approaches. *Communication Theory, 17*, 302–328.

Dutta, M. J. (2008). *Communicating health: A culture-centered approach.* Cambridge, UK: Polity Press.

Dutta, M. J. (2015). Decolonizing communication for social change: A culture-centered approach. *Communication Theory, 25,* 123–143.

Dutta, M. J., & Basu, B. (2009). Sex Workers and HIV/AIDS: Analyzing participatory culture-centered health communication strategies. *Human Communication Research, 35,* 86–114.

Dutta, M. J., & Jamil, R. (2013). Health at the margins of migration: Culture-centered co-constructions among Bangladeshi immigrants. *Health Communication, 28,* 170–182.

Gao, H., Dutta, M., & Okoror, T. (2016). Listening to Chinese immigrant restaurant workers in the Midwest: Application of the culture-centered approach (CCA) to explore perceptions of health and health care. *Health Communication, 31*(6), 727–737.

Kandula, N. R., Kersey, M., & Lurie, N. (2004). Assuring the health of immigrants: What the leading health indicators tell us. *Annual Review of Public Health, 25,* 357–376.

Koening, C. J., Dutta, M. J., Kandula, N., & Palaniappan, L. (2012). "All of those things we don't eat": A culture-centered approach to dietary health meanings for Asian Indians living in the United States. *Health Communication, 27,* 818–828.

Lupton, D. (1995). *The imperative of health: Public health and the regulated body.* London: Sage, doi: 10.4135/9781446221976.

Martin, J. N., & Nakayama, T. K. (1999). Thinking dialectically about culture and communication. *Communication Theory, 9*(1), 1–25.

Sastry, S., & Dutta, M. J. (2012). Public health, global surveillance, and the "emerging disease" worldview: A postcolonial appraisal of PEPFAR. *Health Communication, 27,* 519–532.

Spieldenner, A. R., Robinson, T. M., & Woodruffe, A. (2019). The end of AIDS?: A critical examination of the National HIV/AIDS Strategy, in H. Harris (Ed.), *Neorace realities in the Obama Era* (p. 93–105). Albany, NY: SUNY Press.

PART 1

Engaging Interdisciplinary Approaches: Analysis, Interpretation, Critique, and Action

CHAPTER ONE

Health Narratives and Body Politics on the Margins: Proposing Six Principles of "EMBODY" with Cultural Others

BY YEA-WEN CHEN AND SARAH PARSLOE

In her 2016 blog post, "Being Black Looking Good While Chronically Ill," disability advocate and community activist, Rachel Lovejoy, narrates the ways in which her identity as a woman/mother/person of color subjected her to intersecting experiences of marginalization in the U.S. healthcare system. Lovejoy began experiencing chronic headaches, fatigue, and numbness in her arms and legs in the late 1990s, symptoms that were exacerbated by her child's birth. Doctors attributed her symptoms to psychological issues and prescribed "happy pills," following a historical pattern of equating women's health-related complaints with "hysteria." When she left the maternity ward, an elderly female volunteer advised her, "Be sure to use protection, your people are known to get pregnant fast" (Lovejoy, 2016, para. 4). As a new mother with a biracial child, she experienced frequent microaggressions—subtle, commonplace, and relentless verbal, nonverbal, and/or environmental assaults, insults, or invalidations (e.g., Pierce, 1974). "Door to door salesmen addressed me as the nanny or housekeeper," Lovejoy recounts. "Other moms at home assumed I was lost when I went to our local park .... I was perceived as a social-racial anomaly or other and I felt pretty isolated" (para. 4).

When Lovejoy's mysterious symptoms complicated delivery of her second child, healthcare providers refused to respond to her requests for pain medication. "An anesthesiologist said I was too fat for an epidural," Lovejoy recalls. "Who says that to a pregnant woman? Oh wait, I'm black" (para. 5). Lovejoy blacked out repeatedly over the course of four-and-a-half hours and hemorrhaged enough to require two blood infusions, yet the nurse initially accused her of exaggerating her pain. Even as Lovejoy's symptoms worsened, healthcare providers discounted her complaints. One doctor claimed that she must be bored, suggesting that taking a job would help her to feel better. Insurance companies refused to cover her medical exams. Eventually, when Lovejoy lost vision in her right eye, she was bandied about between "vague, patronizing specialists" (para. 7). When a likely explanation—multiple sclerosis (MS)—finally emerged, her neurologist withheld diagnosis. "He said, 'Your tests show markers of this disease,'" Lovejoy remembers. "I'm not diagnosing you with it. (Scoffing sigh,) I only know white patients with this disease. And YOU'RE BLACK!" (para. 8).

Like many individuals with relatively invisible chronic conditions, Lovejoy found that others believed she looked too good to be sick. In Lovejoy's case (and, likely, in the cases of people of color generally), others' disbelief is augmented by implicit or unacknowledged racism. For example, Lovejoy writes that, when she parks in an accessible stall, there is often "a slow-talking, over-annunciating person ready, white-splaining to me why I, a disabled, college educated, licensed driver who's blackity-black and isn't in a wheelchair, can't park there" (para. 13).

Outraged by her continued mistreatment, Lovejoy became an advocate for persons with disabilities. Frequently, she found that she was the only person of color included on community boards and in national initiatives. In her blog post, Lovejoy expresses frustration with her continued tokenization: "I'm traumatized by the passive-aggressive, clueless (racist) nature of non-profit organizations pulling in money to address POC's needs and who aren't prepared to seek out POC professionals and pay them to work on it" (para. 12).

Lovejoy's narrative reflects intersectional experiences of Othering based on sex and gender, race, and ability in healthcare, public, and advocacy-related settings. Sexism undergirds paternalistic encounters with health experts and flippant dismissals of her invisible chronic pain. Racism fuels biased judgments that she is a promiscuous, lazy drug-seeker whose black body cannot satisfy white diagnostic criteria—or else, that she is a passive, token black person in need of white charity. Ableism (re)enforces disciplining notions of what disability "should" look like. Lovejoy's narrative underscores the necessity of adopting a critical perspective in exploring and better understanding health narratives on the margins—both narratives told by patients, and (meta)narratives internalized by healthcare providers and the general public. Thus, in this chapter, we synthesize intercultural theorizing and health narrative literature to conceptualize "EMBODY"—six guiding principles for centering the health narratives with cultural Others.

(Counter)Storying across Cultural Margins

"We write as an Other, and for an Other" (Boylorn & Orbe, 2014, p. 15). A number of intercultural communication scholars have storied lived experiences and intersectional identities on the margins as critical reflections, (critical) autoethnography, (counter)narratives, and others (e.g., Boylorn & Orbe, 2014; Chen, 2014; Griffin, Ward, & Philips, 2014). Even though there are serious health implications of living with social, political, and communicative processes as cultural Others, the topic of health has rarely been a focus of (counter)storytelling in intercultural communication scholarship. The tradition of (counter)storytelling has much to offer in (re)thinking and broadening health narratives to be more inclusive of individuals and communities on the margins. In particular, the (counter)storytelling tradition within intercultural communication scholarship not only privileges stories of bodies living on/with/in-between the margins, but also highlights the ways in which health narratives are always already raced, gendered, classed, and intersected. In the section below, we synthesize how intercultural communication scholars have considered—and/or can revision—the stories of the Others and their health encounters.

First and foremost, research on health (status) disparities has established particular ways in which cultural Others (such as racial and ethnic minorities, women of color, and low-income immigrants) differentially experience health access, care services, outcomes, and more (e.g., Dutta & Jamil, 2013; Oetzel, DeVargas, Ginossar, & Sanchez, 2007; Williams & Collins, 2001). For instance, Williams and Collins (2001) evidence that "racial residential segregation is a fundamental cause of racial disparities in health," especially for African Americans, due to lower socioeconomic status that determined access to education and employment opportunities, which in turn limited availability of health care access and services (p. 404). Consistently, scholars across disciplines have argued for the need to unpack how social, cultural, and economic factors (also known as determinants) impact health; moreover, they have urged academics to (re)imagine more equitable, heuristic, and collaborative approaches to reduce disparities such as community-based participatory research (e.g., Dutta, 2007; Wallerstein & Duran, 2016). Considering that cultures in a variety of functions, formations, and contestations play important roles in health (disparities), we echo Oetzel's call that "intercultural scholars need to engage actively with interdisciplinary collaborators and community collaborators to address key issues and particularly inequalities in society" such as health disparities (Alexander et al., 2014, p. 71). In particular, (counter)storytelling from and with cultural Others can shed light on and/or point out fruitful directions for examining how interlocking social and cultural structures (re)produce health disparities vis-à-vis everyday communication choices and practices.

Among sociocultural determinants that impact health, intercultural communication scholarship, in particular, highlights racism as an urgent local and global problem. This can be evidenced by two recent special issues on race(ing) intercultural communication edited by Moon and Holling (Holling & Moon, 2015; Moon & Holling, 2015), and various autoethnographic research and (composite) (counter)storytelling regarding race relations across contexts (e.g., Boylorn & Orbe, 2014; Griffin et al., 2014). Collectively, (critical) intercultural communication research on race indicates the centrality of race and power of white supremacy in orchestrating intercultural communication interactions. Holling and Moon (2015) observe that more intercultural communication scholars have focused on race in media, academia, and vernacular discourses than any other contexts. They continue to call for close analyses of race (especially through intersectional and comparative lenses), critiques of post-racial discourses, and tactics of intervention. Furthermore, race-based (counter)storytelling indicates that narrative is a powerful and more accessible and compelling avenue/method/vehicle for "inviting readers into the lived experienced of a presumed 'Other' and to experience it viscerally" (Boylorn & Orbe, 2014, p. 15). Three of the thirteen chapters in Boylorn and Orbe's (2014) book are written about health-related topics: making place with cancer by Mingé and Sterner; negotiating privilege/disadvantage as a student and faculty member with a nonvisible disability by Morella-Pozzi; and surviving lymphoma by Crawley. They all depict layered, contextual, and nuanced experiences with health and illness at the intersection of various identities and subjectivities. Together, these insights suggest two directions of interweaving health narratives and (critical) intercultural communication: (a) a continued call for privileging analyses of the contours of race, racial logic, and race relations within health care contexts as intersecting with other relevant identity positions; and (b) a need for systematically documenting the labors and health impacts of confronting/surviving/resisting racism and other unequal systems via (counter)storytelling.

Considering the body as a site of knowledge and "a powerful set of signifiers in social relations," Yep (2013) urges intercultural communication scholars to engage in queering/quaring/kauering/crippin'/transing Other bodies not just in terms how they are read but also how they become constructed, translated, and disembodied as foreign (p. 118). Thus, Yep (2013) promotes the practice of queering/quaring/kauering/crippin'/transing Other bodies as "embodied translation" in intercultural communication research that asks for whom are Other bodies translated and under what power relations (Chávez, 2009, p. 25). Yep argues that "Embodied translation can help intercultural communication scholars queer/

quare/kauer/crip/trans bodies through its attention to, and unpacking of, the cultural perspectives and the constructions of normativity of their projects" (2013, p. 123). Yep's approach offers a valuable lens to consider ways of queering/quaring/kauering/crippin'/transing health narratives across cultural margins.

In the very spirit of (counter)storytelling, the culture-centered approach (CCA) (to health) leads the way for promoting marginalized cultural voices and communities and their health needs across local and global contexts. Departing from top-down and message-based behavior approached to health communication, CCA focuses on structural inequalities and conditions that constitute health disparities in the first place (Dutta, 2007; Dutta & Jamil, 2013). More importantly, CCA champions for the agency of cultural voices on the margins to articulate their own health needs and also for spaces for them to be heard on their own terms. While CCA affirms and reinforces the ethos of intercultural communication scholarship, CCA remains more influential in the study of health communication than intercultural communication research. Extending Holling and Moon's (2015) question of "What institutions do we neglect, and why?" we wonder if uncommon (counter)stories about health and illness by intercultural communication scholars who are often people of color only evidence the power of racism. Thus, our theorizing is guided by CCA to bring together health institutions, (counter)storytelling, and (inter)cultural communication.

Landscaping Health Narratives

People live in and through idiosyncratic bodies. Yet, while embodied experiences are inherently individual, they are also social; we draw on cultural discourses of health, illness, and wellness as we attach meaning to our own and others' bodies (Sharf & Vanderford, 2003; Yamasaki, 2009). As Frank (2006) writes:

> [People's] bodily awareness is constantly being reshaped by health as ideals and evaluations … What I notice about my body, what I attend to or disregard, how I act on what I notice, what I worry about and what I take satisfaction in—all these are being informed by the flow of stories that affect my embodied sense of health. (p. 423)

These stories—or *health narratives*—constitute health by storying (un)healthy bodies and (un)healthy practices. Thus, health narratives are inherently ideological; they inform both a private and a public "mindset" about who/what counts as (un) healthy (Harter, Japp, & Beck, 2005).

Frank (2006) equates health narratives to "plug-ins." They serve as sense-making programs or scripts, which direct individual patients to engage in specific health-related practices, including practices of self-care, decision-making and treatment, and risk assessment and avoidance. Narratives gain weight as they are re-told and re-affirmed by families, communities, and institutions, solidifying into cultural "collections of normative meanings" embedded in "myths, fairy tales, histories, and other stories" (Harter et al., 2005, p. 20). For instance, Manoogian, Harter, and Denham's (2010) research on Appalachian family health legacies of type 2 diabetes described how participants acted as "intergenerational lynchpins" or "intergenerational buffers," telling or silencing stories of family members' past experiences to shape current disease management strategies and assessments of risk. Over time, we become "anchored" in particular narratives that guide our reasons for (not) acting (Harter & Bochner, 2009). In doing so, we develop a "health consciousness" (Frank, 2006)—otherwise known as a metanarrative, master narrative, or grand narrative of health—that encourages us to reject competing stories in the process of cultivating a set of taken-for-granted assumptions about health.

In the West, the biomedical model has taken hold as the dominant master narrative of health. The narrative of biomedicine "reduces disease to a biological mechanism of cause and effect that can be effectively diagnosed and treated through science and technology" (Harter et al., 2005, p. 22). In doing so, it both constitutes an ideal, "normal" body and reinforces dichotomous ways of thinking about embodiment: bodies are normal/pathological, healthy/sick, able-bodied/disabled, and more. The biomedical narrative conscripts individuals into participating in the "sick role" (Parsons, 1951); sick persons are always expected to seek out and follow medical expertise, engaging in "narrative surrender" (Frank, 1995) as they story their experiences using the "voice of medicine" rather than the "voice of the lifeworld" (Mishler, 1984). By privileging expert knowledge over embodied ways of knowing/feeling/sensing, the biomedical model discounts narratives that attach personal and cultural significance to the physical experiences of pain, nausea, fatigue, etc. Further, the biomedical model individualizes illness, disconnecting individual patients from communal experiences—and structural causes—of suffering and healing.

Clearly, while biomedicine has produced important advances in treating disease and remedying physical and cognitive impairment, the biomedical master narrative can function as a type of "narrative imperialism" (Frank, 2004), particularly when it stigmatizes Other bodies and discounts Other ways of understanding/doing *health*. Indeed, Western health practitioners engage in this kind of imperialism as they build NGOs and develop and implement health campaigns across the Global South. Neoliberal health organizing (Dutta, 2015) works to silence narratives that link health threats to colonization and market-driven exploitation, focusing instead on offering/selling technological solutions to illness. Even within

Western cultures, the biomedical narrative obscures social determinants of health in ways that perpetuate racism, classism, (hetero)sexism, and ableism. In the following sections, we explore how bodies are Othered and/or resist Othering in the contexts of (a) diagnostic narratives and the medical encounter, (b) illness narratives and identity construction, and (c) narratives of advocacy/activism.

Diagnostic Narratives and the Medical Encounter

In the context of medical encounters, patients and healthcare providers tell/elicit *diagnostic narratives*, translating embodied sensations using the languages of symptomology and pathology. Such translations run the risk of reducing bodies to biology at the expense of biography, ignoring the idea that people live in/through bodies that are situated in relational and cultural contexts. In contrast, "narrative medicine recognizes that the central events of health care are the giving and receiving of accounts of self" (Charon, 2009, p. 120). Healthcare providers act as witnesses, listening both to patients' accounts of their lived experiences and to accounts provided by the patient's "self-telling body" (Charon, 2009). Langellier (2009) proposed a performative approach to narrative medicine that requires "listening out loud"—attending to the "gestures of hands and posture, glances and gazes, inflections of voice" and silences that accompany patients' verbal accounts. She notes that, by focusing on the Other's body, healthcare providers can listen empathically while maintaining the distance of disidentification necessary to avoid appropriating the Other's story.

Yet, while narrative medicine attempts to fulfill an ethical obligation to listen to and affirm patients' stories, narrative scholars must also recognize that listeners are always "embedded in socio-political contexts that shape the boundaries of story accessibility, listening, and interpretation" (Matthews & Sunderland, 2017, p. 125). In the case of medicine, diagnostic narratives are constructed from diagnostic criteria that, historically, have been developed in reference to white/Western/male/cisgender/neurotypical bodies. Additionally, stereotypes attached to Othered bodies may shape clinicians' listening in ways that cause them to make attributional errors (Groopman, 2007). Thus, we argue that it would be fruitful for critical health and (inter)cultural scholars to consider the ways in which bodies are and/or become Othered in experiences of remaining undiagnosed, being misdiagnosed, or underdiagnosed, where doctors correctly identify only some of the patient's symptoms.

Even the process of "listening out loud" is shaped by cultural expectations; Langellier (2009) notes that patients' narratives are embodied via routinized "habits of the body" (p. 153)—repertoires of gesture and voice cultivated through repeated social interactions. When cultural Others' verbal accounts and embodied performances of illness do not conform to dominant expectations of how a sick person "should" act, their health concerns might be ignored. Worse, they might be accused of malingering or "crying wolf" (Thompson, Lin, & Parsloe, 2017) about their health. As such, critical health and (inter)cultural scholars might explore the concepts of epistemic injustice, a "specific kind of injustice done to someone in their capacity as a knower" of their own body (Blease, Carel, & Geraghty, 2016, p. 3); and testimonial injustice, when individuals' prejudices make them unlikely to listen to, acknowledge, or act on a person's narrative (Carel & Kidd, 2014; Matthews & Sunderland, 2017). Research might draw particularly interesting connections between Othered bodies and poorly understood, contested health conditions, such as myalgic encephalomyelitis (also known as chronic fatigue syndrome; Blease et al., 2017). For example, Jennifer Brea's 2017 documentary, *Unrest*,[1] depicts her journey as a mixed-race (black and white) woman who was told that her ME symptoms were "all in her head." In creating and sharing this narrative, Brea both re-authors her illness identity and engages in health activism.

Illness Narratives and Identity Constructions

While *health* narratives guide cultural understandings of what counts as (un) healthy, *illness narratives* emerge as individuals respond to the epistemic threats of impairment. When people become sick, they (co-)construct illness narratives in the process of re-authoring fractured identities and re-stor(y)ing ruptured life trajectories. Through emplotment, narratees impose temporal structure on the jumbled morass of their lived experiences (Bosticco & Thompson, 2008; Sharf & Vanderford, 2003). Selecting and ordering life events allows narratees to engage in self-authorship, to gain a sense of control over emotional experiences, and to situate themselves in relation to motivated characters and in meaningful contexts. Frank (1995) proposed three primary illness narratives—the chaos narrative, the quest narrative, and the restitution narrative. Chaos narratives emphasize the uncertain, unpredictable, and inexplicable experience of illness; they are "antinarratives in that they are told from within dehumanized time—time without order and thus without meaning" (Frank, 2004, p. 213). Quest narratives emphasize resilience, epiphany, and self-change (Frank, 1993). Finally, restitution narratives focus on recovery and cure, often emphasizing a reliance on medical treatment and technology.

Constructing an illness narrative is an inherently dialogic activity. Individuals story their lives within specific social and cultural contexts, and in collaboration with real and imagined listeners. Thus, narratives are (co)-created within discursive boundaries; we tend to tell stories that will likely be understood and accepted by a specific audience. For this reason, illness stories often participate in dominant (biomedical) narratives, constituting "truth discourses" (White & Epson, 1990) about the nature of health and illness. Individuals experience deep personal distress when they are forced to participate in dominant narratives that "allow insufficient space for the performance of the person's preferred stories" (White & Epson, 1990, p. 14). As critical health and (inter)cultural scholars, we must ask: how do (intersecting) experiences of Othering (racism, sexism, ableism, classism, and heterosexism) by story listeners shape tellers' illness narratives? How might experiences of inaccessible, inadequate, and culturally insensitive healthcare permeate chaos narratives and preclude restitution narratives? How might stereotypes trap individuals in particular quest narratives, that is, the expectation that a "strong black woman" with breast cancer should always enact the warrior identity of pink ribbon culture (Madlock Gatison, 2016)? For instance, individuals may participate in dominant narratives that blame them for their illnesses, rather than narrating lived experiences of oppression that contribute to health inequities. Additionally, illness narratives that endorse a biomedical perspective preclude telling empowering *disability narratives.* Such narratives frequently adopt the social model of disability, which focuses on the ways in which ableism and stigma oppress individuals with physical and cognitive differences (Shakespeare, 2013). Empowering disability narratives reframe disability as culture, and as a politicized collective whose members must organize to protect the community's rights (Cardillo, 2010; Coopman, 2003). For instance, some autistic individuals share narratives that reframe and reclaim autism "symptoms" as positive aspects of their collective identity (Parsloe, 2015), organizing via social media to resist calls for a cure (Parsloe & Holton, 2017).

By producing self-policing, "docile bodies,"—as well as inhospitable audiences—dominant narratives obscure "subjugated knowledges," or the local, indigenous, regional, or "subaltern" knowledges that "are currently in circulation but are denied or deprived of the space in which they could be adequately performed" (White & Epson, 1990, p. 26). Dutta (2015) used the term "communicative inequality" to describe the idea that oppressed members of a society tend to have less access to technologies of story production and circulation. In other words, "the media" tend to represent white/heterosexual/cisgender/upper-middle class/able-bodied perspectives.

Yet, subjugated knowledge persists in stories told at the margins of society, emerging as *counternarratives* or *counterstories* that resist or disrupt archetypal plots (Lindemann Nelson, 1996). Marginalized storytellers gain narrative agency as they identify and story "unique outcomes" (White & Epson, 1990)—details of their own lived experiences that do not fit with or conform to norms and expectations specified by the dominant narrative. With the advent of the Internet and social media, marginalized storytellers gained the ability to circulate counternarratives more widely. Indeed, Matthews and Sunderland (2017) define *digital storytelling* as "life-story telling in a variety of mediated forms deployed to prompt social change" (p. 4). Initially, the digital storytelling movement involved creating and curating discrete stories, often composed of 3–5 minute video and/or audio clips with first-person narration such as those curated by organizations like StoryCorps.[2] In contrast, contemporary digital storytelling is often accomplished through "fragmented, collaboratively compiled narratives, like a Twitter feed" (Matthews & Sunderland, 2017, p. 5), offering complex, "polyphonic" (or many-voiced) (Kreuter et al., 2007) accounts of illness- and disability-related experiences. By engaging in digital storytelling, members of marginalized communities tell counternarratives as part of health advocacy and activism initiatives. Yet, while digital and technological advancements have made available more and more counternarratives, the availability of counternarratives does not guarantee that they are or will be heard.

Advocacy/Activism Narratives and Health (in)Equities

By defining health problems, locating their causes, and selecting and justifying particular solutions, health narratives offer rationales for collective (in)action, including health advocacy, health activism, and policymaking (Yamasaki, Geist-Martin, & Sharf, 2017; Guttman, 2000; Zoller, 2005). Health advocacy relies on expert knowledge to work within the medical establishment, supporting biomedical definitions of health, illness, and disability (Brown et al., 2004). In contrast, health activism makes use of lay stories to challenge oppressive power structures that create and preserve health inequities. Health activists disrupt the status quo by targeting "social norms, embedded practices, policies, or the dominance of certain social groups" (Zoller, 2005, p. 344). For instance, health activists' narratives might undergird health social movements designed to reveal the ways in which racism, (hetero)sexism, ableism, and classism intersect to (a) block access to quality healthcare, (b) produce layered sources of stigma that exacerbate illness- and disability-related challenges, and (c) create social conditions that lead to health problems. Zoller (2005) encourages critical health scholars to study how these health narratives facilitate identification. For instance, shared stories of racism and cultural insensitivity in healthcare contexts support a politicized collective identity (Brown et al., 2004) among (immigrant) patients of color, mobilizing self-organizing for social change. By incorporating these narratives in public appeals, health activists might recruit allies to their cause.

However, telling a counternarrative for health activism does not guarantee that policymakers will actually listen. For instance, Matthews and Sunderland (2017) noted that patient stories told as part of healthcare provider training, or in an attempt to transform healthcare organizations' problematic practices, are frequently selected and/or edited for listenability/palatability by institutional gatekeepers. They observed that "the 'management' of raw emotion in these narratives, and the shaping of their affective power, might be seen as instances of professionals and organizations refusing to listen or limiting their listening to certain conditions" (Matthews & Sunderland, 2017, p. 95).

Similarly, in the process of becoming mediated, digital stories are often "moved beyond the direct 'reach' or control of the storyteller" (Matthews & Sunderland, 2017, p. 8). While "story caretakers" act to ensure the ethical use and reuse of mediated stories, "story curators" actively fit mediated stories into a larger collection to support a metanarrative for a specific purpose (i.e., to generate PR for a hospital; to generate revenue for a media organization). As Matthews and Sunderland (2017) emphasize, "the power of editing is equated with a capacity, and perhaps willingness, to harm the storyteller" (p. 105). Critical health and (inter)cultural scholars might study the ways in which health activism narratives told by members of marginalized groups are altered and exploited through the process of mediation. For instance, rather than listening to raw stories' bids for social change, institutions might share edited stories as evidence of commitment to "diversity." Similarly, media professionals might reinforce the biomedical model by producing "inspiration porn"—stories that frame disability as an inherently pitiable condition that can and should be overcome through personal effort and/or medical intervention (Young, 2014).

Matthews and Sunderland (2017) define listening itself as a process of mediation, which involves "inevitable dislocations and transformations of meaning and agency" (p. 7). Similarly, Frank (2006) describes stories as "out-of-control" in the sense that they are perpetually being re-decontextualized by different listeners situated in different listening contexts. For instance, Frank (2006) notes that *unbearable health stories*, or stories of times when healthcare is unavailable or inaccessible, might be heard either as calls for activism or as reasons to more firmly disavow personal responsibility for another person's health. He describes a similarly divided response to *stories of strategic health*, where people gain access to (or are denied access to) health resources based on their ability to learn and enact self-advocacy strategies. Frank (2006) explains:

> Some readers will take these stories as good advice, and others will see such stories as indicators of the sickness of a health care system that requires people to be strategic and favors patients who are capable of strategic action. (p. 425)

Critical health and (inter)cultural scholars might study the ways in which storytellers and story curators cultivate contexts for listening that encourage audiences to "read" narratives in particular ways. We begin this work by theorizing EMBODY—six principles for centering the health narratives of cultural Others.

"EMBODY" Culture-Centered Health Narratives

Guided by the CCA, we build on previous scholarship on (counter)storytelling and health narratives to propose an approach of **EMBODY**-ing culture-centered health narratives for activism. In the CCA's spirit of creating spaces for—while recognizing the agency of—cultural voices to articulate their health needs, our proposal theorizes six guiding principles: (a) Exposing dichotomous and hegemonic "health consciousness"; (b) Mobilizing voices from below; (c) Bearing witness to the Other's "exile narratives"; (d) Othering the cultural self; (e) Disrupting diagnoses in the medical encounter; and (f) (excavating) "Yin-yang." Ultimately, the goal of EMBODY-ing cultural voices in health narratives is open up and create new spaces for cultural voices to embody their stories as much as their stories embody them (Rodriguez, 2015).

Exposing Dichotomous and Hegemonic "Health Consciousness"

The process of creating spaces for culturally-informed/embodied health narratives begins with a critical response to willingly see, understand, and expose how our normalized grand narratives of health—or what Frank (2006) calls "health consciousness"—routinely and habitually reject such cultural voices. The hegemonic master narratives normalize dichotomous thinking/feeling/knowing of bodies as either normal or pathological, same or different, healthy or sick, able-bodied or disabled, etc., which then render any alternative worldviews inferior, undesirable, and/or incompetent. Further, the dichotomous health consciousness is (re)enforced in/by the biomedical model and (re)produces the status quo of Western imperialism and whiteness both inside and outside medicine. Thus, to interrupt the dichotomous and hegemonic heath consciousness starts with questioning, challenging, and unpacking what stories of/about health have been taken for granted, and what underlying assumptions they hold true about health and illness.

Exposing hegemonic health narratives itself will not automatically lead to honoring cultural voices that have long been ignored, neglected, and/or silenced in the face of racism/(hetero)sexism/ableism/classism. Also, undoing hegemonic narratives—or the routinized habits of consenting to certain stories over others—takes more than just one-time effort, but also sustained vigilance and critical self-reflexivity at individual and communal levels. This is one of the first and necessary step(s) toward creating new vocabulary, tools, and spaces for honoring the dignity and humanity of cultural voices and bodies that have long struggled to feel, know, speak and be heard on their own terms (Chen, 2018).

Mobilizing Voices from Below

In response to the Other being spoken for and written about, the CCA advocates for "writing theory from below" through engaging with voices that have traditionally been silenced (Dutta, 2007, p. 311). Writing/Thinking/Theorizing from below is not a linear nor straightforward process. Considering that racism/(hetero)sexism/ableism/classism/xenophobia thrives through strategies of dividing and conquering, we argue for a necessary initial step of political mobilization from below. Mobilizing from below seeks to create spaces for individuals and communities that have long battled/survived injustices to connect, (re)learn, and embrace their cultural legacies without having to defend them. Such spaces might serve as enclaves for reconnecting with one's body, allowing one's body to breathe/be/think/feel freely, and possibly for healing and more. By doing so, mobilizing from below strives to move from individualized to collectivized voices for readying to do the work ahead.

Bearing Witness to the Other's "Exile Narratives"

Rodriguez's (2015) notion of the "exile narratives" speaks to stories that become "narratives in exile" struggling to find home in a mainstream space that is ideologically, epistemologically, and/or stylistically unaccustomed to such narratives (p. 105). Moreover, Rodriguez argues that it is possible to find home in exile as home and exile are not mutually exclusively for the Others. Recognizing the Others' full agency to speak their truth(s) and embody their stories, the challenge falls on the listeners who are witnessing exile narratives. Boler (1999) argues that, in contrast to spectating, witnessing "is a process in which we do not have the luxury to seeing a static truth or fixed certainty … as a witness we undertake our historical responsibilities" (p. 186). That is, witnessing is an embodied experience of savoring the visceral experiences of the Other while attending to the luxury of our privileged positions. Unlike spectating, witnessing entails ethical responsibilities and responses and adds to Langellier's (2009) idea of "listening out loud" with the Other.

Othering the Cultural Self

Dutta (2007) explains that the act of othering—the process of reducing, objectifying, and making one into the Other—"does violence to the culture by fixing it in terms of static characteristics" (p. 316). While the Other is more accustomed to looking at one's self through the eyes of others, individuals and members from privileged positions are rarely, if ever, required to do so. The asymmetry of having to or not engaging in what W. E. B. DuBois calls "double-consciousness" poses great challenges for (counter)storytelling and intercultural communication. Hence, we argue that the practicing of othering one's self especially for individuals from more privileged positions is a productive exercise that can increase one's capacity for empathy. In addition, we argue that moments of encountering the Other can become a space with intimate distance to better understand one's taken-for-granted cultural values, beliefs, and assumptions.

Disrupting Diagnoses in The Medical Encounter

Groopman (2007) cautions that all the unexamined stereotypes and implicit biases medical professionals carry in their minds can lead to making attribution errors that become misdiagnoses. This begs the question of how to disrupt the racism/(hetero)sexism/ableism/classism/xenophobia that are always already embedded in the medical encounter. Groopman (2007) suggests that patients might prompt their doctors to reconsider diagnoses by asking questions such as: "What else could it be?", "Is there anything that doesn't fit?", and "Is it possible I have more than one problem?". Tervalon and Murray-García (1998) advocate for inculcating "cultural humility" in physical education that incorporates "a lifelong commitment to self-evaluation and self-critique, to redressing the power imbalances in the patient-physician dynamic" (p. 117). Further, we suggest employing counterstorytelling as a method in the medical encounter in which physicians are not just valuing their patients as vital partners but are required to honor cultural Others' capacity as a thinker/feeler/knower of their own bodies.

(Excavating) "Yin-Yang"

Circling back to our initial principle of exposing dichotomous "health consciousness," it calls for different approaches to (re)considering the relationship between health and illness. The Chinese theory of "yin-yang" serves as one approach. Essentially, yin-yang describes dynamic interplays of two forces in the universe that are both opposing and co-depending. Reality as seen through the lens of yin-yang "takes a fundamentally paradoxical formation" in that the contradictory elements coexist, depend on, and illuminate each other in consistent, permeant, and universal patterns (Luo & Chen, 2017). When applying the yin-yang logic to health, it suggests that health and illness are not contradictory and absolute, but rather interdependent, organic, and constantly shifting. This view is more consistent with an embodied approach to health narratives in capturing the dynamic, humanizing, and liberating potentiality of storying the knowing/feeling/thinking body that is always already raced/gendered/classed in the face of both health and illness. To illustrate our six EMBODY principles, we return to Lovejoy's narrative from the opening of this chapter to explore the potentials and challenges of digital (counter)storytelling through this lens.

Applying "EMBODY" to Intersecting Case Studies

Lovejoy's narrative appears as a guest blog post on the website, the Disability Visibility Project.[3] Created by disability activist, Alice Wong, the Disability Visibility Project (DVP) is "an online community dedicated to recording, amplifying, and sharing disability media and culture" (Wong, 2016, para. 1). As the site's curator, Wong assembles multi-media narratives—oral histories recorded via the StoryCorps app, blog posts, podcast episodes, tweets, and a disability photo project—to promote a disability justice perspective. This perspective opposes the biomedical master narrative, which equates disability with illness and suggests individualized, techno-medical solutions. Rather, the disability justice perspective emphasizes the oppressive impact of ableism, leveraging collective disability pride to demand rights for a disenfranchised community. Wong, and those who contribute to the DVP, employ personal narratives to <u>E</u>xpose the hegemony of biomedicine. In particular, the DVP aims to resurrect the "subjugated knowledges" of disability communit(ies) through preserving and amplifying its/their histor(ies). In an interview with the second author, Wong explained:

> Many people [with disabilities], they don't realize that we as a larger group have a history and culture .... They see themselves, they see the way they navigate the world, but they don't see how we all created this culture that's really important and really meaningful. I think that's where ableism plays in, where it's very difficult for our people to recognize and embrace our history and culture. I think as more people actually discover their own history and culture and that connection with other larger groups, a long line of history of decades of people all over the world doing this stuff, that's when you start realizing, "Wow, I am just small of this. And I'm part of something bigger."

For Wong and others, the process of <u>E</u>xposing hegemony and unearthing subjugated knowledges is closely tied to cultivating a (politicized) collective identity.

Additionally, Lovejoy's narrative participates in efforts to Mobilize voices from below. Specifically, Lovejoy crafted her narrative to participate in the hashtag movement, #DisabilityTooWhite. Created by Vilissa Thompson, founder of the disability equality organization, Ramp Your Voice,[4] #DisabilityTooWhite emerged to critique mainstream media for its tendency to whitewash stories about disability, except in calls for charity. When asked to explain what the hashtag meant to her, Vilissa responded:

> I think the lack of representation hinders our abilities to feel like we belong, to feel like our lives and our stories are important. We feel isolated and outcast when you don't see people who look like you, not just racially but disability-wise. (Blahovec, 2016, para. 7)

The Mighty is one such mainstream media outlet—a digital publishing platform that solicits and publishes stories from contributors writing about experiences with disability, chronic illness, mental health conditions, and rare diseases.[5] As part of her dissertation research, the second author interviewed several of the site's contributors who identified as people of color. Contributors like Sakari noted that *The Mighty* featured few stories from different racial and cultural perspectives. "As a mixed disabled person, my ethnicity I think has played a big role in some of my really toxic interactions with the health care system," Sakari explained. "I'm not going to erase that from the conversation because that's just ludicrous. *The Mighty* is truly white."

In developing digital spaces designed to elicit, curate, and host marginalized stories of disability and chronic illness, Wong and Thompson Bear witness to the Other's "exile narratives." As people of color themselves, their witnessing equates to an act of intersectional solidarity. Importantly, however, hashtag movements such as #DisabilityTooWhite demand that privileged allies also act as ethical witnesses to raced/queer/poor narratives. For instance, disability activist, Alaina Leary, described how #DisabilityTooWhite caused her to engage in self-reflection. She wrote:

> As a white disabled ally, I'm grateful for Vilissa's #DisabilityTooWhite and her overall body of work as an activist. It's important for me to recognize my privilege every time I'm tackling as issue as a writer or activist, because my experience is not the only valid disability experience. (Leary, 2017, para. 9)

Mainstream venues like *The Mighty* have also become more conscious of the need to curate diverse narratives. For instance, in a June 2018 email newsletter entitled, "Why Does Diversity Matter in Mental Health Anyway?" *Mighty* editors showcased articles written by contributors with different racial, cultural, and gender identities. Further, they invited additional contributions: "I'll be the first one to say our Mighty community isn't as diverse as it needs to be. If you're someone who feels like you're not represented, please don't hesitate to submit your story." Yet, *Mighty* contributors have noted the challenge of persuading mainstream audiences to listen to such narratives. For instance, Sakari noted that when *The Mighty* published articles about race, commenters frequently asserted that experiences of mistreatment weren't "about race." "You come to the conclusion, 'Wow, I don't know [that] this is the audience,'" Sakari explained. "I don't see that I can help people like that; those aren't the people I'm talking to."

Frank (2006) notes that people are often active consumers of narratives, silencing stories that threaten the taken-for-granted-ness of their health consciousness. Still, exposure to stories like Lovejoy's might have a gradually transformative effect. As Frank (2006) writes, "people are routinely ambushed by stories that they have not put themselves in a position to hear, and these stories affect their lives; electronic media seem to increase the possibilities of such ambush" (p. 434).

Through digital storytelling tactics like the use of Twitter hashtags, activists of color like Lovejoy, Wong, and Thompson implore privileged witnesses to engage in the process of <u>O</u>thering the cultural self. For instance, Lovejoy's narrative asks readers to acknowledge the ways that they might participate in similar microaggressions in their own community. Further, she asks would-be allies to consider how they continue to exclude people of color when developing advocacy initiatives. Using #DisabilityTooWhite, Thompson asks journalists to consider how they participate in the silencing and marginalizing of disabled people of color. Similarly, using the hashtag #CrippingtheMighty, Wong compelled the editors of *The Mighty* to consider how the perspectives of able-bodied editors and parent contributors had decentered the perspectives of people with disabilities. In an interview with the second author, Wong compared writing about disability from an able-bodied perspective to "non-Black people creating a site about the Black community." "How weird is that?" she asked. "And yet we don't see there's any problem about non-disabled people telling people what disability is about." Through #crippingthemighty, Wong compelled *The Mighty*'s staff to acknowledge the silencing impact of appropriation, and to focus on hiring disabled editors and recruiting disabled contributors.

Clearly, Lovejoys narrative participates in <u>D</u>isrupting diagnoses in the medical encounter. Stories like hers discredit the certainty of medical expertise, reminding readers that the *practice* of medicine is an imperfect art, influenced by providers' assumptions and biases. By publishing and circulating narratives such as this one, authors like Lovejoy speak back to epistemic injustice, reclaim knowledge of their own bodies, and empower others to engage in self-advocacy during doctor-patient interactions.

Finally, these intersecting case studies illustrate the importance of (excavating) "Ying-yang" to disrupt dichotomous categories. Sites like the DVP disrupt dichotomous notions of (un)health and (ab)normalcy by showcasing the ways in which people live well while being disabled. Additionally, by sharing Lovejoy's story of chronic illness on the Disability Visibility Project, Wong blurs the lines between illness, health, and disability. Finally, by curating stories of chronic pain, fatigue, and physical deterioration alongside stories of disability pride, sites like DVP suggest that individuals can embrace a positive disability identity while still struggling with physical impairments. Disrupting this dichotomy is particularly important for disability activists of color, who both resist the medicalization of their differences and fight for equitable access to healthcare. Overall, analyzed through the six principles of EMBODY, the processes of (counter)storytelling for disability rights, pride, and inclusion are always already complicated and contested along intersecting power lines of racism/(hetero)sexism/classism/ableism.

Conclusion

As Rachel Lovejoy has so insightfully stated in "Being Black Looking Good While Chronically Ill," health narratives for bodies living on/with/in-between the margins are always already intersectional. Lovejoy's decision to foreground "Being Black" in her blog post title echoes intercultural communication scholars' (Holling & Moon, 2015) call for close analyses of race in the context of lived health experiences and encounters in the medical spaces. We purposefully propose six principles of "EMBODY" for culture-centered health narratives to underscore the critical issue of (dis)embodiment in how we tell and/or listen to racially, socially, and cultural stratified health experiences. We join Dutta and the CCA researchers in affirming the agency of cultural Others to speak their truths. What is currently missing is a critical listening environment that simultaneously honors storytelling voices while accounting for the audience's (in)capacity to listen.

Notes

1. See https://www.unrest.film/
2. See https://storycorps.org/
3. See https://disabilityvisibilityproject.com/about/
4. See http://rampyourvoice.com/
5. See https://themighty.com/

References

Alexander, B. K., Arasaratnam, L. A., Flores, L. A., Leeds-Hurwitz, W., Mendoza, S. L., Oetzel, J., … Halualani, R. T. (2014). Our role as intercultural scholars, practitioners, activists, and teachers in addressing these key intercultural urgencies, issues, and challenges. *Journal of International and Intercultural Communication*, 7, 68–99. doi: 10.1080/17513057.2014.869526

Blahovec, S. (2016, June 28). Confronting the whitewashing of disability: Interview with #DisabilityTooWhite creator Vilissa Thompson. Retrieved from https://www.huffingtonpost.com/sarah-blahovec/confronting-the-whitewash_b_10574994.html

Blease, C., Carel, H., & Geraghty, K. (2016). Epistemic injustice in healthcare encounters: Evidence from chronic fatigue syndrome. *Journal of Medical Ethics, 43*, 549–557. doi:10.1136/medethics-2016-103691.

Boler, M. (1999). *Feeling power: Emotions and education*. New York, NY: Routledge.

Bosticco, C., & Thompson, C. (2008). Let me tell you a story: Narratives and narration in health communication research. In H. M. Zoller & M. J. Dutta (Eds.), *Emerging perspectives in health communication* (pp. 39–62). New York: Routledge.

Boylorn, R. M., & Orbe, M. P. (Eds.). (2014). *Critical autoethnography: Intersecting cultural identities in everyday life*. New York, NY: Routledge.

Brown, P., Zavestoski, S., McCormick, S., Mayer, B., Morello-Frosh, R., & Altman, R. G. (2004). Embodied health movements: New approaches to social movements in health. *Sociology of Health & Illness, 26*, 50–80.

Cardillo, L. W. (2010). Empowering narratives: Making sense of the experience of growing up with chronic illness or disability. *Western Journal of Communication, 74*, 525–546. doi: 10.1080/10570314.2010.512280

Carel, H., & Kidd, I. J. (2014). Epistemic injustice in healthcare: A philosophial analysis. *Medicine, Health Care and Philosophy, 17*, 529–540. doi:10.1007/s11019-014-9560-2.

Charon, R. (2009). Narrative medicine as witness for the self-telling body. *Journal of Applied Communication Research, 37*, 118–131. doi: 10.1080/00909880902792248

Chávez, K. R. (2009). Embodied translation: Dominant discourse and communication with migrant bodies-as-text. *The Howard Journal of Communications, 20*, 18–36. doi: 10.1080/10646170802664912

Chen, Y.-W. (2014). "Are you an immigrant?": Identity-based critical reflections of teaching intercultural communication. *New Directions for Teaching and Learning, 138*, 5–16. doi: 10.1002/tl.20091

Chen, Y.-W. (2018). "*Why don't you speak (up), Asian/immigrant/woman?*": Rethink silence and voice through family oral history. *Departures in Critical Qualitative Research*, 7(2), 29–48. doi: 10.1525/dcqr.2018.7.2.29

Coopman, S. J. (2003). Communicating disability: Metaphors of oppression, metaphors of empowerment. In P. Kalbfleisch (Ed.), *Communication yearbook* (Vol. 27, pp. 337–394). Mahwah, NJ: Lawrence Erlbaum.

Dutta, M. J. (2007). Communicating about culture and health: Theorizing culture-centered and cultural sensitivity approaches. *Communication Theory, 17*, 304–328. doi: 10.1111/j.1468-2885.2007.00297.x

Dutta, M. J. (2008). *Communicating health: A culture-centered approach.* Cambridge, UK: Polity Press.

Dutta, M. J. (2015). *Neoliberal health organizing: Communication, meaning, and politics.* New York, NY: Routledge.

Dutta, M. J., & Jamil, R. (2013). Health at the margins of migration: Culture-centered co-constructions among Bangladeshi immigrants. *Health Communication, 28*, 170–182. doi: 10.1080/10410236.2012.666956

Frank, A. W. (1995). *The wounded storyteller: Body, illness, and ethics.* Chicago, IL: University of Chicago Press.

Frank, A. W. (2006). Health stories as connectors and subjectifiers. *Health: An Interdisciplinary Journal for the Social Study of Health, Illness and Medicine, 10*, 421–440. doi: 10.1177/1363459306067312

Griffin, R. A., Ward, L., & Phillips, A. R. (2014). Still flies in buttermilk: Black male faculty, critical race theory, and composite counterstorytelling. *International Journal of Qualitative Studies in Education, 27*(10), 1354–1375. doi: 10.1080/09518398.2013.840403

Groopman, J. (2007). *How doctors think.* Boston, MA: Houghton Mifflin.

Guttman, N. (2000). *Public health communication interventions: Values and ethical dilemmas.* Thousand Oaks, CA: Sage.

Harter, L. M., & Bochner, A. P. (2009). Healing through stories: A special issue on narrative medicine. *Journal of Applied Communication Research, 37*, 113–117. doi: 10.1080/00909880902792271

Harter, L. M., Japp, P. M., & Beck, C. S. (Eds.). (2005). *Narratives, health, and healing: Communication theory, research, and practice.* Mahwah, NJ: Erlbaum.

Holling, M. A., & Moon, D. G. (2015). Continuing a politic of disruption: Race(ing) intercultural communication. *Journal of International and Intercultural Communication, 8*, 81–85. doi: 10.1080/17513057.2015.1025326

Kreuter, M. W., Green, M. C., Cappella, J. N., Slater, M. D., Wise, M. E., Storey, D., … Woolley, S. (2007). Narrative communication in cancer prevention and control: A framework to guide research and application. *Annals of Behavioral Medicine, 33*, 221–235. doi: 10.1007/BF02879904

Langellier, K. M. (2009). Performing narrative medicine. *Journal of Applied Communication Research, 37*, 151–158. doi: 10.1080/00909880902792263

Leary, A. (2017, June 14). Reflecting on the impact of #DisabilityTooWhite. Retrieved from https://www.rootedinrights.org/reflecting-on-the-impact-of-disabilitytoowhite/.

Lindemann Nelson, H. (1996). Sophie doesn't: Families and counterstories of self-trust. Hypatia, 11, 91–104. doi.org/10.1111/j.1527-2001.1996.tb00508.x.

Lovejoy, R. (August 9, 2016). Guest blog post: Being black looking good while chronically ill. Retrieved from https://disabilityvisibilityproject.com/2016/08/09/guest-blog-post-being-black-looking-good-while-chronically-ill/comment-page-1/

Luo, G., & Chen, Y.-W. (2017). Communication as paradox and paradox as communication: An interparadigmatic proposal of coexisting cultural epistemologies. *China Media Research, 13*(3), 71–82.

Madlock Gatison, A. D. (2016). *Health communication and breast cancer among black women: Culture, Identity, Spirituality, and Strength.* Lanham, MD: Lexington Books.

Manoogian, M. M., Harter, L. M., & Denham, S. A. (2010). The storied nature of health legacies in the familial experience of type 2 diabetes. *Journal of Family Communication, 10*, 40–56. doi: 10.1080/15267430903385826

Matthews, N., & Sunderland, N. (2017). *Digital storytelling in health and social policy*. New York, NY: Routledge.

Moon, D. G., & Holling, M. A. (2015). A politic of disruption: Race(ing) intercultural communication. *Journal of International and Intercultural Communication, 8*, 1–6. doi: 10.1080/17513057.2015.991073

Oetzel, J., DeVargas, F., Ginossar, T., & Sanchez, C. (2007). Hispanic women's preferences for breast health information: Subjective cultural influences on source, message, and channel. *Health Communication, 21*(3), 223–233.

Parsloe, S. M. (2015). Discourses of disability, narratives of community: Reclaiming an Autistic identity online. *Journal of Applied Communication Research, 33*, 336–356. doi: 10.1080/00909882.2015.1052829

Parsloe, S. M., &Holton, A. E. (2017). #Boycottautismspeaks: Communicating a counternarrative through cyberactivism and connective action. *Information, Communication & Society, 6*, 1–18. doi: 10.1080/1369118x.2017.1301514

Parsons, T. (1951). *The social system*. Glencoe, IL: Free Press.

Pierce, C. (1974). Psychiatric problems of the Black minority. In S. Arietie (Ed.), *American handbook of psychiatry* (pp. 512–523). New York, NY: Basic Books.

Rodriguez, A. (2015). The exile narratives. In D. Chawla & S. Holman Jones (Eds.), *Stories of home: Place, identity, exile* (pp. 105–112). Lanham, MD: Lexington Books.

Shakespeare, T. (2013). The social model of disability. In L. J. Davis (Ed.), *Disability studies reader* (pp. 214–221, 4th ed.). New York, NY: Routledge.

Sharf, B. F., & Vanderford, M. L. (2003). Illness narratives and the social construction of health. In T. L. Thompson, A. Dorsey, K. I. Miller, & R. Parrott (Eds.), *Handbook of health communication* (pp. 9–34). Mahwah, NJ: Erlbaum.

Tervalon, M., & Murray-García, J. (1998). Cultural humility versus cultural competence: A critical distinction in defining physician training outcomes in multicultural education. *Journal of Health Care for the Poor and Underserved, 9*(2), 117–125. doi: 10.1353/hpu.2010.0233

Thompson, C. M., Lin, H., & Parsloe, S. (2017). Misrepresenting health conditions through fabrication and exaggeration: An adaptation and replication of the false alarm effect. *Health Communication, 33*, 562–575. doi: 10.1080/10410236.2017.1283563

Wallerstein, N. B., & Duran, B. (2006). Using community-based participatory research to address health disparities. *Health Promotion Practice, 7*(3), 312–323.

White, M., & Epson, D. (1990). *Narrative means to therapeutic ends*. New York, NY: W.W. Norton & Company.

Williams, D. R., & Collins, C. (2001). Racial residential segregation is a fundamental cause of racial disparities in health. *Public Health Reports*, *116*(5), 404–416.

Wong, A. (2016). About. Disability Visibility Project. Retrieved from https://disabilityvisibilityproject.com/about/.

Yamasaki, J. (2009). Though much is taken, much abides: The storied world of aging in a fictionalized retirement home. *Health Communication*, *24*, 588–596.

Yamasaki, J., Geist-Martin, P., & Sharf, B. F. (2017). *Storied health and illness: Communicating personal, cultural, and political complexities*. Long Grove, IL: Waveland Press.

Yep, G. A. (2013). Queering/Quaring/Kauering/Crippin'/Transing "other bodies" in intercultural communication. *Journal of International and Intercultural Communication*, *6*, 118–126. doi: 10.1080/17513057.2013.777087

Young, S. (2014). I'm not your inspiration, thank you very much. Retrieved from https://www.ted.com/talks/stella_young_i_m_not_your_inspiration_thank_you_very_much/transcript?language=en

Zoller, H. M. (2005). Health activism: Communication theory and action for social change. *Communication Theory*, *15*, 341–364. doi: 10.1111/j.1468-2885.2005.tb00339.x

CHAPTER TWO

Queer(ing) Spaces: Sexualities as Critical Intersections among Health and Intercultural Communication

BY SHINSUKE EGUCHI

Health communication continues to grow as an academic discipline … Health communication scholars have brought an interdisciplinary lens to a broad range of health issues such as HIV, cancer, obesity, alcohol abuse and dying. Health communication has demonstrated value in examining a full spectrum of health …. within institutions and among individuals— (Spieldenner & Anadolis, 2017, p. 97).

[C]ritical intercultural communication research ….engages a complex and context-oriented interrogation of power that (re)produces and is (re)produced through our intercultural encounters ….communication [is] a primary means of rearticulation to explore how meanings, practices, structures, and discourses are developed and negotiated—(Toyosaki & Eguchi, 2017, p. 4).

*****

It is around the middle of May after the end of 2017s spring semester. I am reflecting how I have taught a graduate seminar required for doctoral students, titled *Theorizing about Culture and Communication*. I am trying to make sense of some comments that a couple of students have mentioned to me throughout the semester. One student, focusing on Health Communication emphasis, was nervous about taking my class. They were not familiar with Intercultural Communication and

Critical/Cultural studies related literatures. Also, another student had just realized how recognizing the intersections among culture, identity, and power helps expand their research on Health Communication. Still, these comments, which are supposed to be compliments, reflect how a traditionally defined boundary of the fields between Health and Intercultural Communication remains practiced. There is a material reality of division between Health and Intercultural communication fields, which have separately emerged and evolved into the discipline of Communication. However, I never really understand such academic divisiveness. As a transnational Asian/American queer man of color, I find that both the health and the intercultural have been and are always already my everyday life concerns.

*****

From this personal account, I intellectually and politically move to critique that the discipline of Communication historically produces a stable, fixed, and essentialized border between sub-fields of Health and Intercultural Communication in this theoretical essay. For a long time, Communication scholars, working on both the Health and the Intercultural, are simultaneously marginalized from these two fields. They are often constructed as if they are not really Health or Intercultural Communication scholars. Nakayama and Corey (2003) have critiqued, "Academia is not short on disciplinarians. Academics demonstrate their mastery of the field by carefully guarding its boundaries and the proper production of knowledge" (p. 328). At the same time, there are some disruptions against such a categorical boundary in recent years. It has become so much clearer than before that Intercultural Communication issues such as identity, space/place, and/or power explicate, elucidate, and elaborate some aspects of Health Communication concerns such as depression, healthism, able-bodiedness, disability, and/or HIV/AIDs (e.g., Calafell, 2017; Eguchi, 2019; Halberstam, 2018; McRuer, 2006; Puar, 2017; Snorton, 2017; Yep, 2002). Together, discursive and material executions of Health Communication awareness, education, campaign, and/or intervention require fundamental aspects of Intercultural Communication scholarships accounting the hierarchal productions and constitutions of differences (e.g., Dutta, 2015; Elwood, Greence, & Carter, 2003; Ginossar & Nelson, 2010; Spieldenner & Castro, 2010). Intersections among Health and Intercultural Communication are always already vital. Thus, here I once again remake such movements disrupting the field borders between Health and Intercultural Communication.

With this scholarly goal, I reaffirm that sexualities are indeed critical intersections among Health and Intercultural Communication. As Yep (2003) has asserted, "sexuality has been, until recently, largely a neglected area of inquiry in the communication discipline" (p. 14). This line of thought suggests the way in which compulsory heterosexuality are always already at play behind the theorizing of Health and/or Intercultural Communication. The gendered and sexualized knowledge and practices, embedded in the material realities of queer and transgender people, remain overlooked (Chávez, 2013; Eguchi & Asante, 2016; Yep, 2013). The institutional practices, discourses, and structures of heterosexuality as the normative body of knowledge strategically organize what we are supposed to know about processes of communication in and across Health and Intercultural contexts. Consequently, there remain a lot of spaces that require becoming and being queer(ed). By queer, I mean an intellectual and political commitment to problematize historical productions and existing constitutions of sexual and gender categories along with race, ethnicity, nationality, language, coloniality, class, and the body (Eguchi & Long, 2019; Yep, 2013).

The movement of queer(ing) destabilizes the accepted and unchallenged ideas and social relations such as desire, intimacy, relationship, family, and kinship rooted in the simultaneous technologies of heteronormativity. That is, also intersecting with whiteness, patriarchy, cis-genderism, able-bodiedness, capitalism, and colonialism/imperialism. So, possibilities for alternative modes of living can be visualized, imagined, and hopefully practiced. The major goal of queer(ing) is to make spaces of futurity toward transgressive modes of living through which everyone can be who they want to be. Still, I reject the theoretical and methodological implication of queer(ing) solely rooted in individualism, agency and sexual freedom. As a number of interdisciplinary scholars (Johnson, 2001; Lee, 2003; McRuer, 2006; Stryker, 2006) have argued before, queer(ing) must carefully account how historically contingent forces of power relations operate as impossibilities for queer and transgender people becoming and being who they want to be. The material realities of heteronormativity, producing "the equation 'heterosexual experience = human experience'" (Yep, 2002, p. 167), matter in everyday personal, institutional, and cultural experiences. Consequently, queerness continues to be an ideality that allows us to recognize failures fixed by the hetero-colonialist mappings of the present time (Eguchi, Files-Thompson, & Calafell, 2018; McCune, 2014; Muñoz, 2009; Snorton, 2017). Thus, the intellectual and political engagement of queer(ing) is to keep critiquing the present time revised and revised again for capitalistic and profit-making inclusions of queer and transgender people into the nation-state (Eng, 2010). Therefore, queer(ing) spaces where celebrate transgressive modes of living for the future can be temporaily sustained.

Drawing the genealogy of queer critique described above, I showcase my argument, that is, the conception of sexualities as critical intersections among Health and Intercultural Communication. More specifically, I pay attention to two different cases related to male same-sex cultural performances. By cultural performances, I mean "an all-encompassing aspect of our daily being, inclusive of rituals, customs, policies, and procedures, as well as those performances of self related to sex, gender, class, and race" (Alexander, 2012, p, 87). The examples of cultural performances, which I pay attention to, are: (1) raw sex and (2) intimate partner violence (IPV). I examine how such sexual cultural performances differently explicate, elucidate, and elaborate the complexities and contradictions of male same-sex sexual desire in and across power lines of race, gender, sexuality, class, and the body. Just to clarify my scholarly goal, I do not equate these two cultural performances at all. Instead, I am interested in showcasing how intersections among sexuality, desire, and power are differently circulated, materialized, and performed in and across two cases. Pérez (2015) reminds us, "Queer critique must investigate the circulation of homosexual desire within the erotic economics of both capitalism and the nation in order to guard against its cooptation into neoliberal and colonial projects" (p. 3). By this means, I hope to remake queer(ing) spaces that connect among Health and Intercultural communication fields. In what follows, I introduce the conceptions of sexualities as intersectional productions of historical and existing power relations.

The Politics of Sexualities as Intersectional

Some may think that sexualities are just individuals' sexual preferences. However, sexualities have never been apolitical products in and across various global and transcultural contexts. Indeed, sexualities are the discursive and material products of historical and existing power relations that symbolize and affirm the hierarchal structures of differences (Butler, 2006). Until 1973, the American Psychological Association (APA) considered the condition of homosexuality as a *medical disorder* (Halberstam, 2018; McRuer, 2006). Even after the APA removal of homosexuality from their *Diagnostic and Statistical Manual of Mental Disorders* (DSM), the inferiority of homosexuality to heterosexuality has been always already a part of the mainstream cultural discourse about same-sex sexual and romantic desires in the U.S. The public recognition of HIV/AIDS has widely reinforced the stigmatization of homosexuality by identifying the male-to-male anal intercourse as a major transmission route of the disease (Spieldenner & Castro, 2010). Such perception has also promoted on-going representations of men who engage in same-sex sexual and romantic relations as casual, promiscuous, and irresponsible (McCune 2014; Snorton, 2014). At the same time, such male-centered discourses about same-sex sexual and romantic desires have also ignored, erased, and/or marginalized the presences of women who engage in same-sex sexual and romantic relations. This gendered situation mirrors the way in which the politics of sexualities privilege the masculinist power of phallus as the central gaze (Shimizu, 2012). Accordingly, the politics of sexualities cannot easily separate from the politics of genders (Butler, 2006).

Case in point, the U.S. gay sexual cultures value the scripts of gender resembling and reformatting performative characteristics of hegemonic masculinity. According to Eguchi (2009), men are considered to be attractive and desirable when they show off their physical strengths through their upper body muscles and forces. In addition, physical traits such as short hairs, facial hairs, tanned skin colors, and deep voices add to the layers of gay male physical attractiveness and sexual desirability. Moreover, the large size of a penis is idolized as a hypersexual masculinist sign of power. Such normative messages of gay male ideal body images however, marginalize men being read as *feminine*. In a New York's gay club scene Muñoz (2009) has observed, "those who break the gay-clone edict to act like a man are de-eroticized and demoted to second-class citizenship" (p. 77). Such hatred toward effeminate men insinuates how gay sexual cultural remakings of hegemonic masculinity reconstitute social and performative aspects of anti-femininity and homophobia rooted in heteronormativity and patriarchy (Han 2015; Hoang, 2014). Because patriarchal societies degrade and devalue femininities, men participating in gay sexual cultures are ideologically pressured to overcome the stereotypes of effeminacy as a logo of homosexuality. Accordingly, youthful, healthy, athletic, cis-gendered, and able-bodied representations of masculinity, exhibiting the logics of compulsory heterosexuality, signify the U.S. advancement and progressivity of gay sexual cultures that are no longer stigmatized as a disorder (Eng, 2010; McRuer, 2006; Puar, 2007).

Still, such *healthy* embodiments of U.S. gay sexual exceptionalism are not equally available to men of color who are always already racialized and gendered in and across the historical and ideological contexts. Cis-gendered white men are given privileges to get away with racial and ethnic stereotypes since whiteness operates as a cultural norm (Eng, 2010). For example, Asian/American men are almost always positioned as the sexual fetish category of *feminine Others* for the older white male as a historical consequence of U.S. American racial paradigms (Eguchi, 2019). Oftentimes, younger and helpless Asian men coming from foreign countries, who are capitally in needs of help, mostly constitute such sexually fetish stereotypes (Fung, 2005). Accordingly, when Asian/American men accomplish hyper-masculine images, they are repeatedly emasculated in opposition to the white masculine ideal (Han, 2015). At the same time, black/African American men are commodified as hypersexual and aggressive beings with large endowments (McCune, 2014; Snorton, 2014). When they do not conform to such eroticized images for the white gaze, they experience complex and contested layers of stigmatization rooted in the intersection of racism, cis-genderism, anti-femininity, and classism (Snorton, 2017). Simultaneously, the white (gay) sexual imagination represents the images of cis-gendered brown male able-bodies as hypersexual and hyper-masculine sites of eroticization and desirability (Pérez, 2015). These ideas are often associated with Latino, Arab, and Mediterranean men. While the aforementioned examples are not comprehensive representations, men of color are positioned to be unable to freely imitate, embody, and naturalize youthful, healthy, athletic, cis-gendered, and able-bodied representations of (white) gay masculinity. The body matters in such processes of communication. The macro-structural realities of race and racism are always parts of micro/meso-acts and processes of communication through which men of color develop and negotiate their proximities to gay sexual cultures rooted in whiteness as a compulsory (hetero)sexuality (Eguchi et al., 2018; Han, 2015; Pérez, 2015).

From this perspective, I approach the politics of sexualities as intersectional in this essay. I take into account that the politics of sexualities are always already racialized and gendered together. Yep and colleagues (2017) advocate for the necessity of transing the politics of racialized gender. The engagement of trans(ing) allows communication researchers to interrogate "how gender is contingently assembled and reassembled with other attributes and structures of bodily being, such as race and the body type" (Yep et al., 2017, p. 57). Trans(ing) complicates the intersectional notions of sexualities as gendered and genders as sexualized. Such intellectual move helps locate race, class, the body, and other social positionings as well. Elaborating this political mission of trans(ing), I situate my intellectual move to remake *queer(ing) spaces* grounded in the conception of intersectionality. That is, a method and methodology for accounting simultaneous functions of race, gender, sexuality, and other differences in and across historical and ideological contexts (Crenshaw, 1989, 1991; Muñoz, 1999). However, I also recognize the critical evaluation of intersectionality. As Puar (2007) has mentioned, intersectionality evaporates major points of critique as they simultaneously pay attention to multiple sites of differences. Scholars can easily and unintentionally obfuscate, erase, and restore the reproductive power of whiteness as a normative identity, discourse, system, and knowledge through their methodological utilizations of intersectionality (Bilge, 2014). To minimize such contradiction, I privilege to identify and critique the intersectionalities of heterosexism, homophobia, cis-genderism, and racism as referencing points toward remake *queer(ing) spaces*. So, I offer a queer critique that complicates the politics of sexualities as intersectional productions of historical and existing power relations.

Toward Queer(ing) Spaces in and across Health and Intercultural Communication

Now, I interrogate two different cases of male same-sex cultural performances to help visualize *queer(ing) spaces* in and across Health and Intercultural Communication. I first showcase the ways in which male-to-male performative engagements in raw sex explicate, elucidate, and elaborate the politics of sexualities as intersectional. Then, I interrogate how the politics of sexualities as intersectional are differently implicated by occurrences of male-to-male IPV. In so doing, my goal is to showcase a queer critique allows us as communication scholars to comprehensively move toward praxis.

Case One: Raw Sex

As a consequence of the HIV/AIDS epidemic, since early 1980s the U.S. cultural discourses have almost always reinforced the stigmatizations of male-to-male raw sex, that is, an anal intercourse without a condom. This sexual act is considered as one of the major social interactive sites of spreading HIV/AIDS (Yep, Lovaas, & Pagonis, 2002). Spieldenner (2016) maintains, "ASOs [AIDS Service Organizations], media, and health departments have invested heavily into campaigns and initiatives meant to normatize the use of condoms for gay men" (p. 1692). This Health Communication promotion of condom use and HIV/AIDS prevention identify that men from various racial and ethnic backgrounds, who do not label themselves as gay or bisexual, also engage in anal sexual intercourses (Lewis & Ketzener, 2003). Sexualities are fluid and dynamic constructs in and across cultural and ethnic backgrounds. Such finding influences the media and popular cultural productions and circulations of men on the down low (DL), that is, heterosexually identified black/African American men who sleep with men in early 2000s (McCune, 2014; Snorton, 2014).

The scientific advances in HIV, decreasing the infectiousness of the disease, significantly helps visualize a possibility to end AIDS while HIV is not yet fully curable (Spieldenner, 2016). The relatively recent introduction of HIV pre-exposure prophylaxis (PrEP) also changes the dynamic of HIV prevention and uses of condom (Dieffenbach & Fauci, 2011). Taking PrEP allows sexually active users to reduce the risks of contracting HIV virus when they engage in raw sex. Yet, concerns regarding the costs of HIV medications suggest that everyone is not capitally given equal accessibility to such a resource (Spieldenner, 2016). Still, performative implications and consequences of male-to-male raw sex are changing.

In this current landscape, I call for queering complexities and contradictions of male same-sex sexual desire as it relates to raw sex. The one of most challenging tensions among sexuality, desire, and performance is that what we say we do is performatively different from what we actually do (Bailey, 2016; Yep et al., 2002). Multiple societal stigmatizations of sexual acts and behaviors often create and recreate performative sites through which sexual desires, performances, and pleasures are paradoxically visualized, materialized, and satisfied outside of the cis-heterosexual norms. Still, Rubin (1998) has reminded that "sexuality that is 'good,' 'normal,' and 'natural' should be ideally heterosexual, martial, monogamous, reproductive, and non-commercial … Any sex that violates these rules is 'bad,' 'abnormal' and 'unnatural'" (p. 108). Yet, such hetero-colonialist legacies of good sexual norms rooted in healthism and patriarchy always already cause the paradox of risk, pleasure, and satisfaction. People often get aroused out of being sexually risky to resist and/or feel free from the social and structural constraints. In order to make this line of my queer(ing) argument clear, I will focus on black/African American gay and bisexual men next.

The black gay vernacular of *catching nut*—someone ejaculating his semen inside of his sex partner's anus—symbolizes queer (read as abnormal and unnatural) performances of resistance against multiple layers of social and structural oppressions (Bailey, 2016). The (white-centered) gay sexual cultural concept of barebacking is a decisive and deliberate performance of male-to-male raw sex. Yep et al. (2002) maintain that barebacking can be seen as "reinforcement of sexual identity, resistance to imposed behavioral norms, creation of a new sexual and political identity, or a continuation of practices unaffected by organized messages aimed at stopping such practices" (p. 4). This notion of barebacking goes against the health communication promotion of HIV/AIDS prevention. Its embodied performance challenges the hetero-colonialist definition of *good sex* rooted in the patriarchy and healthism. Accordingly, barebaking can symbolize and affirm the queer politics of resistance. At the same time, Bailey (2016) further complicates such conception of barebacking as it relates to black/African American gay and bisexual men. He suggests, "Although it is well known that unprotected anal intercourse is the primary mode of HIV infection for all MSM [meaning, men who have sex with men], the high HIV prevalence among black men is a result of a variety of social factors that interacts with sexual behavior and that increase their vulnerability to infection" (p. 242). The historical and existing power relations such as racism, classism and heterosexism produce and reproduce how black/African American gay and bisexual men are imagined and represented to have high-risk sex (Scott, 2010).

According to Bailey (2016), there are three major historical and structural constraints for them. First, black/African American gay and bisexual men are identified to have sex within less wider social and sexual networks. Blackness has been historically constructed as undesirable and unattractive particularly in and across white middle-upper class centered gay sexual cultures (Raymond & McFarland, 2009). Second, the historical legacy and contemporary reality of racial segregation affect such less wider social and sexual networks where black/African American gay and bisexual men are materially positioned. Third, the material realities of historically racialized capital inequalities, not limited to but including unemployment, homelessness, mental illness, violence, and sexual abuse, play as additional layers of complications for particularly low-income and working-class black/African American gay and bisexual men. Furthermore, such series of macro-structural constraints point out certain types of social and communal pressures affecting black/African American gay and bisexual men.

In fact, the notion of homosexuality, "effectively 'theorized' as a 'white disease' that had 'infected' the black community" (Johnson & Henderson, 2005, p. 4), is a part of their everyday lives. The communal misperception of being black/African American gay and bisexual men is that they want to act and behave like *white men* (Eguchi et al., 2018). This discursive and ideological condition suggests the way in which black/African American men are historically pressured to embody and perform heteronormative constructs of hypermasculinity. So, they are able to fight against the feelings of powerlessness produced by white surveillance (e.g., McCune, 2014; Snorton, 2014). The racialized, cis-gendered, and sexualized aspects of hypermasculinity, rooted in the hetero-patriarchal repudiation of femininity, eradicate any social and performative symbols suggesting male same-sex sexual and romantic desires. Male same-sex desire becomes and is a performative sign of weakness. Black/African American gay men and MSMs are historically punished and penalized for becoming and being sissy (Snorton, 2017). There has been a very narrow definition of cis-gendered manhood available for black/African American men.

Under such conditions, the phrase, *catching nut*, signifies more than a just resistance. Black/African American gay and bisexual men make bare material barricades (or condoms) that weaken queer possibilities of sexual, romantic, and intimate connections with other (black/African American) men (Bailey, 2016). Engaging in raw sex, they become and are both emotionally and physically vulnerable. They temporaily crave for feeling desired and wanted by other men. Subsequently, they long for deep intimacies of male-to-male anal sex that temporarily interrupt and/or escape from racialized, cis-gendered, and sexualized feelings of powerlessness rooted in the historical continuum of white dominance (Bailey, 2016). This queer of color politics, exhibiting complexities and contradictions of male same-sex sexual desire, calls attention to the intersections among semen, sperm, and ejaculation as phallic symbols of power in the patriarchal societies.

The performative aspects of ejaculation, generating semen exchange, are major sources of struggle through which the stigmatized representations of male-to-male raw anal penetration continue to take place in the post-HIV epidemic context. In fact, the rhetoric of HIV prevention, promoting the use of condom and the introduction of PrEP, literarily reinforces the anal exchange of semen as a highly risky site of transmission (Spieldenner, 2016). In addition, the current societal discourse about viral load, which is the amount of HIV virus in blood system, illuminates how to scientifically determine levels of healthiness for people living with HIV. The lower vital load is suppressed by HIV medication(s), the more one is considered to be less infectious (Spieldenner, 2017). Still, the relational and communicative practice of serosorting, which is "actively choosing sex and intimate partners based on common HIV-status" (Spieldenner, 2017, p. 125), take place. Such sexual choice making process reforms and reconstitutes the marginalization of HIV positive men as *the Others* in and across gay sexual cultures (Bailey, 2016; Spieldenner, 2017; Yep et al., 2002). Thus, the social and performative aspects of semen exchange as a highly risky site of transmission are not disrupted yet. The exchanges of semen regulate ideological and material boundaries, including but not limited to desirability-undesirability, pleasure-displeasure, satisfaction-dissatisfaction, safety-risky, healthy-unhealthy, and/or undetectability-infectiousness. Therefore, discursive intersections among semen, sperm, and ejaculation remain powerfully operating through contexts of male-to-male raw sex today.

With the case of *catching nut* described above, I have demonstrated that performances of raw sex explicate, elucidate, and elaborate complexities and contradictions of male same-sex sexual desire working within the complex and contested paradoxes of risk, pleasure, and satisfaction in and across differences. Here, the queer(ing) politics of male same-sex sexual desire is to call into question historical and existing power relations that not only affect social and performative negotiations of sexuality, gender, identity, and space/place but also generate material consequences of sexual acts and behaviors. Next, I showcase this line of queer(ing) intercultural health critique with a case of intimate male same-sex partner violence.

Case Two: Intimate Partner Violence (IPV)

IPV among men who participate in sexual and romantic relations with men has been one of the major interpersonal and dyadic issues (Stiles-Shields & Carroll, 2015). Still, such relational violence has not been given enough attention as a result of the socially expected gender role (Frankland & Brown, 2014). That is, men are not supposed to be IPV victims. The mainstream discourse of IPV frequently visualizes heterosexual relationships as they relate to men as IPV perpetuators

(Woodyatt & Stephenson, 2016). At the same time, other relational dyad violence and abuse such as female against female, female against male, and male against male remain overlooked today (Seelau & Seelau, 2005). Accordingly, when male-to-male IPV is reported, some officials such as police officers and health providers may not respond to such critical incident appropriately (Brown & Groscup, 2009). However, some officials must recognize the contemporary political and economic spheres that promote the rapid increase of male same-sex couples making their relational status public. Eng (2010) maintains, "While gays and lesbians were once decidedly excluded from the normative structures of family and kinship, today they are re-inhabiting them in growing numbers in increasingly public and visible ways" (p. 3). In 2015 the federal legalization of same-sex marriages further normalizes the institution of same-sex couplings as similar to the heterosexual ones in U.S. America. Gays and lesbians, who are particularly white, cis-gender, and/or affluent, are becoming and being constructed as *almost heterosexuals* when they replicate, embody and perform the heteronoromative scripts of marital, monogamous, and non-commercial relationship through their same-sex desires (Eguchi et al., 2018). The visibility of same-sex parenting is also increasing (Oakley, Farr, & Scherer, 2017). Thus, exploring the Health and Intercultural issues involved in intimate same-sex partner violence is timely.

Accordingly, I argue for queering complexities and contradictions of male same-sex sexual desire in the contexts of IPV. The one of the most challenging IPV issues is that a number of complex, contested, and ambivalent layers of abuses such as the physical, the sexual, the emotional, the social, and/or the spiritual are simultaneously at play (Woodyatt & Stephenson, 2016). The historical and structural variables such as racism, (hetero)sexism, homophobia, cis-genderism, ableism, and/or classism can complicate the occurrences of IPV for men who participate in sexual and romantic relations with men (Poon, 2000). For example, threatening to *out* a partner who is discreet of one's same-sex desire has been one of the intimate same-sex partner violence occurrences (Burke & Owen, 2006). In addition, performing overtly hypermasculinity has been a way to exercise control and power over a partner who displays more effeminate than masculine characteristics (Sandfort, Melendez, & Diaz, 2007). At the same time, a simplistic notion of binary between a victim and a perpetuator, rooted in the heteronormative paradigm, cannot represent the material consequences of IPV among men who participate in sexual and romantic relationships with men. Its cause and effect is much more complicated. In order to exemplify such particular messiness, I will explicitly elaborate cultural and performative aspects of Asian/American male identity next.

The 2016s LGBTQ and HIV-affected IPV report, published by the National Coalition of Anti-Violence Groups (2017), demonstrates that Asian/Americans remain to be the one of underreported racial groups. This underrepresentation may implicate the historical and structural complexity of Asian/Americans through which multiple cultural differences such as nationality, ethnicity, citizenship, migration status, language, class, and skin color are strategically ignored and erased for the white superiority, dominance, and power. However, there are small numbers of Asian/Americans who report their IPV experiences. To make sense of such underreports, Poon (2000) has strongly warned the following risky and vulnerable cultural factors in which Asian/American men who participate in interracial same-sex sexual and romantic relationships cope with their IPV experiences.

Some Asian/American men may embody and perform their ethnic family values of one's obedience or subservience to their partners. Then, some of them may hope that violence and abuse will disappear in the future when they remain being quiet. In addition, some Asian/American men may not seek help relationally within and beyond their ethnic cultures because of everyday power circulations of heterosexism and homophobia. Due to the lack of familial and communal supports, there is a possibility in which some Asian/American men are in sexual and romantic relationships with men who own higher economic privileges and/or cultural capitals than them. The material realities of financial dependency and/or unemployment do not easily allow some Asian/American men to separate from their abusive partners. Simultaneously, Asian/American men may be also isolated from the gay sexual cultures because of anti-Asian racism (Poon, 2006).

The global gay sexual cultures, emphasizing the (white) masculine ideal, almost always represent desexualized images of Asian/American men as *feminine* and *sexually subservient foreigners*. Consequently, the Asian/American male is racially imagined as a sexually exotic fetish label for the older white male who cannot find their sexual and romantic partners otherwise because of ageism (Fung, 2005; Lim, 2014). This stereotype is known to reproduce sexual undesirability of Asian American men in and across western gay sexual cultures (Hoang, 2014). Han (2015) maintains that Asian/American men continue to "report feeling physically inadequate in the larger gay community where Eurocentric displays of physical beauty are constantly touted" (p. 105). Still, there have been increasingly emerging images of hypermasculine Asian/American men that temporarily disrupt such feminized positionality (Eguchi, 2019). Yet, this counter-hegemonic performance takes place through a historically racist logic, which Asian American masculinities symbolize their physical failures to meet the gay cultural expectation of white masculinity as the sexual modernity (Shimizu, 2012). In consequence, some Asian/American men, who are fear of becoming and being single, may not easily break up with their abusive partners.

Considering such complex layers of social isolation possibly taking place for Asian/American men in the occurrences of IPV, I call attention to the contradictions of same-sex sexual and romantic desire constructing such vulnerable path for Asian/American men who engage in male same-sex sexual and romantic relationships. More specifically, I reflexively raise the following questions to the rest of Asian/American queer male fellows regardless of IPV experiences. Aren't we all attracted to men who perform (toxic) hypermasculinity because they are considered as sexually desirable? Aren't we all ironically helping sustain the cultural reproductions of male violence and aggression? Aren't we all a part of the problem? In order to collectively take steps to answer these questions, I turn our attention to what Muñoz (2009) has pointed out before is the metrosexualization of male same-sex sexual and romantic desires.

We collectively must recognize the gay sexual desirability of men as the resemblances of dominant imprint. That is, a (cis-gender, able-bodied, and white) masculine ideal. The historical multiplicities of male same-sex desire, embracing queer and trans possibilities of gender, sexuality, and sex, are being repeatedly homogenized for the sake of gay male assimilative politics. Today, gay men are increasingly acting, behaving, and performing as if they are *almost* heterosexual males. Simultaneously, such embodied performances of imitating the dominant imprint without the doubt reproduce and reconstitute cis-heteronormative aspects of toxic masculinity rooted in the cultural developments and promotions of male violence and aggression. The traditionally idealized characters of masculinity historically stress social and performative aspects of powerfulness, toughness, and competitiveness that require the subordination of women and queer and trans people and the repudiation of femininities (Eguchi, 2009, 2019). This discursive adjustment remakes the hierarchical politics of masculinity ranking men according to differences such as sexuality, race, class, gender performance, nationality, and the body (Eguchi et al., 2018; Yep et al., 2017). Then, the counter-hegemonic performative aspects of desiring for and being attracted toward the (toxic) masculine ideal never ever allow men engaging in same-sex sexual and romantic relations to be completely free from the paradoxes of power, violence, and abuse. Thus, the heterosexualization of male same-sex sexual and romantic desires re-secures the centrality of toxic masculinity as a symbol of power. Therefore, it is the time for us to revise and change what we desire for. Otherwise, male violence and aggression being reproduced in gay sexual cultures never ever come to an end.

Consequently, I reiterate that the conception of male same-sex sexual and romantic desire as it relates to IPV requires queer intercultural health critiques further. I recognize that studying visible and invisible connections among such desire, power, and violence can be very complex and controversial. It points out unreasonable, irrational, illogical, and socially taboo aspects of human interactions and relationships according to the institutional norms, rules, and laws. The messy interplays between power, domination, and subordination always already represent the performative paradoxes of sexual desire (Butler, 2006; Cruz, 2016). This controversial topic illuminates the ways in which material consequences of power, desire, and violence explicate, elucidate, and elaborate performative negotiations of sexuality, gender, identity, and space/place. In view of that, unpacking such interrelatedness offers a *queer(ing) space* to find ways to work with culturally specific incidences of intimate male same-sex partner violence in and across historical and ideological contexts.

In Closing

In this theoretical essay, I have attempted to draw a queer critique to demonstrate possibilities to examine the conception of sexualities as critical intersections among Health and Intercultural Communication. More specifically, I have paid attention to two different cases of male same-sex cultural performance in and across the lines of differences. One is raw sex. Another one is IPV. These two different cases are extremely complex, contested, and culturally sensitive. The reasons behind micro/meso-acts and processes of such critical incidents can be never clearly defined. There always already remain spaces for confusion, ambiguity, and/or inconsistency.

Simultaneously, this is the reason why I have called for queering culturally specific performances of male same-sex sexual and romantic desire. The socially and culturally acceptable ideas and relations cannot solely provide details of such micro-communication acts and behaviors. Understanding comprehensive pictures of the incidents requires queer(ing) thoughts that resist the sets of (hetero)normative ideas and relations organizing everyday personal, institutional, and political lives. So, alternative and additional possibilities to work out the material consequences, produced by the paradoxes of male same-sex sexual and romantic desire, can be imagined. Still, there remains a long and long way to get to a society where people will be free of historical and existing power relations. Consequently, in the meantime I advocate for a queer critique interrogating, challenging, and transforming the field boundaries of Health and Intercultural Communication. Such divisive disciplinary boundary limits and/or disables potential emergences of different sets of knowledge.

Thus, I once again remind the readers that the discipline of Communication has been always already interdisciplinary since the beginning. The discipline of Communication has been that way for a long time. Yet, most Communication scholars carry on and perform their academic trainings that explicate the assumed boundaries of the field and its appropriate productions of knowledge. We, as Communication scholars who are interested in working on both the health and intercultural, must be critically self-reflexive of our own trainings that may constraint us to work toward *(im)proper* productions of interdisciplinary knowledge. There remain intellectual and political spaces for us to recognize and disrupt our own internalizations and reproductions of disciplinary boundaries. So, each of us will help build stronger and thicker bridges to intersect among Health and Intercultural Communication, which have been mostly treated as two different fields of Communication Inquiry. Therefore, I end this essay with the following statement. *Let's start from ourselves!*

References

Alexander, B. K. (2012). *The performative sustainability of race: Reflections on black culture and the politics of identity*. New York: Peter Lang.

Bailey, M. M. (2016). Black gay (raw) sex. In E. P. Johnson (Ed.), *No tea no shade: new writings in black queer studies* (pp. 239–261). Durham, NC: Duke University Press.

Bilge, S. (2014). Whitening intersectionality: Evanescence of race in intersectionality scholarship. In W. D. Hund & A. Lentin (Eds.), *Racism and sociology: Racism analysis yearbook 5* (pp. 175–205). Berlin: Lit Verlag/Routledge.

Brown, M. J., & Groscup, J. (2009). Perceptions of same-sex domestic violence among crisis center staff. *Journal of Family Violence, 24*(2), 87–93.

Burke, T. W., & Owen, S. S. (2006). Same-sex domestic violence: Is anyone listening? *Gay & Lesbian Review Worldwide, 13*(1), 6–7.

Butler, J. (2006). *Gender trouble: Feminism and the subversion of identity* (3rd ed.). New York: Routledge.

Calafell, B. M. (2017). When depression is in the job description #realacademicbios. *Departures in Critical Qualitative Research, 6*(1), 5–10.

Chávez, K. R. (2013). Pushing boundaries: Queer intercultural communication. *Journal of International and Intercultural Communication, 6*(2), 83–95.

Crenshaw, K. (1989). Demarginalizing the intersection of race and sex: A black feminist critique of antidiscrimination doctrine, feminist theory, and antiracist policies. *The University of Chicago Legal Forum*, 139–167.

Crenshaw, K. (1991). Mapping the margins. *Stanford Law Review, 43*, 1241–1299.

Cruz, A. (2016). *The color of kink: Black women, BDSM, and pornography*. New York: New York University Press.

Dieffenbach, C. W., & Fauci, A. S. (2011). Thirty years of HIV and AIDS: Future challenges and opportunities. *Annals of Internal Medicine, 154*, 766–771.

Dutta, M. J., & Acharya, L. (2015). Power, control, and the margins in HIV/AIDS intervention: A culture-centered interrogation of the "Avahan" campaign targeting Indian truckers. *Communication, Culture, & Critique*, *8*(2), 254–272.

Eguchi, S. (2009). Negotiating hegemonic masculinity: The rhetorical strategy of 'straight-acting' among gay men. *Journal of Intercultural Communication Research*, *38*(3), 193–209.

Eguchi, S. (2019). Queerness as strategic whiteness: A queer Asian American critique of Peter Le. In D. M. McInthosh, D. G. Moon, & T. K. Nakayama (Eds.), *Theorizing communicative power of whiteness* (pp. 29–44). New York: Routledge.

Eguchi, S., & Asante, G. (2016). Disidentifications revisited: Queer(y)ing intercultural communication theory. *Communication Theory*, *26*(2), 171–189.

Eguchi, S. & Long, H. (2019). Queer relationality as family: Yas fats! yas femmes! Yas Asians! *Journal of Homosexuality*, *66*(11), 1589–1606.

Eguchi, S., Files-Thompson, N., & Calafell, B. M. (2018). Queer (of color) aesthetics: Fleeting moments of transgression in VH1's *Love & Hip-Hop: Hollywood Season 2. Critical Studies in Media Communication*, *35*(2), 180–193.

Elwood, W. N., Greene, K., & Carter, K. K. (2003). Gentlemen don't speak: communication norms and condom use in bathhouses. *Journal of Applied Communication Research*, *31*(4), 277–297.

Eng, D. L. (2010). *The feeling of kinship: Queer liberalism and the racialization of intimacy*. Durham, NC: Duke University Press.

Frankland, A., & Brown, J. (2014). Coercive control in same-sex intimate partner violence. *Journal of Family Violence*, *29*(1), 15–22.

Fung, R. (2005). Looking for my penis: The eroticized Asian in gay video porn. In R. Guins & O.Z. Cruz (Eds.), *Popular culture: A reader* (pp. 338–348). London: Sage.

Ginossar, T., & Nelson, S., (2010). La comunidad habla: Using internet community-based information interventions to increase empowerment and access to health care of low-income Latino/a immigrants. *Communication Education*, *59*(3), 328–343.

Halberstam, J. (2018). *Trans: A quick and quirky account of gender variability*. Oakland: University of California Press.

Han, C. W. (2015). *Geisha of a different kind: Race and sexuality in gaysian America*. New York: New York University Press.

Hoang, N. T. (2014). *A View from the Bottom: Asian American masculinity and sexual representaion*. Durham, NC: Duke University Press.

Johnson, E. P. (2001). "Quare" studies, or (almost) everything I know about queer studies I learned from my grandmother. *Text and Performance Quarterly*, *21*(1), 1–25.

Johnson, E. P., & Henderson, M. G. (Eds.). (2005). *Black queer studies: A critical anthology*. Durham, NC: Duke University Press.

Lee, W. (2003). Kauering queer theory: My autocritography and a race-conscious, womanist, transnational turn. In G. A. Yep, K. E. Lovaas, & J. P. Elia (Eds.), *Queer theory and communication: From disciplining queers to queering the discipline(s)* (pp. 147–170). Binghamton, NY: Harrington Park Press.

Lewis, L. J. & Kreutzer, R. M. (2003). Toward improved interpretation and theory building of African American male sexualities. *The Journal of Sex Research*, *40*(4), 383–395.

Lim, E.-G. (2014). *Brown boys and rice queens: Spellbinding performances in the Asias*. New York: New York University Press.

McCune Jr. J. Q. (2014). *Sexual discretion: Black masculinity and the politics of passing*. Chicago, IL: University of Chicago Press.

McRuer, R. (2006). *Crip theory: Cultural signs of queerness and disability*. New York: New York University Press.

Muñoz, J. E. (1999). Disidentifications: Queers of color and the performance of politics. Minneapolis: University of Minnesota Press.

Muñoz, J. E. (2009). *Cruising utopia: The then and there of queer futurity*. New York: New York University Press.

Nakayama, T. K., & Corey, F. C. (2003). Nextext. In G. A. Yep, K. E. Lovaas, & J. P. Elia (Eds.), *Queer theory and communication: From disciplining queers to queering the discipline(s)* (pp. 147–170). Binghamton, NY: Harrington Park Press.

National Coalition of Anti-Violence Programs (NCAVP). (2017). *Lesbian, gay, bisexual transgender, queer, and HIV affected intimate partner violence in 2016*. New York: Emily Waters.

Oakley, M., Farr, R. H., & Scherer, D. G. (2017). Same-Sex parent socialization: Understanding gay and lesbian parenting practices as cultural socialization. *Journal of GLBT Family Studies*, *13*(1), 56–75.

Pérez, H. (2015). *A taste for brown bodies: Gay modernity and cosmopolitan desire*. New York: New York University Press.

Poon, M. K.-L. (2000). Inter-racial same-sex abuse. *Journal of Gay & Lesbian Social Services*, *11*(4), 39–67.

Poon, M. K.-L. (2006). The discourse if oppression in contemporary gay Asian diasporal literature: liberation or limitation? *Sexuality and Culture*, *10*(3), 29–58.

Puar, J. K. (2007). *Terrorist assemblages: Homonationalism in queer times*. Durham, NC: Duke University Press.

Puar, J. K. (2017). *The right to maim: Debility, capacity, disability*. Durham, NC: Duke University Press.

Raymond, H. F., & McFarland, W. (2009). Racial mixing and HIV risk among men who have sex with men. *AIDS Behavior*, *13*(4), 630–637.

Rubin, G. S. (1998). Thinking sex: Notes for a radical theory of the politics of sexuality. IN P. N. Nardi & B. E. Schneider (Eds.), *Social perspectives in lesbian and gay studies: A reader* (pp. 100–133). London, England: Routledge.

Sandfort, T. G. M., Melendez, R. M., & Diaz, R. M. (2007). Gender nonconformity, homophobia, and mental distress in Latino gay and bisexual men. *Journal of Sex Research*, *44* (2), 181–189.

Scott, D. (2010). *Extravagant abjection: Blackness, power, and sexuality in the African American literacy imagination*. New York: New York University Press.

Seelau, S. M., & Seelau, E. P. (2005). Gender-role stereotypes and perceptions of heterosexual, gay and lesbian domestic violence. *Journal of Family Violence*, *20*(6), 363–371.

Shimizu, C. P. (2012). *Straight sexualities: Unbinding Asian American manhoods in the movies*. Stanford, CA: Stanford University Press.

Snorton, C. R. (2014). *Nobody is supposed to know: Black sexuality on the down low*. Minneapolis: University of Minnesota Press.

Snorton, C. R. (2017). *Black on both sides: A racial history of trans identity*. Minneapolis: University of Minnesota.

Spieldenner, A. R. (2016). PrEP whores and HIV prevention: The queer communication of HIV Pre-Exposure Prophylaxis (PrEP). *Journal of Homosexuality*, *63*(12), 1685–1697.

Spieldenner, A. R. (2017). Infectious sex?: An autoethnographic exploration of HIV prevention. *QED: A Journal in LGBTQ Worldmaking*, *4*(1), 121–129.

Spieldenner, A., & Castro, C. F. (2010). Education and fear: Black and gay in the public sphere of HIV prevention. *Communication Education*, *59*(3), 274–281.

Spieldenner, A. R., & Anadolis, E. (2017). Bodies of dis-ease: Toward the re-conception of 'health' in health communication. In M. S. Jeffress (Ed.), *Pedagogy, disability and communication: Applying disability studies in the classroom* (pp. 97–110). New York: Routledge.

Stiles-Shields, C., & Carroll, R. A. (2015). Same-sex domestic violence: Prevalence, unique aspects, and clinical implications. *Journal of Sex and Marital Therapy*, *41*(6), 636–648.

Stryker, S. (2006). (De)subjugated knowledges: An introduction to transgender studies. In S. Stryker & S. Whittle (Eds.), *The transgender studies reader* (pp. 1–17). New York: Routledge.

Toyosaki, S., & Eguchi, S. (2017). Powerful uncertainty for the future of Japan's cultural diversity: Theorizing Japanese homogenizing discourses. In S. Toyosaki & S. Eguchi (Eds.), *Intercultural communication in Japan: Theorizing homogenized discourse* (pp. 1–23). New York: Routledge.

Woodyatt, C. R., & Stephenson, R. (2016). Emotional intimate partner violence experienced by men in same-sex relationships. *Culture, Health, & Sexuality*, *18*(10), 1137–1149.

Yep, G. A. (2002). From homophobia and heterosexism to heteronormativity. *Journal of Lesbian Studies*, *6*(3–4), 163–176.

Yep, G. A. (2003). The violence of heteronormativity in communication studies: Notes on injury, healing, and queer world-making. In G. A. Yep, K. E. Lovaas, & J. P. Elia (Eds.), *Queer theory and communication: From disciplining queers to queering the discipline(s)* (pp. 11–59). Binghamton, NY: Harrington Park Press.

Yep, G. A. (2013). Queering/quaring/kauering/crippin'/transing "other bodies" in intercultural communication. *Journal of International and Intercultural Communication*, *6*(2), 118–126.

Yep, G. A., Lovaas, K. E., & Pagonis, A. V. (2002). The case of "riding bareback." *Journal of Homosexuality*, *42*(4), 1–14.

Yep, G. A., Russo, S. E., Allen, J. K., & Chivers, N. T. (2017). Uniquely Glee: Transing racialized gender. In R. A. Lind (Ed.), *Race and gender in electronic media: Content, context, culture* (pp. 55–71). New York: Routledge.

CHAPTER THREE

The Construction of Women and Their Health across Cultures

BY KATIE D. SCOTT AND TINA M. HARRIS

Across the globe, the female body is simultaneously constructed through and regulated by varied cultural expectations for womanhood and wellness. Any attempt to understand women's health issues absent of a cultural and intercultural context is at best deficient and at worst counterproductive. In fact, communication about women's health is inextricably linked to cultural gender roles, an expectation for female bodies to reproduce, and a historical trend of prioritizing others' (especially men's) health and comfort over women's well-being. These interconnected forces are produced and reproduced across many levels of communication, from interpersonal provider-patient interactions to mass mediated health campaigns. To emancipate women from the negative health outcomes resulting from these forces, and to empower them to take control of conversations concerning their bodies, it is first necessary to understand the way these culturally embedded and often opaque forces conspire in the construction of the female body and what it means for that body to be "healthy."

This chapter begins with a broad overview of the social construction of health and womanhood. We explain that, while cultures vary in their understanding of each, this socially constructed view of women's health is also subject to cross-cultural influence that shapes the intersection of health and womanhood to form a shared experience for many women in the 21st century. Then, using a critical feminist lens (Wood, 2015), we use menstruation as a focal point for viewing the disguise of hegemonic behavioral regulations as critical health imperatives that are imposed upon women, often without regard for their lived experience and to their ultimate detriment. To do this, we search existing reports from social science and humanities literature for discourse for reflections of themes that feminist rhetorical and discursive scholars have critiqued for decades. To conclude, we offer suggestions for the improvement of future research on intercultural communication regarding women's health issues.

Before we begin our essay, we think it important to clarify our use of the phrases "women" and "women's health." There is a commonly made distinction between sex, seen as a largely biological construct, and gender, seen generally as a social construct. We subscribe to this notion, embracing Lorber's argument that "bodies differ in many ways physiologically, but they are completely transformed by social practices to fit into the salient categories of a society" (2003, p. 13). In other words, any physiological differences between female and male bodies are only socially important when "social practices transform [these differences] into social facts" (Lorber, 2003, p. 19). Thus, while truly "pure" categories of sex and gender do not exist, societies attempt to identify characteristics of sex and gender categories to reduce ambiguities; both sex and gender are socially constructed. And while communication scholars have been aware of the inadequacy of this particularly pernicious binary for some time (e.g., Condit, 1992), the traditional understanding of healthcare within the bounds of a female-male sex binary remains widely unchallenged by medical practitioners, health communication scholars, and lay persons alike.

This binary excludes intersex and non-cisgender individuals by failing to acknowledge the social construction of gender and sex. Particularly when discussing healthcare conducted in gender- or sex-segregated facilities (i.e., women's health clinics), we see trans, agender, and nonbinary individuals face erasure through "a politics of recognition regarding being in the appropriate place or possessing the correct anatomy to be provided service" (Bauer et al., 2009, p. 355). Some inclusivity efforts are beginning to address these concerns; for example, the World Health Organization released a bulletin in 2017 on the need to address health inequities for transgender and non-gender binary individuals (Thomas et al., 2017). Yet despite such efforts, the imposition of the existing binary remains salient in health interventions, public policy, and cultural expectations placed upon those persons labeled biologically female.

Thus, we use the phrase "women's health" to refer to health issues that affect individuals who tend to fit society's salient categories of "female" or "woman." For example, individuals who menstruate may not identify as women but nevertheless will face societal repercussions for experiencing a bodily condition affiliated with femaleness and womanhood. It is to be expected that menstruation would come with additional stressors if one's gender identity marginalized their experience further, but such a discussion is not within the scope of this chapter.

Our final task before beginning the bulk of this chapter is to acknowledge our subjectivities as authors, which is a common practice in feminist scholarship. We find that, in the discussion of cultures, bodies, and identities other than our own, disclosing our standpoints could be beneficial for readers interpreting the content that follows. Katie Scott is a White, cis-gender woman who was raised exclusively in the Southeast United States. As a graduate student, she uses a critical feminist lens to research communication about women's health issues such as chronic pelvic pain, menstruation, and gynecologic health disclosures. Her interest in this area of study stems from personal dissatisfaction in her experiences with women's healthcare, including a lengthy delay in diagnosis of chronic pelvic pain that she attributes to a systemic failure in understanding and prioritizing women's health issues. Dr. Tina Harris, although by all appearances African American, has a rich ethnic heritage, including grandmothers of Native American and European descent. She was raised in Rota, Spain for a several of her formative years and still feels connected to Spanish culture. Although known best for her work on interracial communication, she also does work with intersecting identities including religion, race, ethnicity, and gender. Together, the authors' interests in culture, gender, and health communication respectively shape the remainder of this chapter.

The Social Construction of Health and Womanhood

Health as a Social Construct

Conceptualizing health as a social construct will likely seem odd to those individuals who conceive of health as a state of being that is identifiable through detectable biological characteristics. Nevertheless, it is important to realize that health extends beyond purely material concerns like body mass index, the functionality of vital organs, and the presence or absence of an infectious disease. Although these markers can be indicative of health status, health and illness are also *ideas*, constructed and experienced through the communication of cultural beliefs, values, and attitudes (Kleinman, Eisenberg, & Good, 2006). Presently, we unpack this approach to conceptualizing health in two ways: the way culture shapes understandings of healthiness and healthcare, and the role of culture in individuals' (un) healthy behaviors.

To appropriately account for this social construction of health in research and theorizing about *intercultural* health communication, we must thoughtfully consider the balance between unique and shared cultural values. Each culture has a rich and interesting history that has shaped the way people in that culture understand health. We see this exemplified in the prevalence of fatalistic attitudes among African-American Evangelical Protestant women in the southern United States, who have historically placed control of difficult situations—including important health outcomes—into God's hands (Mansfield, Mitchell, & King, 2002; Peek, Sayad, & Markwardt, 2008). Still, given the history of international influence and our increasingly globalized world, we can look for generalizable characteristics across some cultures (e.g., commonalities in perceptions of womanhood that create intercultural agendas for "women's" health issues).

However, it is vital that we understand the risk of looking for and employing generalizations in health communication research. One risky generalization in the literature is the common differentiation between "Eastern" and "Western" understandings of health (see du Pré, 2014). This differentiation depicts Western conceptualizations of health as science- and evidence-oriented and Eastern conceptualizations as nature- and harmony-oriented. While Western medicine is typified as prioritizing the discovery of health-compromising forces and a fight-the-enemy approach to healthcare, Eastern medicine is described as coping-focused with a preference for less aggressive treatments.

Although this geographic binary might serve as a productive starting point for understanding that cultures differ in perceptions of health and the history that shapes those differences (e.g., in du Pré's textbook for an undergraduate health communication course, published 2014), making generalizations aligning geography with cultural values risks erasing important cultural differences and reproducing power structures based in stereotypes or prejudice. For example, the problematics of the East-West binary for Asian Americans (e.g., Orientalism; Said, 1978) has been explored in psychology literature. Research notes that collectivism, face-saving, and other "Eastern" behavioral phenomena are implicitly and explicitly ascribed to Asian Americans by mental health professionals (Okazaki & Saw, 2011). Critically, the result is that Asian American behavior is interpreted through a cultural deficit lens, privileging explanations that would credit "Eastern" ethnic heritage and "foreigner" status for behaviors that contrast with dominant European American behavioral patterns (Uba, 2002). Considering these criticisms of the East-West binary and other essentializing theorization on culture, we will attempt to cautiously avoid similar problematics in our efforts to draw connections between (and differentiate) cultures' views of health and women.

Culture not only constructs conceptions of health and illness, but also influences the context in which people engage in "healthy" or "unhealthy" behaviors. In a recent critique of how culture is used in global public health policy creation, which often frames culture as an *obstacle* to objective and efficient health interventions, Mohan Dutta (2016) explains that when considering cultural context in research and praxis we must account for practices and resources like sports, dances, spirituality, cuisine, and artistic expression that can *positively* impact physical and mental well-being. Cultural context, in tandem with structural features such as access to affordable healthcare, can both improve and detract from the health of individuals within a community. Social scientists and health practitioners who recognize this are working to integrate culture more effectively in their work, although with varying levels of success.

Unfortunately, international and cross-cultural health initiatives often forsake genuine consideration of such cultural health resources for "lip service to cultural insiders," while prioritizing "objective" biomedical expertise when designing health interventions (Dutta, 2016, p. 6). To address this, Basu and Dutta advocate the use of culture-centered participatory health communication work, which would center the needs of at-risk populations "by highlighting the voices of cultural participants and by offering community participation" in health communication praxis (2009, p. 86). They have demonstrated the value of such an approach by working with commercial sex workers in Sonagachi and Kalighat, India to design solutions to increase safer sex practices.

While a traditional, biomedical health intervention would likely have centered educating women about the risks of unprotected sex and teaching them how to request that clients use a condom, the participatory approach used by Basu and Dutta (2009) discovered that the underlying motivation for having unprotected sex was not a lack of health information or assertiveness with clients. Rather, a key obstacle for using barriers was the need for stable income; that is to say, women who needed the income to support their families felt that their financial dependence on clients gave the client the power to decide whether or not to use a condom. The participatory approach to culture-centered health intervention accounted for the women's lives outside of their risk-status and occupation as sex workers. This acknowledged the women's agency, humanity, and role in their communities while also finding a solution that addressed the root of the health concern (economic resources) rather than defaulting to teaching communication strategies or health information.

It is vital that we consider the socially constructed aspects of health, as well as who is represented in the spaces where conceptualizations of health are discussed and agendas for global health initiatives are created. Discrepancies in understanding health, healthiness, and healthcare have the potential to both reveal rich cultural differences and impede intercultural health communication. As nations and cultures become increasingly interconnected, opportunities for productive intercultural communication about health issues grow in importance. Understanding and respecting cultural forces linked to the idea of health will be imperative to the successful navigation of international health initiatives.

Womanhood as a Social Construct

Although we acknowledged earlier the problems in labeling certain health concerns and behaviors "women's health" issues, we feel the need to supply further clarification on what we mean by "womanhood" in the following section. This chapter aims to address similarities and differences in women's health issues from cultures across the globe, so we have approached our discussion of the social construction of health and womanhood broadly. Nevertheless, even necessary breadth and generalizability risks essentializing claims of what "womanhood" is. Essentialism places static and inescapable identities upon groups of individuals (i.e., women or females) without accounting for personal or cultural differences (Collins & Bilge, 2016). Thus, we advise readers to keep in mind that the following critical analysis of womanhood makes claims about how many cultures understand women and the female body *generally*, but does not exhaustively account for the nuanced differences in societies across the world. Specific cultures are discussed more later in this chapter.

Across cultures, womanhood is often synonymous with motherhood, and the female body is inextricably linked with its presumed heterosexual reproductive potential. In an interdisciplinary book analyzing the rhetoric of infertility in the United States and Europe, Robin Jensen notes that "although men and male bodies play a central role in the process of conception, the female body and its ability to conceive and carry a child to term have remained the primary focus of medical and societal discussions" (2016, p. 8). Said another way, while the female body cannot procreate alone, it is the subject of significantly more attention from medicine and politics than the other (male) body in the procreation equation. Jensen goes on to narrate a history in which women are the near-exclusive focus of research on infertility and remain discursively the sole agents responsible for failure to conceive children. While the current chapter does not center infertility as a topic of inquiry, Jensen's thesis reveals one understanding of womanhood shared by many cultures: the female body alone is medically and morally responsible for reproduction.

Linking womanhood to motherhood, and in turn to reproduction, also constructs the female body as inherently sexual, but this sexuality lacks the agency for sexual desire (Tolman, 2003). Rather, the female body is a sexual object, on display for beholders to enjoy but not for its own benefit and pleasure. We should mention here that some female bodies are perceived to be more sexual and/or less motherly than others; for example, within the United States, the *hyper*sexualizing of Black bodies has constructed Black women as sexually voracious and deviant (Collins, 2000). As an object, the female body requires constant attention to maintain its appeal to those who gaze upon it. Dominant discourse demands ongoing cosmetic improvement, which can be accomplished "by buying certain products that … make 'the most girl parts' of them socially legitimized and accepted" (Levine, 2002, p. 37). These products range from various diets, to makeup, to discrete menstrual hygiene products, to cosmetic surgery. One sinister yet convincing interpretation of societal emphasis on female body presentation posits that increasing preoccupation with outward appearance "represents the ways society has responded to the gains of marginalized groups through 'distractions' that focus energy on the body and its management" (Shaw & Lee, 2007, p. 231). Womanhood demands a presentable body for the public, creating an exhausting agenda for the individual who must behave according to cultural expectations, maintain a proportional figure, and conceal natural body processes (e.g., menstruation or body hair growth).

Womanhood is a social construction that has developed throughout time with an expectation—at least in patriarchal societies—that women will submit to men as their superiors. And across modern societies, the echo of this patriarchal construction can be heard at the structural level, of which culture is part and parcel. Historically, laws have defined women as property, justice systems have permitted husbands to abuse their wives as a form of behavioral correction, and doctors have willingly experimented on women's bodies to treat spurious afflictions such as "rebelliousness" (Weitz, 2003). One might be inclined to label these examples of patriarchal control as matters of the past, or argue that such blatant sexism is not a systemic issue in modern "developed" cultures. Yet, social trends set into motion by those preceding us can have lasting effects on our lives and well-being. As this chapter will demonstrate, many societies still perpetuate implicit and explicit gender roles—now ingrained in our cultures—which can be manipulated to justify excessive demands upon the "female body" for the sake of maintaining a body that fits the socially constructed criteria for healthiness.

The Intersection of Health and Womanhood

Communication both within and across cultures constructs not only the idea of womanhood—including which people are recognized as women and how women should use, or not use, their bodies—but also the perceptions of the unique health issues faced by women. In early writings about the politics of sex, Foucault (1990) argued that societal influencers strategically discipline bodies and regulate populations in part through the medicalization of women's bodies and sex.

The reproductive potential of women—or those society deems women—is used to enforce moral responsibility for their own health outcomes in addition to the health and stability of their children, family, and society. By connecting women's sexuality to these responsibilities, "sex became a crucial target of a power organized around the management of life rather than the menace of death" (Foucault, 1990, p. 147). This sort of coercive control over women in the name of responsible "management of life" (i.e., healthcare) is still manifest today.

By acknowledging the socially constructed nature of health, we can understand how medicine and medical language could be used to regulate bodily behaviors. Medicalization—present at linguistic, interpersonal, and institutional levels—both ascribes medical meaning to behaviors or conditions and prescribes medical care "for eliminating or controlling problematic experiences that are defined as deviant for the purpose of securing adherence to social norms" (Riessman, 2003, p. 48). Particularly with women's health issues, medicalization has the potential to estrange individuals from their bodies by making natural states of the female body (such as menstruation) incompatible with the social demands of womanhood (concealment of all bodily fluids). Riessman (2003), among other critical scholars, faults medicalization for stigmatizing individuals with "deviant" conditions, removing agency and self-efficacy from laypeople, and risking iatrogenic (i.e., harm done by a health provider or service) effects. Both childbirth (Riessman, 2003) and infertility (Jensen, 2016) have been identified as examples of the medicalization of women's health within the United States and Europe. Because of multiple parties' vested interest in reproductive success, it was not difficult for societies to justify moving the female body and its procreation potential from the privacy of homes (with midwives and close relatives) to controlled settings such as hospitals and clinics.

Through the medicalization of women's health issues, the healthcare industry and others invested in the management of women's behavior gain considerable control over the female body, even prior to pregnancy. While we do not mean to suggest that all women's health concerns are unnecessarily medicalized, we do argue that health communication often addresses women's health in a way that decenters the (sometimes medical) needs of women and prioritizes the comfort of the elite—often male—individuals present in crafting public health policy and health campaigns. Put another way, public health agendas have historically been men-centric (i.e., centering male interest and privilege) at the societal, national, and global levels (Barker et al., 2010). Women are underrepresented in agenda-setting spaces and, when they do have access to those spaces, may not be in positions of power to confront problematic cultural practices. This prevents women from challenging proposed "solutions" for health concerns that actually reinforce "notions of purity and hygiene [that] are often harmful to [their] health" (Sen, Östlin, &

George, 2007). A review of the literature will reveal that few societies escape culpability for perpetuating a rhetoric of the healthy female body that places societal expectations for reproduction and etiquette above women's actual health needs.

Menstruation Across Cultures: The Medicalization of the Female Body's Fluids

Thus far, we have reviewed health and womanhood as socially constructed ideas that both vary and share similarities across cultures. We explained that people interpret their health in ways that surpass the knowledge we can glean from objective biomedical markers. To elaborate, we mean that health is socially constructed through cultural beliefs that affect "how we communicate about our health problems, the manner in which we present our symptoms, when and to whom we go for care, how long we remain in care, and how we evaluate that care" (Klcinman et al., 2006, p. 141). In addition, we drew upon the work of feminist scholars to reveal a discourse that aligns womanhood with motherhood, motherhood with reproductive potential, and reproductive potential with sexuality. We argued that this sexuality is implicitly and explicitly regulated through society's excessive demands of the female body, some of which are masked as well-intentioned health initiatives.

Given what we have detailed about the social construction of health and womanhood across cultures, we will now discuss how menstrual hygiene initiatives across cultures reflect dominant discourses commonly used to exercise control over the female body. We choose menstrual hygiene as a topic of interest for two reasons: first, because of its multicultural affiliation with fertility, menstruation is a health topic closely tied to discourses of womanhood, motherhood, and sexuality; second, because United Nations officials have recognized menstrual health and hygiene inequity as a human rights violation (Every woman's right to water, sanitation and hygiene, 2014). As mentioned before, the socially constructed aspects of health can be harnessed to make natural states of the female body incompatible with the social demands of womanhood; local and international menstrual hygiene initiatives often exemplify this manufactured incompatibility.

Using a critical feminist lens to analyze how women are asked to maintain "healthy" bodies while menstruating, we can see that the standards for managing this natural process prioritize reducing societal discomfort with menstrual fluids over protecting individuals' health while menstruating. As we investigate policies, initiatives, and research on menstrual hygiene, we acknowledge that the forces at play represent gender and health norms that have been socially constructed both within and across cultures. Although most research studies focus on a single nation or culture, even these single-culture reports implicitly reflect discourses shared through a history of colonization and globalization.

The Stigmatization and Medicalization of Menstruation

In 1978, Gloria Steinem authored a short essay titled *If Men Could Menstruate.* Attempting to guess at the hypothetical outcomes of men dealing with menstruation, she posits that "menstruation would become an enviable, boast-worthy, masculine event … Boys would mark the onset of menses, the longed-for proof of manhood, with religious ritual and stag parties … [and] Sanitary supplies would be federally funded and free" (Steinem, 2019, p. 151). Although Steinem's essay is written with the United States in mind, her critique—that menstruation is taboo by virtue of its affiliation with the female (rather than the male) body—reflects an understanding of the stigmatization and medicalization of menstruation that crosses national boundaries. Such cross-cultural similarities, and intercultural differences, in the perception of menstruation and menstrual hygiene are at play in agenda-setting to address menstrual hygiene as a global human rights issue. Before we look at specific global and local initiatives, we must review historical understandings of menstruation that continue to circulate in conversations about women's health issues.

While experts on the rhetoric of menstruation acknowledge that "there can be no fixed framework for the analysis of the treatment of menstruation from a cultural point of view," certain historical discourse surrounding menstruation is relevant to present expectations of women who are menstruating (Newton, 2016, p. 42). For instance, several foundational religious texts (e.g., the Bible, the Quran, and the Jewish code of law, *Halakha*) depict a menstruating woman as sinful or unclean and compel her to remove herself from certain settings (Bhartiya, 2013; Newton, 2016). Early medical thinking, documented in records from the Hippocratic school and Aristotle's writings on natural science, purported that the accumulation of menstrual blood in the body could have negative health outcomes and described menstruation as a release of bodily toxins (Newton, 2016). Some cultures even connected menstruation to cosmology (Delaney, 1988) and witchcraft (Delaney, Lupton, & Toth, 1988), with menstrual blood symbolizing women's destructive power. Whether because it was unseemly, unholy, or unsanitary, women throughout history and across cultures were expected to conceal menstrual bleeding (Newton, 2016). This imperative to hide menstrual blood—interpreted in some cultures as needing to hide the menstruating individual altogether—is a salient and significant similarity in cultures' attitudes towards menstruation. We will ultimately argue that this imperative is representative of attitudes towards women's health issues more broadly, which often marginalize women in the name of self- and societal-care.

Stigmatizing Menstruation in the Name of Hygiene

The construction of menstruation as an unhygienic, and even deadly, process stigmatizes menstruating individuals. Goffman (1963) proposes three categories of stigma—bodily abominations, character blemishes, and visible inclusion in marginalized groups—and, as Johnston-Robledo and Chrisler (2013) write, menstrual blood fits within each category. First, menstrual blood—like other bodily fluids (Curtis & Biran, 2001)—could, if visible, trigger disgust and be classified as a bodily abomination. Second, menstrual blood leaks violate expectations for female characters to be in control of their bodily processes, because "through the proper [behavior or] choice of products, she *should* have kept the evidence of her menses out of sight" (Johnston-Robledo & Chrisler, 2013, p. 10). Finally, menstruation, and any visible mark of it, is connected to the socially constructed category of "woman." Thus, a person revealed to be menstruating is included—or reminded of their inclusion—in the near-universally marginalized status of *woman*. This stigma contributes to modern expectations for the management and concealment of menstrual blood; examples of such expectations in specific cultures will be discussed later.

Unfounded skepticism and stigma towards menstruation remains prevalent; and, although most modern health initiatives may not align menstruation with magic, they continue to justify their demands of bleeding female bodies in the name of protecting individual and community health. Behavioral expectations during menstruation puts the menstruating person's well-being at risk—from adolescents stressing about keeping tampons hidden (Kissling, 1996) to women isolating themselves in outdoor buildings while bleeding (Bhartiya, 2013)—for the sake of not discomforting others with visible menstrual blood or menstrual hygiene products.

While menstrual blood may not be considered witchcraft today (with the exception of some countries; e.g., Yaprak, 2011), it is still seen as both inherently sexual—"a crucial signifier of reproductive potential and thus embodied womanhood" (Lee, 2003, p. 84)—and unsanitary. Though some cultures are exceptional—for instance, Sikhism "condemns the taboos surrounding menstruation and post-partum pollution … [it is regarded] as an essential and natural process" (Bhartiya, 2013)—practices like isolating menstruating individuals in a secluded part of their home or blocking women from education, religious sanctuaries, and the workplace continue today (Newton, 2016). In many cultures, it is still normal for menarche—one's first menstrual cycle—to signal a removal of girls from the public sphere (i.e., the classroom) to begin their lives as women in the private sphere (i.e., their marital home).

Even cultures that do not explicitly practice isolating menstruating women from certain spaces continue to systemically impede the achievement of their own societal norms for concealment. Despite global health officials' agreement that access to menstrual hygiene products is essential (Every woman's right to water, sanitation and hygiene, 2014), most countries (e.g., the United States, United Kingdom, Malaysia, Australia, Hungary, Denmark, Sweden, Norway, Greece, Italy, and France) continue to tax sanitary products, maintaining financial barriers that seem to conflict with their hygiene initiatives (Phelan, 2015). Thus, women are socialized to see their menstrual body as unhygienic and repulsive to others, yet they are rarely given easy access to the resources they need to meet concealment norms and maintain the image of controlled femininity often demanded by social constructions of womanhood.

Medicalization and the Concealment of Menstrual Blood

So far, we have demonstrated that menstrual stigma perpetuates gender inequity, from social isolation to the taxing of products deemed a human right. Now, we will discuss how health initiatives medicalize menstruation, a natural bodily process, in an attempt to resolve the health disparities that result from menstrual stigma. Continuing, at first, to discuss cross-cultural similarities, we begin by explaining how concealment imperatives are used to justify health interventions which do not address the root cause of the health concerns (i.e., the concealment imperative). We then analyze specific cultures' treatment of menstruation and menstrual hygiene as examples of how the social construction of women's health imposes hegemonic behavioral regulations that are often detrimental for those it purports to help.

Medicalization, or using medical language and medical care to discourage "deviant" behaviors (Riessman, 2003), incentivizes conformity to social norms with healthiness. At linguistic, interpersonal, and institutional levels, menstruation is medicalized by incentivizing the concealment of menstrual blood with the reward of social acceptability; that is to say, by concealing menstrual blood women conform to acceptable norms of healthiness and womanhood. The conflation of concealment and healthiness constructs menstruation "as something that [is] happening *to* [women], as something *outside* of themselves" which can only be regulated through pharmaceuticals or sanitation devices (Lee, 2003, p. 87; our emphasis). Women, absent of medical or natural interference, must then anticipate the equivalent of a monthly *illness* that arises naturally from their seemingly traitorous body; the treatment for this illness: concealment. While cultures vary in preferred concealment measures and intensity of consequences for failure to conceal menstrual blood, they typically share healthiness as a justification for menstrual hygiene norms.

The identification of menstrual hygiene as a global health concern and human rights issue confirms its medicalization generally (Every woman's right to water, sanitation and hygiene, 2014). More specifically, menstruation is medicalized at a linguistic level when rhetoric surrounding the natural process makes use of medical vocabulary, such as sanitation and hygiene (Riessman, 2003). The treatment of menstruation as a process for medical intervention occurs at both an institutional level—in the adequate provision of menstrual hygiene products and clean water sources—and at an interpersonal (i.e., patient-provider) level when oral contraceptives or other medications are prescribed. This is not to say that medical interventions are wholly bad. The introduction of tampons and other menstrual hygiene products has helped women—or at least those with access to such products—reclaim some freedom "to carry on life as normal," and remain active as long as they used the proper tools to conceal their menstrual blood (Newton, 2016, p. 110). In addition, contraceptive prescriptions can be sexually liberating and make a significant improvement in menstrual pain for some.

Nevertheless, the medicalization of menstruation rests upon, and accordingly upholds, the imperative to conceal signs of menstruation. Often, advertisements for menstrual hygiene products, such as tampons, frame the products as tools for maintaining a socially acceptable female body during unsanitary biological cycles. For example, original Tampax ads acknowledged and perpetuated the perception of menstruation as unfeminine and unsanitary—and in need of concealment—by emphasizing that an applicator is used to insert tampons, so that people who menstruate do not have to physically touch their "most girl parts" (Linton, 2007). The very marketing of hygiene products reinforces the concealment imperative that contributes to ongoing gender inequity.

Cultures' Menstrual Attitudes and Practices

While this chapter has touched broadly on the social construction of key concepts (i.e., health and womanhood); the role of stigma in creating a concealment imperative for menstruating individuals; and how medicalization makes that concealment imperative a matter of personal and public health, we now turn our analysis to individual cultures. We look at menstrual practices and health initiatives together to understand how different culture reflect or deviate from the hegemonic behavioral regulations discussed thus far. To be clear, the following analyses should be read and interpreted within their intended scope. The authors are scholars who work primarily with health communication, interracial communication, and critical gender and race theories contextually situated in the United States, and they do not claim expert knowledge of all cultures. So, the analyses should be read as brief reviews of preexisting research, deductively coded for the themes discussed in this chapter. It is our hope that this specific analysis of a broad selection of literature will provide a launching pad for future investigations into specific intra- and intercultural communication about menstruation.

Menarche and ama-Xhosa women

The tensions that arise as a result of medicalizing menstruation can be observed in cultures' treatment of menarche and menstruating in public. Menarche, often seen as a marker of sexual maturation, can be both a period of celebration and a time to initiate bodily discipline. Interviews with South African women in the ama-Xhosa ethnic group reveal examples of this duplicitous experience (Padmanabhanunni, Jaffer, & Steenkamp, 2017). A quarter of those interviewed disclosed that their families had, either with or without consent, sought contraceptive medications upon menarche to reduce the interviewee's risk of extramarital pregnancy. Although this practice was normal to the ama-Xhosa women, they also noted that it indicated a lack of trust in their ability to remain sexually inactive prior to marriage. Yet, even as they found their sexual agency being questioned, a few of the participants reported that menarche and following menstrual cycles were welcome indicators of womanhood, fertility, and "feeling alive." Post-menarche, though, women must continue the management of their recurring condition in a society that deems their menstruation, even when concealed, unclean (Padmanabhanunni et al., 2017). Within these menarche narratives, we can see how the interviewees' culture connected menstruation to womanhood, womanhood to sexuality, and sexuality to a need for bodily regulation.

As the women explained, menarche indicated a transition into womanhood and fertility. While their culture encouraged celebration of this new life stage, the women had mixed feelings about the implications that this new experience had for their bodies. Almost immediately, menarche was connected with reproductive potential and a demand for self-control. In addition to concealing menstrual cycles after the menarche celebration, the women were expected to exercise discipline over presumed sexual desires and avoid premarital pregnancy. The decision some families made—to purchase contraceptives—reflects medicalization at the interpersonal level, as close relations seeking medical intervention upon menarche communicated their desire for the women to regulate behaviors and avoid potentially shameful outcomes. Though fear of pregnancy may have mediated the relationship between medical intervention and menstruation, the use of contraceptives still serves a dual function—extramarital pregnancy would be a visible reminder that the women are capable of menstruating, in addition to an admission of unmarried sex.

Water and Concealment: India and Tanzania

Having toilets and running water, though taken for granted in some countries, has a significant influence on the experience of menstruation and gender equity. Many women in rural India and Tanzania are still deeply influenced by menstrual taboos (Thérèse & Maria, 2010), which makes concealment of marks that would identify someone as actively menstruating essential for maintaining personal and familial dignity (arora, 2017). In families with more traditional attitudes toward menstruation, an individual caught with a visible blood stain could bring shame to themselves and their family. Although women in more urban areas may face little restriction to their mobility during menstruation (Kumar & Srivastava, 2011), women in very rural areas may have to support each other in retrieving water from far-away sources to clean their bodies and menstrual rags, as the risk of cramping while walking or staining one's clothes renders the walk unsafe or unmanageable (arora, 2017). Similar concerns are present elsewhere.

In many countries, girls still struggle to manage their menstrual cycles while in school (e.g., arora, 2017; Sommer, 2013). An in-depth study in Tanzania found that students felt uncomfortable discussing their menstrual cycle with teachers or nurses at the school. Teachers reinforced menstrual taboos, electing themselves to visit nearby colleagues' homes to change menstrual products during the school day. Nurses were also known to criticize students seeking help with menstrual discomfort because menstruation "is not a disease" (Sommer, 2013, p. 338). The same study's students explained that they felt unequipped to manage their menstrual hygiene privately at school, as an organization donated toilets to their school's dorms rather than pit latrines. Because the toilets required running water, students were afraid of leaving blood stains in toilets during water shortages and might instead opt to manage their menstrual hygiene products in a way that was more private but less clean.

In both India and Tanzania, women living under the pressure of traditional taboos go to extreme lengths to conceal signs of menstruation, including imposing limits on their own mobility and sacrificing cleanliness for privacy. While some health interventions treat medicalization as the remedy for stigma, the Tanzanian study shows that international efforts made to remedy disparities in nations' access to menstrual sanitation and hygienic resources should avoid dependence on medicalization as a solution. Many international efforts lack effective cross-cultural communication and fail to meet the needs of the people they aim to help, as seen in the donation of toilets rather than pit latrines to a Tanzanian school where water shortages are common. Perhaps consideration of the stigmatizing cultural discourses that enforce concealment—rather than a medicalized lens that presumes running-water toilets are inherently more hygienic than pit latrines—would have resulted in a more suitable intervention.

Alternative Interpretations of Menstrual Attitudes

Within cultures, there are activists, researchers, laypeople, and policy makers who challenge dominant discourse and attempt to improve gender equity and human rights. We will provide two examples of this. First, we will discuss the menstrual equity movement in the United States. This feminist-driven movement hopes to increase access to menstrual hygiene products for women of various socioeconomic backgrounds in the U.S. Second, we review one researcher's reinterpretation of menstrual taboos in ancient Egypt for an alternative understanding of the common concealment imperative. The inclusion of these nations as exemplars of alternative attitudes provides contrasting interpretations of the discourse previously charged with medicalization and stigmatization. Selection of each resulted from access to scholarly and popular literature that supported alternative readings of the cultures' treatment of menstruation, not to forward either as more or less progressive in their approach to menstrual hygiene and gender equity.

The U.S.'s Tampon Tax and Menstrual Equity Movement

While the discourse about access to feminine hygiene resources—from water, to tampons, to menstrual cups—varies across the globe, one recurring controversy in the U.S. is the "tampon tax." Although medicalizing menstruation creates a demand for the use of feminine hygiene products, like tampons, to contain unsanitary fluids, in the U.S. tampons are not universally exempt from taxes as other non-luxury necessities are (Hillin, 2015; Paquette, 2016). National activists and policy drivers have dubbed the fight for increased access to menstrual products "menstrual equity" (Weiss-Wolf & Burns, 2016). Although the fight for menstrual equity and ending the tax on tampons is not new, recent events—Donald Trump's remarks on menstruation during a presidential debate (Weiss-Wolf, 2015), Barack Obama's call for women to organize at state-level against the sales tax (Weiss-Wolf,

2016), and the introduction of the Dignity for Incarcerated Women Act in 2017 (Weiss-Wolf & Bozelko, 2017)—have renewed national attention to menstrual rights.

The menstrual equity movement in the U.S. uptakes the medicalization of menstruation to fight for better access to menstrual hygiene products, from ending the tampon tax in all states to increasing availability of products for homeless and incarcerated women. Although this upholds the concealment imperative, it is differentiated by its somewhat counter-culture leadership. Menstrual equity is forwarded as a movement by women outside of the dominant culture, including menstrual policy advocate, Jennifer Weiss-Wolf, and legal strategist, Laura Strausfeld, Period Equity is "the [United States'] first law and policy organization fighting for menstrual equity" (Period Equity, n.d.). Additionally, in their vocal arguments for their cause menstrual equity advocates bring menstruation into the public sphere for conversation, challenging stigma and the need to conceal all reminders of menstruation as they argue for the right to access products that would equip them to maintain their menstrual hygiene.

Menstrual Customs to Protect Women in Egypt

Challenging assumptions that all cultural practices that temporarily remove women from society are based in perceptions of menstruation as evil or impure, Frandsen (2007) examines ancient Egyptian rules for (not) interacting with menstruating women for alternative explanations for the rules. Through an investigation into Egyptian writings on the anatomy, physiology, and religious meaning of reproduction, Frandsen concludes that "'the menstrual taboo' as such does not exist. Rather, what is found … is a wide range of distinct rules for conduct regarding menstruation that bespeak quite different, even opposite, purposes and meanings" (2007, p. 81)

According to Frandsen (2007), prescribed behavior for *men* in ancient Egypt told them to avoid their place of work while their wives or daughters were menstruating. However, the women were also directed to leave their village while menstruating. The bidirectional expectation for isolation during times of menstruation appears to maintain a concealment imperative based in stigma, but perhaps a less sexist or inequitable imperative. Ultimately, Frandsen's explains that human reproduction—including the menstrual cycle—was simply too "mundane" to taint sacred spaces (i.e., tombs) where men worked. Though we believe this cosmological interpretation—as opposed to a medicalization interpretation—still reflects a view of menstruation as impure, we do find the outlining of proactive steps for men to contribute to the maintenance of the tomb's purity interesting.

Moving Forward

If health experts continue to define health and design initiatives with minimal, obligatory attention to cultural insiders, then the change-making potential of effective intercultural health communication is wasted (Dutta, 2016). In the words of Mahon and Fernandes, "There is a cyclical causal relationship between the neglect of menstrual hygiene within development initiatives … and low levels of awareness among communities, practitioners and policymakers … The negative effects of this neglect are far-ranging on the lives of girls and women, and on the achievement of wider development goals" (Mahon & Fernandes, 2010, p. 103). The low levels of awareness referenced by Mahon and Fernandes are particularly malicious in their ability to unintentionally create health initiatives that serve the goals of the agenda-setters—who often represent the dominant discourse—rather than the individuals the agenda is meant to help. As those invested in improving health communication move forward, we must not applaud ourselves for intercultural communication between international biomedical experts, elite representatives or policy makers from different countries, or even superficial interactions with laypeople from a culture not our own. Until it becomes the norm for health communication research to incorporate culture, gender, and even the global transmission of hegemonic discourse, true progress will be consistently impeded.

In addition to the consideration of culture and discourse in health communication research, it would be beneficial for future studies to regularly engage the international historical, political, and social power underlying women's health issues. Cultures were not formed, and do not exist now, in a vacuum. While health communication scholars and practitioners tend to consider a single culture broadly, perhaps with the addition of that culture's treatment of gender—a criticism this chapter does not escape—rarely do we thoughtfully investigate the rich *global* history that has shaped a culture historically and presently. By beginning to do so, we may learn to appreciate the importance of culture as more than an obstacle for biomedical interests to overcome when addressing health issues (Dutta, 2016). In addition, sensitizing ourselves to the multifaceted and complex history of cultures and gender inequity within them will enable us to conduct research and propose solutions that do not reflect, reproduce, or reinforce problematic power structures.

Conclusion

Intercultural communication has shaped the social construction of health, womanhood, and the intersection between the two. Policy, campaigns, and research are often intercultural in nature, particularly when addressing global health concerns. Of note, intercultural communication is also prevalent in changing the way we understand women's health issues. The nature of our interconnected world provides us with a way to know when injustice is occurring, as well as networks to hold those who perpetuate inequity accountable. The future of good health communication research must be cognizant of intercultural influence from the past and present if we are to proceed with contributing meaningful knowledge and successful health outcomes through our work. While healthcare is not often connected to social justice, a global shift in the understanding of the role health experts play in challenging or perpetuating social inequity is vital if the medical field is truly invested in the well-being of those affected by its actions. To conclude this chapter, we suggest a starting point for envisioning a future for global women's healthcare that is truly culturally sensitive and feminist in nature.

References

arora, N. (2017). Menstruation in India: Ideology, politics, and capitalism. *Asian Journal of Women's Studies, 23*(4), 528–537. doi: 10.1080/12259276.2017.1386817

Barker, G., Greene, M., Goldstein-Siegel, E., Nascimento, M., Segundo, M., & Pawlak, P. (2010). *What men have to do with it: Public policies to promote gender equality*. Washington, DC: International Center for Research on Women. Retrieved from https://www.icrw.org/wp-content/uploads/2016/10/What-Men-Have-to-Do-With-It.pdf

Basu, A., & Dutta, M. J. (2009). Sex workers and HIV/AIDS: Analyzing participatory culture-centered health communication strategies. *Human Communication Research, 35*(1), 86–114. doi: 10.1111/j.1468-2958.2008.01339.x

Bauer, G. R., Hammond, R., Travers, R., Kaay, M., Hohenadel, K. M., & Boyce, M. (2009). "I don't think this is theoretical; this is our lives": How erasure impacts care for transgender people. *Journal of the Association of Nurses in AIDS Care, 20*(5), 348–361. doi: 10.1016/j.jana.2009.07.004

Bhartiya, A. (2013). Menstruation, religion and society. *International Journal of Social Science and Humanity, 3*(6), 523–527. doi: 10.7763/IJSSH.2013.V3.296

Collins, P. H. (2000). The sexual politics of Black womanhood. *Black feminist thought: Knowledge, consciousness, and the politics of empowerment* (pp. 123–148). New York, NY: Routledge.

Collins, P. H., & Bilge, S. (2016). Intersectionality and identity. In *Intersectionality: Key concepts* (pp. 114–135). Malden, MA: Polity Press.

Condit, C. M. (1992). Post-Burke: Transcending the sub-stance of dramatism. *Quarterly Journal of Speech, 78*, 349–355. doi: 10.1080/00335639209384002

Curtis, V. A., &Biran, A. (2001). Dirt, disgust, and disease: Is hygiene in our genes? *Perspectives in Biology and Medicine, 44*, 17–31. doi: 10.1353/pbm.2001.0001

Delaney, C. (1988). Mortal flow: Menstruation in Turkish village society. In T. Buckley & A. Gottlieb (Eds.), *Blood magic: The anthropology of menstruation* (pp. 75–93). Berkeley: University of California Press.

Delaney, J., Lupton, M., & Toth, E. (1988). The miracle of blood: Menstrual imagery in myth and poetry. In *The curse: A cultural history of menstruation* (pp. 186–199). Urbana: University of Illinois Press. (1st edn. 1976. New York: Dutton).

du Pré, A. (2014). Cultural conceptions of health and illness. In *Communicating about health: Current issues and perspectives* (pp. 166–197). New York, NY: Oxford University Press.

Dutta, M. J. (2016). Cultural context, structural determinants, and global health inequities: The role of communication. *Frontiers in Communication*, *1*(5), 1–9. doi: 10.3389/fcomm.2016.00005

Every woman's right to water, sanitation and hygiene. (2014, March 14). *Office of the United Nations High Commissioner for human rights.* Retrieved from https://www.ohchr.org/EN/NewsEvents/Pages/Everywomansrighttowatersanitationandhygiene.aspx

Foucault, M. (1990). *The history of sexuality*. New York, NY: Random House.

Frandsen, P. J. (2007). The menstrual "taboo" in ancient Egypt. *Journal of Near Eastern Studies*, *66*(2), 81–105. doi: none.

Goffman, E. (1963). *Stigma: Notes on the management of spoiled identity*. Englewood Cliffs, NJ: Prentice-Hall.

Hillin, T. (2015, June 3). These are the U.S. states that tax women for having periods. *Splinter News*. Retrieved from https://splinternews.com/these-are-the-u-s-states-that-tax-women-for-having-per-1793848102

Jensen, R. E. (2016). *Infertility: Tracing the history of a transformative term*. University Park: The Pennsylvania State University Press.

Johnston-Robledo, I., & Chrisler, J. C. (2013). The menstrual mark: Menstruation as social stigma. *Sex Roles*, *68*, 9–18. doi: 10.1007/s11199-011-0052-z

Kissling, E. A. (1996). "That's just a basic teen-age rule": Girls' linguistic strategies for managing the menstrual communication taboo. *Journal of Applied Communication Research*, *24*, 292–309. doi: 10.1080/00909889609365458

Kleinman, A., Eisenberg, L., & Good, B. (2006). Culture, illness, and care: Clinical lessons from anthropologic and cross-cultural research. *FOCUS: The Journal of Lifelong Learning in Psychiatry*, *4*(1), 140–149. doi: 10.1176/foc.4.1.140

Kumar, A., & Srivastava, K. (2011). Cultural and social practices regarding menstruation among adolescent girls. *Social Work in Public Health*, *26*, 594–604. doi: 10.1080/19371918.2010.525144

Lee, J. (2003). Menarche and the (hetero)sexualization of the female body. In R. Weitz (Ed.), *The politics of women's bodies: Sexuality, appearance, and behavior* (pp. 82–99). New York, NY: Oxford University Press.

Levine, E. (2002). "Having a female body doesn't make you feminine": Feminine hygiene advertising and 1970s television. *The Velvet Light Trap*, *50*, 36–47. doi: none.

Linton, D. (2007). Men in menstrual product advertising—1920–1949. *Women & Health, 46*(1), 99–114. doi: 10.1300/J013v46n01_07

Lorber, J. (2003). Believing is seeing: Biology as ideology. In R. Weitz (Ed.), *The politics of women's bodies: Sexuality, appearance, and behavior* (pp. 12–24). New York, NY: Oxford University Press.

Mahon, T., & Fernandes, M. (2010). Menstrual hygiene in South Asia: A neglected issue for WASH (water, sanitation and hygiene) programmes. *Gender & Development, 18*(1), 99–113. doi: 10.1080/13552071003600083

Mansfield, C. J., Mitchell, J., King, D. E. (2002). The doctor as God's mechanic? Beliefs in the southeastern United States. *Social Science & Medicine, 54*(3), 399–409. doi: 10.1016/S0277-9536(01)00038-7

Newton, V. L. (2016). *Everyday discourses of menstruation: Cultural and social perspectives.* Basingstoke, UK: Palgrave Macmillan.

Okazaki, S., & Saw, A. (2011). Culture in Asian American community psychology: Beyond the East-West binary. *American Journal of Community Psychology, 47*, 144–156. doi: 10.1007/s10464-010-9368-z

Padmanabhanunni, A., Jaffer, L., & Steenkamp, J. (2017). Menstruation experiences of South African women belonging to the ama-Xhosa ethnic group. *Culture, Health, & Sexuality*, 1–11. doi: 10.1080/13691058.2017.1371335

Paquette, D. (2016, March 15). The sudden controversy around the cost of tampons. *The Washington Post.* Retrieved from https://www.washingtonpost.com/news/wonk/wp/2016/03/15/the-sudden-controversy-around-the-cost-of-the-tampons/?utm_term=.d3a5646cb362

Peek, M. E., Sayad, J. V., & Markwardt, R. (2008). Fear, fatalism and breast cancer screening in low-income African-American women: the role of clinicians and the health care system. *Journal of General Internal Medicine, 23*(11), 1847–1853.

Period Equity. (n.d.). Home Page. Retrieved October 3, 2017, from https://www.periodequity.org/

Phelan, J. (2015, August 15). Tampon tax is real. Women everywhere pay their governments extra to have periods. *GlobalPost.* Retrieved from https://www.pri.org/stories/2015-08-15/tampon-tax-real-women-everywhere-pay-their-governments-extra-have-periods

Riessman, C. K. (2003). Women and medicalization: A new perspective. In R. Weitz (Ed.), *The politics of women's bodies: Sexuality, appearance, and behavior* (pp. 46–64). New York, NY: Oxford University Press.

Said, E. W. (1978). *Orientalism.* New York: Vintage.

Sen, G., Östlin, P., & George, A. (2007). *Unequal, unfair, ineffective and inefficient. Gender inequity in health: Why it exists and how we can change it.* Final report to the WHO Commission on Social Determinants of Health. Geneva, Switzerland: World Health Organization. Retrieved from http://www.who.int/social_determinants/resources/csdh_media/wgekn_final_report_07.pdf

Shaw, S. M., & Lee, J. (2007). Inscribing gender on the body. In S. M. Shaw & J. Lee (Eds.), *Women's voices, feminist visions: Classical and contemporary readings* (pp. 229–300). New York, NY: McGraw-Hill.

Sommer, M. (2013). Structural factors influencing menstruating school girls' health and well-being in Tanzania. *Compare: A Journal of Comparative and International Education, 43*(3), 323–345. doi: 10.1080/03057925.2012.693280

Steinem, G. (2019). If men could menstruate. *Women's Reproductive Health,* 6(3), 151–152.

Thérèse, M., & Maria, F. (2010). Menstrual hygiene in South Asia: A neglected issue for WASH (water, sanitation and hygiene) programmes. *Gender & Development, 18*(1), 99–113.

Thomas, R., Pega, F., Khosla, R., Verster, A., Hana, T., & Say, L. (2017). Ensuring an inclusive global health agenda for transgender people. *Bulletin of the World Health Organization*, 95, 154–156. doi: 10.2471/BLT.16.183913

Tolman, D. L. (2003). Daring to desire: Culture and the bodies of adolescent girls. In R. Weitz (Ed.), *The politics of women's bodies: Sexuality, appearance, and behavior* (pp. 100–121). New York, NY: Oxford University Press.

Uba, L. (2002). *A postmodern psychology of Asian Americans: Creating knowledge of a racial minority.* Albany, NY: State University of New York Press

Weiss-Wolf, J. (2015, August 11). America's very real menstrual crisis. *TIME.* Retrieved from http://time.com/3989966/america-menstrual-crisis/

Weiss-Wolf, J. (2016, January 26). Why are we paying sales tax on tampons? *The Nation.* Retrieved from https://www.thenation.com/article/why-are-we-paying-sales-tax-on-tampons/

Weiss-Wolf, J., & Bozelko, C. (2017, July 13). For women in prison, tampons should be free. *The New York Times.* Retrieved from https://kristof.blogs.nytimes.com/2017/07/13/for-women-in-prison-tampons-should-be-free/

Weiss-Wolf, J., & Burns, D. (2016, April 20). Why feminine hygiene product should be free in school. *Newsweek.* Retrieved from http://www.newsweek.com/let-girls-learn-michelle-obama-tampons-pads-education-450244

Weitz, R. (2003). A history of women's bodies. In R. Weitz (Ed.), *The politics of women's bodies: Sexuality, appearance, and behavior* (pp. 3–11). New York, NY: Oxford University Press.

Wood, J. T. (2015). Critical feminist theories: Giving voice and visibility to women's experiences in interpersonal relations. In D. O. Braithwaite & P. Schrodt (Eds.), *Engaging theories in interpersonal communication: Multiple perspectives* (pp. 203–215). Thousand Oaks, CA: SAGE Publications, Inc.

Yaprak, O. (2011). Improving the lives of African women: Proctor & Gamble "No Check No Stain" campaign for Always sanitary pads. *Advertising & Society Review, 11*(4). doi: 10.1353/asr.2011.0002

CHAPTER FOUR

Moving beyond Awareness Social Media in Health and Policy Communication: The Case of the Black Women's Health Imperative's Black Women Vote 2018 National Health Policy Agenda

BY ANNETTE MADLOCK GATISON

> Every woman has a militant responsibility to involve herself actively with her own health. We owe ourselves the protection of all the information we can acquire about the treatment of cancer and its causes, as well as about the recent findings concerning immunology, nutrition, environment, and stress. And we owe ourselves this information **before** we may have a reason to use it.
>
> Audre Lorde The Cancer Journals, 1980

Introduction

The health of individuals, communities, and the population as a whole encompasses a variety of contexts that intersects the political. Littlejohn, Foss, and Oetzel (2017) describe health as a "composite state of physical, mental, and social well-being, not simply the absence of disease (p. 347)." When *Health Communication and Breast Cancer among Black Women Culture, Identity, Spirituality, and Strength* (Madlock

Gatison, 2016b) was written the author was looking for an outlet to empower Black women and give voice regarding the trifecta of strength—the warrior metaphors found in breast cancer and other disease fighting rhetoric, Christian faith talk, and the strong Black women mythology—all of which can influence how some Black women make health care decisions (Madlock Gatison, 2016a). Results from this research indicate that Black women are well aware of breast cancer risks and that Pink Ribbon marketing has done its job. Taking into consideration all that was learned from interviews, focus groups, autoethnography (Madlock Gatison, 2016b, pp. 5–10), and social media (SM) content analysis it was determined that a stronger emphasis for action should include increasing political awareness in addition to the continued focus on the more prominent disease-specific awareness campaigns, such as pink ribbon and breast cancer awareness (Madlock Gatison, 2017, p. 38). For this author political advocacy was chosen as an area of inquire as a disconnect was recognized in the dissemination of information and information seeking in the area of health care policies, legislation, and information beyond the agenda set by the media and political pundits (p. 59). Therefore, this case study draws from both health communication and political communication perspectives within a SM context.

Political Agency and Women's Health Movements

Historically, Black women have been involved politically with many issues and are part of the political discourse. These conversations include health care with an understanding that at times black women and black communities are "othered" with various issues and concerns being relegated to an afterthought if addressed at all. Black women by necessity and care for self and community will set and prioritize their needs and create their own agenda. For this reason, it is important to note that 2017 was a historic moment in time for Black women in America due to two important events: first, First Lady Michelle Obama left the White House and her platforms of healthy eating and advocating for girls education also departed. Second, 2017 was the 40th anniversary of the Combahee River Collective Statement (Harris, 2019), an organization preceded by the National Black Feminist Organization (a grassroots political voice for some Black women). These are strong reminders that Black women are present in the political discourse at various levels in this nation, even as the media landscape is full of contrary representations and narratives. These moments in time and organizations represent spaces where Black women are in conversations that include the health and well-being of Black women, Black girls, and the Black community and are relevant exemplars to much of the social activism that currently takes place.

BWHI was founded in 1983 by activist Bylley Avery. According to the BWHI's Who We Are Page, BWHI is the longest running and the only national organization dedicated solely to improving the health and wellness of 21 million Black women and girls in the United States. With a vision to see Black women enjoy optimal health and well-being in a socially just society. Their mission is to lead the effort to solve the most pressing health issues that affect Black women and girls in the U.S. through investments in evidence-based strategies, delivering bold new programs and advocating for health-promoting policies (BWHI, 2018; Seaman & Eldridge, 2012). The *Black Women's Health Imperative 2018 National Policy Agenda* is one salient strategy to actively engage Black women collectively to politically advocate for their health with a strategic plan. Released on September 14, 2018 the *BWHI 2018 National Policy Agenda* is available free of charge on the internet with an invitation to freely share the document individually and organizationally.

Though the question of connecting political communication and health care information is an often secondary or overlooked part of the awareness messaging targeted towards Black women or the Black community overall. The goal of this chapter is to acknowledge the contributions made by the Black Women's Health Imperative and offer a communication strategy that could be used to help this non-profit as they work to help mitigate this weak informative communication connection between health/disease awareness messaging and health policy through their activism and use of SM.

Health Communication and Political Information Seeking

"Health communication serves as an excellent umbrella to merge researchers across disciplines with community advocates and the lay public at large" (Atkin & Silk, 2009, p. 499). This merging includes the political. Kaid (2009) provides a simplistic definition of political communication in that "political communication is the role of communication in the political process" (p. 457). A process that includes media coverage of political campaigns and events, political debates, political advertising, and varied political rhetoric (Kaid, 2009, p. 466). This case study includes the dissemination of advocacy group political information as part of this process as the BWHI is a source for both health and political information.

When you think about health and politics, what comes to mind? For many it might be the Affordable Care Act (ACA) also known as Obama Care, Medicaid or Medicare, and currently the Opioid crisis. Health communication is directly tied to political issues with the dissemination of both health and political information happening much more across cyberspace (Brubaker, 2010). As much as politics encompasses "private" decision-making that takes place at home, work, or other social spaces how are individuals informed about the issues (Vardeman-Winter, Jiang, & Tindall, 2013; Zoller & Sastry, 2017). By looking at the case of the Black Women's Health Imperative this report will shed some light on this question and raise others as it relates to health information, political information seeking and the internet.

Cyberactivism

As the political climate in the United States continues to take on a divisive tone it is significant to mention that coinciding with the sociopolitical debates taking place on mainstream media news outlets many such discussions are also taking place on SM (Pew Research, 2018). The internet is a beehive of activism regarding sociopolitical issues and civic engagement. Activism itself is about citizens and communities taking action for social and political change (Mahoney & Tang, 2017, p. 177). With the advent of all the political tweeting it became important to take a closer look at SM use and its relationship to health care policy information seeking as a component of disease specific health information seeking by Black women. Specifically, the role of SM and cyberactivism in health information and political information seeking.

Howard (2011) defines cyberactivism as the act of using the Internet to advance a political cause that is difficult to advance offline. BWHI is using SM to inform their audience regarding a variety of health information policy topics with the goal of informing there political choices and mobilizing them to vote by developing a strategy—*Black Women Vote: The 2018 National Health Policy Agenda*—and making the strategy freely available for use offline. BWHI is advancing their policy agenda with the help of the internet.

It was predicted by many health care professionals, communication practitioners and scholars that health communication would not be limited to didactic transactions in medical settings or media messages delivered to passive audiences (Kreps & Thornton 1992; Rus & Cameron, 2016; Whitten, Kreps, & Eastin, 2011). With the rapid evolution of the Internet and online social networking, health communication now incorporates dynamic exchanges of information on a worldwide scale. SM, defined as Internet-based applications that allow for the creation and exchange of user-generated content can boast billions of users. These numbers are only expected to keep growing.

While observing the SM platforms of other international, national, and regional women's health advocacy organizations such as the National Breast Cancer Coalition, the National Women's Health Network, and the International Women's Health Coalition all of which are communicating a political agenda it is evident that policy and health are clear part of their vision and mission. While other organizations such as the Center for Black Women's Wellness focus on providing services with an emphasis on health care access and health equity. All of the afore mentioned organizations SM use included one or more of the following platforms: Facebook, Twitter, Instagram, Pinterest, and discussion forums that can contain host and user-generated information. This observation questions user engagement of the information presented. Therefore, how well did the BWHI engage its followers in regards to their 2018 National Health Policy Agenda? Additionally, does a secondary measurement of health behavior change, political engagement, and social activism need to take place by looking at offline results?

Vardeman-Winter et al. (2013) indicate that "women make health decisions based on how their multiple identities are addressed by policymakers, and they reject important health messages when their intersecting identities are disregarded" (p. 409). As a scholar and women's health advocate the nagging question of—Do Facebook pages targeting Black American women with posts of political health communication is an important question to answer considering the current political climate. As a health care consumer and health information seeker it takes a high level of Internet self-efficacy to persevere in the task of locating relevant health information (Sundar, Rice, Kim, & Sciamanna, 2011), now add the task of locating relevant health care policy information. Offline the African American community has a history of working to shape social and political outcomes in government and society, to bring equity to their community and by default that of other disenfranchised citizens and communities of color as the Civil Rights Movement created a blue print for all to reference and follow.

As many organizations work to disrupt social inequalities what role does policy communication play in public advocacy about health care for Black Women. Policy communication is communicating about health or scientific data in support of policy change, or a new or existing policy and its implementation and evaluation (Schiavo, 2013, p. 265). While public advocacy is defined as the strategic use of communication to affect changes in public opinion and attitudes so that it influences policy makers or other decision-makers and promotes changes in behaviors, social norms, policies, and resource allocation to benefit a community, group, population or organization (Schiavo, 2013, p. 265).

Pew Research Report on Activism in the social media age (July 2018) indicates that certain groups of social media users—most notably, those who are black or Hispanic—view Social Network Sites (SNS) as an important tool for their own political engagement. For example, roughly half of black social media users say these platforms are at least somewhat personally important to them as a venue for expressing their political views or for getting involved with issues that are important to them. This Pew Research Report was relative to the #BlackLivesMatter movement and did not translate to political concerns regarding health disparities.

A sizeable majority of adult Internet users report looking for health information online. We live in a digital age and SNS like Facebook represent a common place to seek information. SNS have been growing in popularity across broad segments of Internet users, and are a convenient means to exchange information and support. Studies have been conducted that investigate how individuals use SNS for support groups and health information seeking related to treatment of diseases such as cancers, diabetes, heart disease, and the common cold. However, very little research exists about the use of SNS and information seeking for health care policy or political health communication and Black women.

Social Media in Health Policy Communication: The Case of the Black Women's Health Imperative

Current trends in health promotion by community and grassroots organizations seek to disseminate not only information related to health disparities, health care, health equity and general health care tips, but also information regarding the policies that influence individual health and health care. Using the case study method as the research strategy this report focused on how the Black Women's Health Imperative used Facebook, Twitter, and Instagram to disseminate their 2018 National Health Policy Agenda.

The BWHI, the single case, is the unit of analysis. Yin (2003) describes the case study as an empirical inquiry that investigates a contemporary phenomenon within its real-life context, especially when the boundaries between phenomenon and context are not clearly evident (Gray, 2018; Yin, 2012, p. 4 as cited in Yin, 2003, p. 18; Yin, 2018). This case study is pertinent as the research is addressing both descriptive questions—"What is happening or has happened?—an explanatory question—"How or why did something happen (Yin, 2012, p. 5; Yin, 2018, p. 12)?" Basically, "a how or why question is being asked about a contemporary set of events over which a researcher has little or no control (Yin, 2018, p. 12)." The case study evidence to answer the following questions will come from the content of the Black Women's Health Imperative social networking sites (Yin, 2018, p. 110).

As 2018 was a contentious midterm election year this study aimed to identify if an African American centered women's health-related organizations political health information messages would engage their key public during the month preceding the midterm election. The question posed earlier in this chapter "How well did the BWHI engage their followers in regards to their 2018 National Health Policy Agenda from the inaugural release on September 14, 2018–November 6, 2018, midterm election?" was reimagined as follows:

> *RQ1*: How does an African American centered health-related organization communicate about health care policy (political health communication information) on their organizational social networking sites such as Facebook, Twitter, and Instagram?
>
> *RQ2:* How do visitors to their social networking sites such as Facebook, Twitter, and Instagram respond to the political health communication information?

Theoretical Framework

This analysis used a grounded theory approach. Facebook Page, Twitter, and Instagram, information was collected without a predefined theory allowing concepts and ideas to emerge naturally. Grounded theory allows the researcher to study human interaction and behavior within its social context (Schreiber & Stern, 2001). For this study the SNS community serves as the larger social context, and the conversations and interactions on the Facebook Page, Twitter, and Instagram, are the studied behavior. The goal was to asses user engagement with BWHI 2018 National Health Policy Agenda via the standard engagement indicators of liking, sharing, or commenting on BWHI posts related to the policy agenda.

Method

Content analysis was the methodology used to examine how BWHI used SNS to inform and engage their key publics related to health care and political awareness messaging. There is much debate in the literature on what is public data the consensus is that the Internet and information posted on SNS is public information in a public space (McKee & Porter, 2009; Parsi & Elster, 2014; Sinclair, 2017). This study did not include any personal identifiers that could link any comment to a particular user. Only the indicators of number of likes, number of follows, or number of comments were used as indicators of engagement.

Results

Briefly stated, the BWHI produced online health policy documents available across all platforms. Information was not segmented by audience or by platform. Research indicates that different demographics use SM differently and use different platforms (Mahoney & Tang, 2017). In order to increase interaction, BWHI could have produced different messages, information and products for the various ways of interacting with constituents.

In the time frame of this study, BWHI social media platforms had various interactions. Facebook followers total 8,380 and 8,302 like the page as of November 10, 2018. There were 56 Facebook posts on Policy Agenda and Voting between September 14–November 6 with a total of 389 likes, 26 comments, 195 shares. Twitter followers total 26.3k and 3,429 likes as of November 10, 2018. There were 28 original organizational Tweets on Policy Agenda and Voting between September 14–November 6 with 76 retweets, 122 likes, and 4 comments. Instagram followers total 3, 375 as of November 10, 2018. There were 14 Posts on Policy Agenda and Voting between September 14–November 6 with 1,058 total likes for 14 posts.

Discussion

In Gordon's 2018 explication of theorizing as a part of the social media promotion framework the author indicates that because using social media infers that one is doing communication some practitioners still have a linear view of communication and perform activities such as posting and tweeting without a theoretical rational for messaging strategy.

While the BWHI has 8,380 followers on their Facebook Page, 26,300 Twitter followers, 667 LinkedIn followers; 3,375 Instagram; and 186 YouTube subscribers at the time of this report (the use of LinkedIn and YouTube were not included). The number of comments, likes, or shares on their posts related to their recently released Black Women Vote: The 2018 National Policy Agenda is minimal in comparison to the number of indicated followers during the time of its inaugural release of September 14, 2018–November 6, 2018, midterm election day. These preliminary findings indicate that while the web is an easily available source of health and policy information it can be hard to assesses true user engagement by just counting comments, likes, and shares alone. BWHI did include community conversations as part of its face-to-face user engagement, however based on the low numbers of likes, shares or comments it would appear that the information is not engaging users online.

This research represents the first attempt to comprehensively describe publicly available policy content and user engagement with political communication on a Facebook Page specifically designed for the health and well-being of Black women and girls. Policy interventions using Facebook will need to be designed to ensure relevant information is easy to find but also include a face-to-face component. The inclusion of an offline user engagement component was part of the BWHI strategy as they hosted workshops and meetings in select cities to introduce the 2018 Policy Agenda to various communities.

After an extensive review it appears that Gordon's social media health promotion framework would be an appropriate analytical guide for future planning and assessment of BWHI SNS. In brief Gordon's (2017) 3T's approach to SM health promotion to communicate BWHI's National Health Policy Agenda and Black Women Vote initiative prior to the next election cycle. This is a structured framework that utilizes theorizing, targeting, and tracking, hence the 3Ts. First, *theorizing* is necessary as it helps to describe communication phenomena, predict possible outcomes of communication interactions, and explain why things happen communicationally in terms of human behavior (p. 166). Second, *targeting* which emphasizes audience segmentation and profile creation which would provide a structure to create audience-centered messages (p. 172). Third, *tracking* the message to asses impact and reach would provide valuable feedback and measure results of the intended message (p. 173). SNS provide an open and informal communication space for the dissemination of information and audience-centered engagement. This author suggests that Gordon's 3T's framework would be of strategic value to BWHI Black Women Vote National Health Policy Agenda initiative as they use SM to engage key stakeholders and other concerned citizens prior to the 2020 election.

Limitations and Future Research

This chapter is a part of a larger study that was based on a content analysis of the original posts to SNS and websites that specifically targeted Black women's health. Future research would include a quantitative study to measure any political or community action that users might have engaged in after exposure to political health communication messaging via online surveys and focus groups of community and sister organizations featured on the subject SNS. Interviewing members of the subject organizations to determine their on ground or face-to-face strategies for user/individual engagement and that of complimentary organizations that have implemented use of the BWHI 2018 Policy Agenda. Over all this would be advantageous to developing health communication campaigns that include a policy component for health care consumers. This line of research merits further investigation to include other organizations but also with the understanding that SNS will continue to evolve over time.

Choosing the quote that began this chapter from Audre Lorde's *Cancer Journal* resonates as these words have relevancy across diseases and health disparities. Our

Table 1. Framework guide of how 3 Ts model may be used to examine social media communication

The 3 Ts	Description	Application to Social Media
Theorizing	Do you have a theoretical framework that is appropriate? • Behavior Change o Social Marketing o Community Mobilization o Behavioral Decision-Making • Interpersonal Communication o Cognitive Dissonance o Communication Privacy Management o Social Networking Are goals identified based on the predictions of the framework? Are behavior change strategies developed based on the framework? Have you developed a specific message/s informed by the framework?	Any platform
Targeting	Have you identified your audience? That is, • By Age • By Geographic Location • By Socioeconomic Status • By Education • By Cultural attitudes and Beliefs • By Social Media Patterns (Which platforms to use to reach whom?)	Choose Relevant Platform
Tracking	Do you have an assessment strategy? That is, • How will you collect data about the campaign? o Frequency (once per week, once per month) o Phases (beginning, middle, and after) • What type of data should you collect? o Who is engaging with the message? o Where are they receiving the message? o When are they engaging with the message? o What are they saying about the message? o To whom are they saying it?	Social Media Metrics

Table 1. *Continued*

The 3 Ts	Description	Application to Social Media
	• What are the data saying? o Am I reaching who I am supposed to? o Do they understand the message? o Are they acting on the message? o Are they acting on the message appropriately? • How will you use data? o Adjust message? o Change/add platforms? o Add/subtract information? o Rephrase main message? o Follow up with secondary messages?	

Table designed by Nickesia S. Gordon, used with permission.

health is political with many situations and contexts that affect the health of individuals, communities, and the national population as a whole. Lorde's words provide a strategic reminder of self-care that includes political agency that must be communicated.

References

Al Mamun, M., Ibrahim, H. M., & Turin, T. C. (2015). Social media in communicating health information: An analysis of Facebook groups related to hypertension. *Preventing Chronic Disease, 12*, E11. http://doi.org.ezproxy.liberty.edu/10.5888/pcd12.140265

Anderson, M., Toor, S.,Rainem, L., & Smith, A. (2018). *Pew Research Internet—Activism in the social media age.*

Anderson, S. C., & Guyton, M. R. (2013). Ethics in an age of information seekers: A survey of licensed healthcare providers about online social networking. *Journal of Technology in Human Services, 31*(2), 112–128. https://doi.org/10.1080/15228835.2013.775901

Atkin, C., & Silk, K. (2009). Health communication. In Stacks, D. W., & Salwen, M. B. (Eds.), *An integrated approach to communication theory and research* (pp. 489–503). New York, NY: Routledge Taylor & Francis Group.

Balatsoukas, P., Kennedy, C. M., Buchan, I., Powell, J., & Ainsworth, J. (2015). The role of social network technologies in online health promotion: A narrative review of theoretical and empirical factors influencing intervention effectiveness. *Journal of Medical Internet Research, 17*(6), e141. http://doi.org.ezproxy.liberty.edu/10.2196/jmir.3662

Bender, J. L., Jimenez-Marroquin, M.-C., & Jadad, A. R. (2011). Seeking support on Facebook: A content analysis of breast cancer groups. *Journal of Medical Internet Research, 13*(1), e16. http://doi.org.ezproxy.liberty.edu/10.2196/jmir.1560

Benetoli, A., Chen, T. F., & Aslani, P. (2017). Consumer health-related activities on social media: Exploratory study. *Journal of Medical Internet Research, 19*(10), e352. http://doi.org.ezproxy.liberty.edu/10.2196/jmir.7656

Birkland, T. A. (2005). *An introduction to the policy process: Theories, concepts, and models of public policy making* (2nd ed.). Armonk, NY: M.E. Sharpe.

Black Women's Health Imperative. (2018). Black Women's Health Imperative publishes its first national health policy agenda to educate and empower Black voters. Retrieved March 23, 2019 from https://www.bwhi.org/2018/09/14/black-womens-health-imperative-publishes-its-first-national-health-policy-agenda-to-educate-and-empower-black-voter/

Bowen, S. A. (2013). Using classic social media cases to distill ethical guidelines for digital engagement. *Journal of Mass Media Ethics, 28*(2), 119–133. https://doi.org/10.1080/08900523.2013.793523

Brubaker, J. (2010). Internet and television are not substitutes for seeking political information. *Communication Research Reports, 27*(4), 298–309. doi: 10.1080/08824096.2010.518906

Buckingham, D. (2013). Representing audiences: Audience research, public knowledge, and policy. *Communication Review, 16*(1/2), 51–60. https://doi.org/10.1080/10714421.2013.757487

Center for Black Women's Wellness. Retrieved February 25, 2019, from https://www.cbww.org/

Chou, W. S., Hunt, Y. M., Beckjord, E. B., Moser, R. P., & Hesse, B. W. (2009). Social media use in the United States: implications for health communication. *Journal of Medical Internet Research, 11*(4), e48. https://doi.org/10.2196/jmir.1249

Conrad, C. (2004). The illusion of reform: Corporate discourse and agenda denial in the 2002 "corporate meltdown". *Rhetoric and Public Affairs,* 7(3), 311–338. Retrieved from http://www.jstor.org/stable/41939925

Cutilli, C. C. (2010). Seeking health information: What sources do your patients use? *Orthopedic Nursing, 29*(3), 214–219. Retrieved from http://ezproxy.liberty.edu/login?url=https://search.proquest.com/docview/613950717?accountid=12085

Facebook News Room. Retrieved November 2, 2018 from https://newsroom.fb.com/company-info/

Facebook Optimization Analyze Results. Retrieved March 3, 2019, from https://www.facebook.com/business/help/735720159834389?helpref=faq_content

Facebook Pages for Business. Retrieved November 1, 2018, from https://www.facebook.com/business/products/pages

Facebook Pages for Nonprofits. Retrieved November 1, 2018, from https://nonprofits.fb.com/topic/create-a-page/

Farnan, J. M. (2014). Connectivity and consent: Does posting imply participation? *American Journal of Bioethics, 14*(10), 62–63. https://doi.org/10.1080/15265161.2014.947823

Glaser, B., & Strauss, A. (1967). *The discovery of grounded theory: Strategies for qualitative research*. Chicago, IL: Aldine.

Gollop, C. J. (1997). Health information-seeking behavior and older African American women. *Bulletin of the Medical Library Association*, *85*(2), 141–146.

Gordon, N. S. (2017). Toward a framework for communicating women's health via social media in Jamaica. In K. Langmia and T. C. M. Tyree(Eds.), *Social media culture and identity*. Lanham, MD: Lexington Books.

Gray, D. E. (2018). *Doing research in the real world.* Thousand Oaks, CA: Sage Publication, Inc.

Hale, T. M., Pathipati, A. S., Zan, S., & Jethwani, K. (2014). Representation of health conditions on Facebook: Content analysis and evaluation of user engagement. *Journal of Medical Internet Research*, *16*(8), e182. http://doi.org.ezproxy.liberty.edu/10.2196/jmir.3275

Harris, D. (2019). *Black feminist politics from Kennedy to Trump*. Cham, Switzerland: Palgrave.

Harris, L. M., Baur, C., Donaldonson, M. S., Lefebvre, R. C., Dugan, E., & Arayasirikul, S. (2011). Health communication and health information technology: Priority issues, policy implications, and research opportunities for healthy people 2020. In T. Thompson, R. Parrott, & J. Nussbaum (Eds.), *The Routledge handbook of health communication*. New York: Routledge.

Howard, P. N. (2011). *The digital origins of dictatorship and democracy: Information technology and political Islam*. Oxford: Oxford University Press.

Instagram Business. Retrieved November 1, 2018 from https://business.instagram.com/

International Women's Health Organization. Priorities page. Retrieved February 25, 2019, from https://iwhc.org/about-us/

Kaid, L. L. (2009). Political communication. In D. W. Stacks and M. B. Salwen (Eds.) *An Integrated Approach to Communication Theory and Research*, 2nd edition. New York, NY: Routledge.

Kim, D. K., Singhal, A., & Kreps, G. L. (Eds.). (2013). *Health communication: Strategies for developing global health programs*. Retrieved from https://ebookcentral.proquest.com

Kreps, G. L. & Thornton, B. C. (1992). *Health communication theory and practice* (2nd ed). Long Grove, IL: Waveland Press.

Lee, S. S.-J. (2017). Studying "friends": The ethics of using social media as research platforms. *American Journal of Bioethics*, *17*(3), 1–2. https://doi.org/10.1080/15265161.2017.1288969

Lefebvre, R. C. (2013). *Social marketing and social change: Strategies and tools for improving health, well-being and the environment*. San Francisco, CA: Jossey Bass.

Lewis, B., & Lewis, J. (2015). *Health communication: A media and cultural studies approach*. New York, NY: Palgrave.

Littlejohn, S. W., Foss, K. A., & Oetzel, J. G. (2017). *Theories of human communication* (11th ed.). Long Grove, IL: Waveland Press.

Lorde, A. (2006). *The cancer journals*. San Francisco, CA: Aunt Lute Books.

Madlock Gatison, A. D. (2016a). *Communicating women's health: Social and cultural norms that influence health decisions*. New York, NY: Routledge Taylor & Francis Group.

Madlock Gatison, A. D. (2016b). *Health communication and breast cancer among black women culture, identity, spirituality, and strength*. Lanham, MD: Lexington Books.

Madlock, G. A. D. (2017). Complicit in Concealing Illness: Black Women, Beauty, Identity, and Breast Cancer. In K. Morant Williams (Ed). *Reifying Women's Experience with Invisible Illness: Illusions, Delusions, Reality*. Lanham, MD: Lexington Books.

Mahoney, L. M., & Tang, T. (2017). *Strategic social media from marketing to social change*. West Sussex, UK: John Wiley & Sons LTD Blackwell.

McKee, H., & Porter, J. E. (2009). The Ethics of Internet Research: A Rhetorical Case-Based Proess. New York, NY: Peter Lang.

Meyerson, B. E., Haderxhanaj, L. T., Comer, K. et al. BMC Public Health. (2018). 18: 700. https://doi.org/10.1186/s12889-018-5617-0

National Breast Cancer Coalition. Success page. Retrieved February 25, 2019, from http://www.breastcancerdeadline2020.org/about-nbcc/nbcc-successes.html

National Women's Health Network. Policy advocacy page. Retrieved from January 26, 2019 https://nwhn.org/our-advocacy-issues/

Paige, S. R., Krieger, J. L., & Stellefson, M. L. (2017). The influence of eHealth literacy on perceived trust in online health communication channels and sources. *Journal of Health Communication*, *22*(1), 53–65. http://doi.org.ezproxy.liberty.edu/10.1080/10810730.2016.1250846

Parsi, K., & Elster, N. (2014). Conducting research on social media—Is Facebook like the public square? *American Journal of Bioethics*, *14*(10), 63–65. https://doi.org/10.1080/15265161.2014.947825

Rus, H. M., & Cameron, L. D. (2016). Health communication in social media: Message features predicting user engagement on diabetes-related Facebook pages. *Annals of Behavioral Medicine*, *50*, 678. https://doi.org/10.1007/s12160-016-9793-9

Schiavo, R. (2013). *Health communication: From theory to practice*. Retrieved November 1, 2018 from https://ebookcentral.proquest.com

Schreiber, R. (2001). New directions in grounded formal theory. In R. Schreiber & P. N. Stern (Eds.), *Using grounded theory in nursing* (pp. 227–246). New York, NY: Springer.

Seaman, B., & Eldridge, L. (2012). *Voices of the women's health movement, volume one and volume two*. New York: Seven Stories Press.

Sinclair, M. (2017). Using social media for research. *Evidence Based Midwifery*, *15*(2), 39.

Sirgy, M. J. (2008). Ethics and public policy implications of research on consumer well-being. *Journal of Public Policy & Marketing*, *27*(2), 207–212. https://doi.org/10.1509/jppm.27.2.207

Stacks, D. W., & Salwen, M. B. (Eds.). (2009). *An integrated approach to communication theory and research* (2nd ed.). New York, NY: Routledge Taylor & Francis Group.

Strach, P. (2016, October 27). Foundations: Cause marketing, breast cancer, and framing in America. In *Hiding politics in plain sight: Cause marketing, corporate influence, and breast cancer policymaking*. New York, NY: Oxford University Press. Retrieved 26 Oct. 2018 from http://www.oxfordscholarship.com/view/10.1093/acprof:oso/9780190606848.001.0001/acprof-9780190606848-chapter-2

Sulik, G. (2014). #RETHINKPINK: Moving beyond breast cancer awareness SWS distinguished feminist lecture. *Gender and Society*, *28*(5), 655–678. Retrieved from http://www.jstor.org/stable/44288182

Sundar, S. S., Rice, R. E., Kim, H., & Sciamanna, C. N. (2011). Online health information: Conceptual challenges and theoretical opportunities. In T. Thompson, R. Parrott, & J. Nussbaum (Eds.), *The Routledge handbook of health communication*. New York: Routledge.

Taylor, J., & Pagliari, C. (2018). Mining social media data: How are research sponsors and researchers addressing the ethical challenges? *Research Ethics*, *14*(2), 1–39. https://doi.org/10.1177/1747016117738559

Thompson, T., Parrott, R., & Nussbaum, J. (Eds.). (2011). *The Routledge handbook of health communication*. New York: Routledge.

Using social media for research. (2017). *Evidence based Midwifery*, *15*(2), 39. Retrieved November 2, 2018 from http://ezproxy.liberty.edu/login?url=https://search.proquest.com/docview/2001309408?accountid=12085

Valdez, R. S., Guterbock, T. M., Thompson, M. J., Reilly, J. D., Menefee, H. K., Bennici, M. S., … Rexrode, D. L. (2014). Beyond traditional advertisements: Leveraging Facebook's social structures for research recruitment. *Journal of Medical Internet Research*, *16*(10), e243. http://doi.org.ezproxy.liberty.edu/10.2196/jmir.3786

Valente, T. W. (2011). Social Networks and Health Communication. In T. Thompson, R. Parrott, & J. Nussbaum (Eds.), *The Routledge handbook of health communication*. New York: Routledge.

Vardeman-Winter, J., Jiang, H., & Tindall, N. T. J. (2013). Information-seeking outcomes of representational, structural, and political intersectionality among health media consumers. *Journal of Applied Communication Research*, *41*(4), 389–411. doi: 10.1080/00909882.2013.828360

Whitten, P., Kreps, G. L., & Eastin, M. (Eds.). (2011). *E-Health: The advent of online cancer information systems*. New York, NY: Hampton Press, Inc.

Yamamoto, M., & Nah, S. (2018). Mobile information seeking and political participation: A differential gains approach with offline and online discussion attributes. *New Media & Society*, *20*(5), 2070–2090. https://doi.org/10.1177/1461444817712722

Yamasaki, J., Geist-Martin, P., & Sharf, B. S. (Eds.). (2017). *Storied health and illness: Communicating personal, cultural, and political complexities*. Long Grove, IL: Waveland Press, Inc.

Yin, R. (2003). Case Study Research: Design and Methods. Newbury Park, CA: Sage Publications.

Yin, R. K. (2012). *Applications of case study research* (3rd ed.). Thousand Oaks, CA: Sage Publications, Inc.

Yin, R. K. (2018). *Case study research and applications: Design and methods* (6th ed.) [VitalSource]. Retrieved from https://bookshelf.vitalsource.com/#/books/9781506336176/

Zoller, H., & Sastry, S. (2017). Communicating the politics of healthcare systems. In , J. Yamasaki, P. Geist-Martin, & Sharf, B. S. (Eds.), *Storied health and illness: Communicating personal, cultural, and political complexities*. Long Grove, IL: Waveland Press, Inc.

PART 2

Engaging Selfhoods: Contextual Complexity between Biomedical and Cultural Narratives

CHAPTER FIVE

"I'm Not Sick, I'm Hairy": Cultural Constructions of Women's Bodies in the Ob/Gyn Exam

BY GLORIA N. PINDI

Introduction

When I moved to the U.S., I did not know that shaving was a criterion of physical attractiveness for women. I was not shaving my body at all, and particularly not my hairy chin. Thus, people often were shocked to see that I do not shave. I remembered one day a conversation about shaving with an old white woman in the bus on my way back home from school.

I was sitting in the bus looking at the windows, lost in my memories after a long day of school when the woman suddenly turned to me and said in a friendly voice "Hi!" I was surprised and automatically responded with "Hi."

"How are you doing today? Very cold day, right!" She continued.

I looked at her with a shy smile and said, "I'm fine, just trying to adjust to the snow." Then I turned to the windows and pursued, "It kept snowing since this morning. Oh my God. This is too much."

"That's Chicago. The windy city," she replied. "Oh, by the way you have a nice accent! Where are you from?" She asked me.

I don't know why I always felt embarrassed wherever people asked me that question. I really don't know why they were all so curious about my identity. Nevertheless, I replied politely "I'm from the Congo, in Central Africa."

"Wow! That is far away! I don't think I ever met someone from the Congo before," she replied looking at me with surprise.

"Ha ha ha! I am not surprised. I meet many people telling me the same thing. Now, you met me." I said laughing.

For one moment, she stopped talking and stared at me strangely. I felt embarrassed trying to understand what her gaze was trying to communicate, but I couldn't get it. "Can I ask you something?" She said suddenly.

"Of course. Go ahead please!" I responded spontaneously hoping that she will finally tell me what I could not interpret from her nonverbal attitude.

"You have hair on your chin? Is it a beard?" She asked me with surprise.

"Yeah!" I replied laughing. Honestly, I did not know what to say. I was thinking maybe she would ask me a trivial question, such as "what is your native language?" or "how long have you been in the U.S.?" I was not expecting a question about hair. I started wondering why she asked me so.

"And why do you keep it? It's nasty and disgusting! You should shave it or get it waxed." She told me.

"No, I can't! It is a sign of beauty in my culture." I replied automatically. I could not understand why this woman, a total stranger, I met in the bus would suggest me to cut what has been one of my most attractive beauty features back home.

"Wow! This is amazing. In the U.S. women won't keep hair on their chin as a sign of beauty. Believe me, honey, with that hair no man will approach you!" She replied.

I was speechless. I didn't know what to say.

"Could you please pull that thing for me, I am getting out at the next stop" She asked me.

"Of course." I replied with a shy smile trying to pull down the bus rope for her.

"Thank you. It was nice talking to you." she said getting out of the bus.

Although the removal of body hair is often taken for granted because of its universal practice in most Western societies (Tiggemann & Kenyon, 1998; Toerien & Wilkinson, 2003; Toerien, Wilkinson, & Choi, 2005), this practice is not trivial or inconsequential. Hope (1982) asserts that "those behaviors which are most taken-for-granted in a culture may well be the most important ones for revealing an understanding of that culture" (p. 93). Likewise, body hair removal is one the most revealing practices for understanding the social construction of gendered norms imposed upon the female body for what is socially, culturally, even medically acceptable or not (Hope 1982; Tiggemann & Hodgson, 2008; Toerien & Wilkinson, 2003). As a transnational Black woman with a hairy body, I've watched how my body has been read in two different cultural contexts: Congolese and U.S.. In the Democratic Republic of Congo (DRC), I was "the beautiful and healthy hairy woman" because female hairiness is considered as a sign of beauty and strength in the Congolese culture. However, since my move to the U.S., my hairy body is constantly perceived as "nasty," "deviant" and even medically "ill" and "abnormal."

In the U.S., female hairy bodies are often "diagnosed as diseased or sick and subject to medical treatment and intervention" (Roach-Anlieu, 2006, p. 359). More precisely, a female hairy body is associated to hirsutism, a body condition of increased hair growth often conceived as a medical condition caused by the polycystic ovarian syndrome (PCOS) characterized mainly by weight gain/obesity, irregular and/or no menstrual cycle, and infertility (Ferrante, 1988; Kitzinger & Willmott, 2002; Lunde & Grøttum, 1984; Simpson, 1986). Although women with increased body hair have been historically associated to hirsutism (Shah, 1957), current research has demonstrated that medical diagnoses of hirsutism are not universal; instead, they may vary with respect to differences among races, ethnicities, and families, and as such should carefully be assessed within specific cultural contexts (Ferrante, 1988; Lunde & Grøttum, 1984; Toerien & Wilkinson, 2003; Simpson, 1986). Critical health communication scholars decry medical diagnoses such as hirsutism operating under the biomedical model for dismissing the role culture plays in the health care system (Dutta, 2008, 2015; Dutta & Basu, 2008, 2009).

In this critical autoethnographic piece, I use Mohan Dutta's culture-centered approach (CCA) to health communication to challenge the social construction of my Black female hairy body in U.S. culture as "sick" and "abnormal." I argue that a diagnosis of my female hairy body as a medical condition is rooted in the hegemonic Eurocentric understandings of health, which does not take into consideration the cultural differences—contexts and values—that shape my subjectivity as a transnational female immigrant from the Congo. Moreover, as a Congolese female immigrant, I claim that the medical pressure on my body as hairless is grounded in the U.S. western cultural and social expectations of the construction of the "appropriately" feminine woman, which in turns result into the disciplining and/or colonizing of my body. Ultimately, as a critical scholar, I use my female hairy body as a site of resistance to challenge such medicalization as an instance of "policing" of a narrow Eurocentric ideal of what is perceived as "healthy," and thereby socially/culturally "acceptable."

A Culture-Centered Approach to Health Communication

CCA is committed to recovering those raced, classed, gendered, and alike marginalized/subaltern voices erased and/or ignored from the elite/epistemic structures in order to create alternative ways of knowing/looking at health and thereby provide new discursive spaces to these marginalized voices (Dutta, 2007, 2015). Inspired by Spivak's notion of "Can the subaltern speak?" CCA takes a move forward and asks: "When the subaltern does speak, how can her or his voice be heard in the elite structures that systematically profit through the erasure of subaltern voices?" (Dutta, 2015, p. 136). CCA explores how the absence and presence of these marginalized voices offers "opportunities for social change by suggesting new interpretations for, and thus challenging, the dominant articulations of social reality and cultural and behavioral norms" (Dutta, 2008, p. 38) within the healthcare system. By doing so, this approach aims to empower the subaltern community in order "to assume autonomy and resist subjugation by the dominant culture, [by] achieving equality of status" (Chai, 2009, p. 77).

Despite the growing scholarship on CCA and immigration, little is still known about the health experiences of African immigrants in the U.S. As argued elsewhere, most CCA research conducted so far focused solely on the experiences of Asian immigrants. Regardless of this shortcoming, these studies provide important insights about how immigrants negotiate their identity in health care settings. Dutta (2008) argues that the CCA questions the exclusion of marginalized voices in the health care system, as such this also points to the lack of voices of African cultures in mainstream health communication research. This chapter aims to expand CCA scholarship on the health experiences of African immigrants living in the U.S. My goal is to use CCA as a theoretical framework to explore how, as a Black Congolese/African female immigrant whose identity navigates at the borderlands of two cultural worldviews (Congolese/African and U.S. American), I negotiate the health meanings associated to my female hairy body at the intersections of the Congolese and U.S. American cultures.

In the next section, I discuss scholarship related to female body hair and its medicalization.

On the Female Hairy Body and Its Medicalization

Research conducted on women and body hair across the globe—in the United States (Basow, 1991; Basow & Braman, 1998; Basow & Willis, 2001), the United Kingdom (Toerien & Wilkinson, 2004; Toerien et al., 2005), Australia (Tiggemann & Kenyon, 1998; Tiggemann & Lewis, 2004; Tiggemann & Hodgson, 2008), and New Zealand (Terry & Braun, 2013)—on different categories of women–professional (Basow, 1991), high school students (Tiggemann & Kenyon, 1998), college students (Tiggemann & Hodgson, 2008; Tiggemann & Kenyon, 1998;

Tiggemann & Lewis, 2004)—has revealed that, with respect to cultural differences among these countries/geographical areas, most women (regardless of their level of education, age, or professional background), shave their body—and precisely their legs, underarms, and bikini line—to conform to norms of femininity and attractiveness. As a socially and culturally normative practice of Western culture rooted in ancient Rome, where "women removed body hair with hot tar and razor-sharp shells" (Basow, 1991, p. 85), body hair removal is widely performed today through more recent methods including, but not limited to: tweezing, shaving, waxing, plucking, bleaching and depilatory creams/gels, cosmetic surgery, electrolysis, lasers, and many more (Simpson, 1986; Tiggemann & Hodgson, 2008; Toerien et al., 2005).

Body hair removal has become so normalized in the U.S. and many other Western cultures that "its normativity points to a socio-cultural presumption that hairlessness is the appropriate condition for the feminine body" (Toerien & Wilkinson, 2003, p. 333). Many of the women shaving their bodies—as early as at 13 years old (Toerien et al., 2005)—have internalized body hair removal as their normal everyday life practice to the extent of rationalizing it as an enhancement of their beauty rather than a gendered norm women are pressured to conform to (Tiggemann & Hodgson, 2008; Tiggemann & Kenyon, 1998). The common belief is that visible body hair on places other than the head—including but not limited to underarms, legs, face (such as mustaches, sideburns, and beard), nipples/breast, stomach, groin area, and toes—is often viewed as superfluous, disgusting, repulsive, ugly, dirty, unhygienic, animal/circus animal appearance, unfashionable, and overall non-attractive (Basow, 1991; Basow & Braman, 1998; Basow & Willis, 2001; Fahs, 2011a; Hope, 1982; Terry & Braun, 2013; Tiggemann & Lewis, 2004; Toerien & Wilkinson, 2004; Toerien et al., 2005). Likewise, studies have shown that women with body hair are often perceived and/or stereotyped as lesbian, feminist, unsociable, unintelligent, unhappy, unruly, more aggressive, vulgar, out of control, witch, and devil (Basow & Braman, 1998; Ferrante, 1988; Toerien & Wilkinson, 2003).

Moreover, Toerien and Wilkinson (2003) assert that the female hairy body has for a long time historically been a site of medical debate, and more particularly on hirsutism. However, research on hirsutism has shown that there is still little medical agreement about what counts as normal or abnormal hair growth (Ferrante, 1988; Lunde & Grøttum, 1984). Likewise, not all women with excess body hair have symptoms of the PCOS, which in turn makes a medical assessment of hirsutism somehow difficult (Ferrante, 1988; Lunde, 1984; Lunde & Grøttum, 1984; Simpson, 1986). Thus, to medically associate any form of increased female body hair growth to hirsutism is to subjectively assume that such body is medically "unfit," "sick," "ill" or suffers from a "medical disorder" and thereby necessitates some type of medical intervention such as hormone and/or cosmetic treatment (Ferrante, 1988; Toerien & Wilkinson, 2003). On the contrary, Lunde and Grøttum (1984) argue, it is important to draw the difference between normal and abnormal "as narrowly as possible in order to select those cases where increased hair growth might be an early sign of underlying disease and also reassure those patients whose hair growth falls within the variation of the normal population" (p. 308).

In their medical assessment of the female hairy body, physicians' main objective is often "to find a means of differentiating between patients whose 'problem' is 'merely' that, culturally, they are defined as having too much body hair, and those whose body hair is associated with a medical condition" (Toerien & Wilkinson, 2003, p. 336). Unfortunately, very often the cultural aspect is neglected and female body hair is automatically diagnosed as a medical condition (Lunde, 1984; Lunde & Grøttum, 1984). However, Ferrante (1988) argues that such medical implications should carefully be questioned because "what lies behind conceptions of abnormality is a biological reality mediated by social constructs and classificatory schema" (p. 220). In fact, historically the medicalization process of the female hairy body involved quantitative measures of hirsutism designed to reach medical objectivity in comparison to male hairiness through the use of a rating scale for the body parts, quality of hair (such as thickness), density and/or quantity of the hair, etc. (Ferrante, 1988; Toerien & Wilkinson, 2003)

Given the complexity of female body hair as not only a socially, culturally, but also medically constructed phenomenon, Toerien and Wilkinson (2003) conclude:

> While increased body hair growth in women can indicate an underlying medical condition, the two are not necessarily linked … In biological terms, body hair growth (including facial hair) is not exclusively associated with men. Indeed, what should count as 'abnormal' female hair growth is not clear even medically. (p. 335)

It can then be inferred that with medical diagnoses of hirsutism, women's bodies become "sites in which, women, both individually and collectively, struggle for autonomy and power vis-à-vis medical dominance" (Roach Anlieu, 2006, p. 360). For instance, Toerien and Wilkinson (2004) revealed that some hairy women felt pressure to perform depilation prior to medical examinations (such as OB-GYN) to avoid negative comments/criticisms as well as unpleasant looks/stares from doctors. Ultimately, in medical encounters, "the presence of hair on a woman's body, then, may be symbolically-and, importantly, socially-problematic irrespective of whether or not it may be defined as a medical concern" (Toerien et al., 2005, p. 400).

Furthermore, Basow and Braman (1998) note that "the norm of 'hairlessness' contributes to women's overall negative body image" (p. 644). For instance,

Toerien and Wilkinson (2003) mention that, among the many negative reactions movie actress Julia Roberts received for appearing to the public with unshaved underarms, the editor of a magazine claimed "from hairy armpits it is only a small step to the Planet Of The Apes" (p. 334). Once again, the use of the term "Apes" calls for attention on the connection often made between hairy body and "animal-like appearance." However, as stated by Fahs (2011a, 2011b), body hair as a socially constructed phenomenon is profoundly complex and can be experienced by women differently at the intersections of various layers of their identity such as race, class, gender, ethnicity, sexual orientation, and more. Ultimately, comments/descriptors referring to "animal like" looks (e.g., "Apes") carry a racist connotation, and particularly when applied to bodies of women's of color such as Black women (Fahs 2011a, 2011b; Toerien & Wilkinson, 2003).

Despite the social pressure women experience about shaving, research has also shown some level of resistance. Whereas women in general start shaving their bodies at puberty due to social norms and/or pressure (Basow, 1991), as they mature (such as in their 30s), they can embrace different stances toward body removal including rejecting the depilation norm for cultural and political reasons including but not limited to feminism (Tiggemann & Kenyon, 1998). For instance, in Basow's study (1991), women claimed not to shave for political purpose because they believed that "women's bodies are fine as they are, that women should not have to remove body hair, and that shaving is stupid" (p. 93). Similarly, Basow and Braman's (1998) study showed that women identifying themselves as feminist rejected shaving because it was seen as oppressive. Along the same lines, Fahs' (2011a, 2011b) research on body hair, intersectionality, and sexuality, revealed that women used their bodies as sites of resistance to challenge homophobia, heterosexism, and racism perpetrated through the hairless norm.

Toerien and Wilkinson (2003) assert that "the literature on women's body hair refers either to women as a homogenous category—overlooking differences such as class and 'race'/ethnicity—or refers specifically to white women" (p. 342). In fact, most research conducted so far has focused on White women only, and particularly middle-class ones, revealing that body hair removal as a sign of middle-class femininity and "appropriate" womanhood against which other types of womanhood (such as Black) have been defined (Basow & Braman, 1998; Hope 1982; Toerien & Wilkinson, 2003). An eloquent illustration is Fahs' studies (2011a, 2011b), which revealed that women of color who went against the hairless norm received more negative comments than their white counterparts because of the color of the skin described as "darker and dirty" in contrast to light white skin; the quality of their hair described as "thick and coarse" in contrast to the "thinner" white hair;

and, their being stereotyped as "poor-working class" women in contrast to "middle/upper-class" white women.

Consistent with the above findings, Toerien and Wilkinson (2003) argue that "the possible existence of alternative body hair norms for black women [women of color] highlights the potential for constructing notions of femininity that challenge the normative assumptions [of white middle-class womanhood]" (p. 342). In fact, Basow's study (1991) revealed than White women shave more than Blacks and this difference is mainly tied to cultural norms as some participants stated "it goes against my cultural background" (p. 89). More precisely, she argues that these women's refusal results from their positioning as members the U.S. second-wave Women's Movement and sub-culture of the 1970s, during which Black women challenged various norms of female physical appearance (e.g., body shaving and adorning their bodies with makeup, girdles, or padded bras) in order to "prove themselves" as different. Thus, further investigation is needed to explore different body hair norms for women from other cultures, and particularly non-Western ones (Toerien et al., 2005). In response to this lacuna, my goal is to use my female hairy body as a site of knowledge to demonstrate how as a transnational female immigrant whose identity is shaped by two different cultural worldviews (Congolese and American), I negotiate the different sociocultural meanings medically assigned to my hairy body across cultures. In the next section, I describe autoethnography as my methodological approach.

Autoethnography: A Methodology of storytelling

Health communication scholars have highlighted the legitimacy of autoethnography as a method of knowing in health-related research (Chang, 2016; Dutta, 2008; Dutta & Basu, 2009, 2018; Richards, 2008; Spieldenner, 2014). Richardson (2000) defines autoethnographies as "highly personalized, revealing texts in which authors tell stories about their own lived experiences, relating the personal to the cultural" (p. 931). Similarly, in this study, I use a critical approach to autoethnography "as a means to enhance existing understandings of lived experiences [of the medicalization of my hairy body] enacted within larger systems of power, oppression, and social privilege" (Boylorn & Orbe, 2014, p. 19) at the intersections of Congolese/African and U.S. American cultures. Relying on intersectionality—"the cultural synergy that is created through the interactions of race/ethnicity, gender/sex, socioeconomic status, sexuality, nationality, age, spirituality, and/or abilities" (Boylorn & Orbe, 2014, p. 16)—I use my own lived experience to examine the intricacies of culture, health, and body hair that play out in transnational/diasporic context in the process of my identity construction as a hairy Black female Congolese/African immigrant living in the U.S.

Ellis, Adams and Bochner (2011) describe personal narratives as "stories about authors who view themselves as the phenomenon and write evocative narratives specially focused on their academic, research, and personal lives" (p. 7). In health communication research, personal narratives are used as "sense-making narratives" (Dutta & Basu, 2008, p. 562) to explore how health and sickness/illness are socially and/or culturally constructed within a particular context as well as the personal beliefs that people hold about such construction (Spieldenner, 2014). In a similar way, I use health narratives as a way of making sense of the medicalization of my hairy body in health settings as a transnational female immigrant from the Congo. Inspired by Richards' (2008) classification of illness narratives, I opted for the "emancipatory discourse" (p. 1722) to break silence on the othering process I have been subject to in health settings in the U.S. Richards eloquently describe this process of coming to voice as follows:

> Emancipatory discourse gives a voice to the voiceless … Emancipatory discourse breaks silence. For people who are othered, this can be a powerful means of improving their position in society. It can allow them to be seen in a more complex way and to show that the group to which they belong is varied and complex—and frequently consists of many people. (p. 1723)

Positioning autoethnography as an embodied practice (Pelias, 2007; Spry, 2011) which "brings forward bodies that are marked differently, have been historically denied speech, and have been unrecognized and unacknowledged" (Pelias, 2007, p. 186), I use my body as a postcolonial subaltern to create spaces/ways for my voice to be heard as I talk back to the medical colonization of my hairy female body in order to claim back my dignity (Dutta & Basu, 2018). Ultimately, I conceptualize autoethnography as "an examination of the self who engages in social justice/responds to social injustice" (Toyosaki & Pensoneau-Conway, 2013, p. 560) in order to promote "critical intervention in social, political, and cultural life" (Holman-Jones, 2008, p. 763). In fact, through the use of autoethnography, "my politically present body demands its rights in behalf of social justice, often placing itself at risk, often becoming a location where others can rally … It asserts its identity, claims its voice, refuses to back away" (Pelias, 2007, p. 186).

In this autoethnographic piece, I posit "the self, the focal point of the study, [as] a member of certain cultural groups connected to others" (Chang, 2016, p. 445) and as such, I believe that "[my] being is both social (in relationship with others) and fluid (capable of changing at any moment), and always already intersubjective" (Toyosaki & Pensoneau-Conway, 2013, p. 565). From this perspective, my personal experience serves as a way to explore/analyze/make sense and theorize on systemic larger sociocultural health issues of oppression and privilege related to the medicalization of the female hairy body (Boylorn & Orbe, 2014; Chang, 2016; Holman-Jones, 2008; Spry, 2011). In other words, I aim to "engage micro-level experience (my experience) as it is intersubjectively embodied within a macro-social context" (Toyosaki & Pensoneau-Conway, 2013, p. 562) of health issues related to hairy women. In order to do so, I use stories to uncover and/or "offer insights into the ways in which the culture [on the medicalization of female hairy body] constitutes its meanings of health, approaches health and illness, and engages in healthcare practices" (Dutta, 2008, p. 14).

In this process of storytelling, I construct a sequencing of events/plots to recount a couple of episodes from my lived experiences that I encountered in health settings as Black Congolese hairy woman whose identity is shaped by two cultural worldviews: Congolese and U.S. American. By doing so, I rely on emotional recall—"the process by which performers imagine being back in a scene by exploring its emotional and physical characteristics" (Fox, 2010, p. 8)—to invite my readers to emotionally relive these events with me (Richardson, 2000). Embracing "practice vulnerability" (Spry, 2011), I position myself as "an intentionally vulnerable subject" (Holman-Jones, Adams, & Ellis, 2013, p. 25) to call attention on the othering process I have been subject to in health settings due to my hairy body. In the next section, I discuss my lived experience as pertaining to the medicalization of my hairy body across the Congolese and U.S. American cultures.

Narratives of My Hairy Body

This section illustrates how I negotiate the medicalization of my female hairy body as a Black female Congolese woman whose identity navigates at the borderlands of two cultural worldviews: Congolese and U.S. American. Relying on a series of episodes contextual to each cultural setting, I discuss the socially constructed meanings assigned to my hairy body at the intersections of four layers of my identity: race, gender, ethnicity, and nationality.

My Hairy Body in the Congo: "The Virile Woman"

In a racially homogenous Black country such as the Congo where female body hair is considered as a sign of beauty, the depilatory norms is quasi nonexistent (Culture of the Democratic Republic of Congo, n.d.). This is to say that apart from eyebrows, armpits, and perhaps pubic area, most women do not shave the rest of their bodies. Hairy body is so praised that sometimes women would use specific beauty products to get hairier (Culture of the Democratic Republic of Congo, n.d.). Thus, growing up in the Congo, my hairy body wasn't really a major concern for me. Like any other girl going through puberty, I started developing body hair around 13 years old. Whereas this was a biological phase to my womanhood, I didn't pay close attention to the fact that I was developing hair on other areas of my body such as chin and chest. And as years passed by, I was getting hairier and hairier.

Unlike in Western culture where hairy women are seen as less and/or not sexually attractive (Basow, 1991; Basow & Braman, 1998; Terry & Braun, 2013; Tiggemann & Hodgson, 2008; Tiggemann & Kenyon, 1998; Tiggemann & Lewis, 2004; Toerien & Wilkinson, 2004; Toerien et al., 2005), hairy women in the Congo are seen as more sexually attractive. Therefore, for the most visible parts (such as chin, sideburns, and legs), my body hair started to cause more attention than usual. For instance, I was always complimented—by men mostly, and sometimes by women—for my hairy body. Some of the comments men particularly made are: "sexy," "attractive," "charming," "enchanting," and "interesting." Ultimately, I got labeled "mwasi ya mandefu/la femme barbue" (the lady with a beard) or "mwasi ya ba poils/la femme velue" (the hairy lady). This is how I slowly came to realize that my hairy body was some sort of "special identity marker" that differentiated me from other women.

Although a "beauty asset" in the Congolese culture, female body hair also carries a lot of sexual connotation. As argued by scholars, the hairy female body has historically been associated to hypersexuality and wantonness (Ferrante, 1988; Toerien & Wilkinson, 2003) probably because "constructed as masculine, hair, when visible on a woman's body, represents a symbolic threat to the gendered social order [as such it] has no rightful place on the feminine body" (Toerien & Wilkinson, 2003, p. 341). Similarly, most men who were after me because of my hairy body often make inappropriate sexual innuendoes to the extent of getting labeled *"mwasi mobali" (a woman-man)*. The tale below illustrates one of these episodes:

> *When I was in College, a man who was chasing me once told me "I can only imagine what it is like to make love to a hairy girl like you. You must be so intense in bed." Because I was still innocent at that time, I didn't know what he meant by that. I asked him and he just laughed at me loud and said "You don't even know that you have this treasure to make a man happy in bed." I was really embarrassed by his inappropriate comments because I couldn't discern the meaning behind it. As I struggled to make sense of his comments, I decided to turn to a person I believed would provide me with more insights on that, a hairy woman like me: my mom. When I got home, I approached my mom and told her the story. Then I asked her: "Mom, why would this man tell me that making love to me will be so intense because I am hairy. I don't understand. What does this mean?" My mother glared at me and just screamed "Shut up. What kind of stupid question is this? Don't you ever ask me such a*

stupid question again! Also, I don't want you to ever get close to that guy again. Stay away from him, do you hear me?" I was so frustrated and couldn't understand what I did or said wrong to make my mom so angry. As a Catholic practicing, I knew my mother to have very strong moral values regarding sexuality. She strove her best throughout her life to raise all her daughters, according to the "cult of purity" (Dyer, 1997). This to me, was probably the reason why asking questions about sexuality was a "taboo topic" to her. Thus, I decided to turn to my mom's sister, who was hairy just like me, but she also told me that "it was a stupid question."

After being silenced by my mom and aunt for who sexuality was probably a "taboo" topic, I still struggled to get the sexual meanings men assigned to my hairy body. However, I didn't know to who I should turn to for such an intimate issue. Thus, I decided to turn to the gynecologist. Doctor X was our family gynecologist. He knew me from a very young age once I started my puberty to the time I left the Congo for the U.S. So he knew my body well and all the metamorphoses I've gone through as a woman. Of a particular interest to me on the agenda of that doctoral appointment day was the link between my hairy body and my sexuality. I was concerned and thought there was something wrong with me. What was supposed to be a usual medical routine turned out to be a particular examination of my hairy body per my request. The narrative below describes this medical visit:

That day as I walked into Dr. X office for my routine exams, I was determined to learn more about my hairy body. As I walked into his medical office, I was greeted by the nurses who after filling out the paperwork gently walked me to his office. I wasn't' a stranger in this place, I felt pretty comfortable. Dr. X welcomed me with a big smile on his face as usual:

"Hi Gloria, how are you, it is good to see you. How is school going?" he said.

"I'm fine, Dr. Good to see you to. School is going well." I replied with a shy smile.

"Please make yourself comfortable," the Dr. said.

Because I was pretty familiar with the routine, I knew what he meant by make yourself comfortable. So, I undressed myself and l laid down on the bed. The doctor started his usual consultation. Once he was done, he asked me to get dressed but I stayed there and started asking him questions:

"So, tell me Dr. is this all hair on my body normal? Is everything okay with me?" I asked referring to different hairy parts of my body.

I could see the surprise on his face as he looked at me and said: "Why are you asking all these questions? Of course you're okay."

"Dr. X, I've been receiving some weird comments from men about my hairy body. They make so many sexual innuendoes about me such has 'making love to me should be so intense.' I just don't understand what this is all about. This is why I am asking." I told him.

"Oh, I see," Doctor X said smiling while looking at different parts of my hairy body.

Then putting on back his serious face of a doctor, he then started this long lecture on female hairy body:

"This is a common stereotype that many men carry about hairy women. Because hairy women like you often have a higher level of male hormone, particularly testosterone, which is socially perceived as a masculine trait, men or even people believe that you are a 'virile woman.' As you probably know, pilosity is a sign of beauty and strength for women in our culture. Thus, my intention is neither to support what these men say nor even to speak on their behalf, but I think that to them this is more of a compliment to you."

Dutta (2008) asserts that "the identities of cultural members play important roles in constituting health experiences of cultural members" (p. 3). Similarly, this explains why Dr. X's medical interpretation of my hairy body was embedded in his cultural background as a Congolese man. His account on "virile woman" explained all the sexual comments I was struggling to make sense of. I also finally understood why some people referred to me as "mwasi mobali" (a woman-man). However, reflecting back to my lived experience as a critical scholar today, I feel revolted by the label of "virile woman." As noted by Toerien and Wilkinson (2003), "given gendered biological labels, to have a hormone balance designated 'female'—too many 'male' hormones, and one's femininity comes into question" (as cited p. 341). Similarly, the label of "virile woman" reinforces a negative stereotype of my hairy body as "hypersexual" while simultaneously dictating what "true" and/or "appropriate femininity/womanhood" should be. I wonder why while body hair is culturally associated to strength and virility for the male body, such association is denied to the female hairy body that is rather perceived as wanton and hypersexual (Ferrante, 1988; Toerien & Wilkinson, 2003).

Because I became more interested in the medical aspect of my hairy body, I asked him for more clarification about the hormone imbalance:

"So, is this hormone imbalance a big issue? Do I need any treatment for this testosterone thing?" I said.

"It is up to you. Some people decide to take pills for hormone imbalance; however, that is a matter of personal choice. I can still prescribe it to you if you want to, but you have nothing to worry about, Gloria. I know your medical record and I can reassure you that you're perfectly fine and healthy and you have nothing to worry about. Indeed, your hairy body is hereditary. Your mom, her sister, and some of your siblings are hairy just like you. Some people might react differently to your body because you are hairy, but always remember that there is nothing wrong with you. Actually, a lot of women in this country would love to be hairy like you, believe me."

Dutta (2008) notes that "cultural meanings provide the locally situated scripts through which structures influence the health choices of cultural participants" (p. 7). So, I found no need for me to take medication for what wasn't a disease since Dr. X just reassured me that all was okay with my body and I had nothing to worry about. Speaking of the medical diagnosis of hirsutism, Lunde and Grøttum (1984) state that "it has been subjectively defined from a socially desirable basis against that which is statistically common or medically normal" (p. 311). Consistent with this argument, Dr. X explained that within the context of Congolese culture and given my family background, my hairy body was not a case of abnormal hair growth with pathology (Ferrante, 1988; Lunde & Grøttum, 1984). Moreover, Dutta (2007) argues that "culture is articulated in the meanings co-constructed by the cultural participants, and these meanings are located within the local context of the culture" (p. 311). Likewise, as demonstrated in the above narrative, Dr. X and I collaboratively worked on the medical meaning assigned to my hairy female body through our respective positionalities—doctor-patient—commonly shaped by the Congolese culture. In other words, regardless of the doctor/patient power dynamics, we engaged in this process as "cultural participants [who] articulate their health problems and co-construct the solutions to these health problems through engagement in dialogue" (Dutta, 2007, p. 321). As a critical scholar, this two-way process of meaning making is particularly important for me because I had the opportunity to voice my opinion on potential medical decisions made about my body and also use my agency in the choices I was comfortable with as a patient.

My Hairy Body in the U.S.: "You Look Like an Animal!"

In a racially diverse country like the U.S., my ethnic identity of African coupled with my national identity of Congolese as well as my racial identity of Black played a major role in the social and medical perception of my female hairy body. Upon my move to the U.S., I started to get criticized by Americans for not shaving my body. While referring to my hairy body, people usually used negative words such as *"nasty," "disgusting," "dirty," "unhygienic," and so forth.* I just could not comprehend how what I was once praised for as "beautiful," became "dirty" in the eyes of American people. The more effort I put into explaining to them what they considered as "negative" was a sign of beauty in my culture, the more people laughed at me. Their ultimate suggestion was that I had to shave my body if I wanted to adjust "appropriately" to the U.S. culture. One particular incident that never left my mind was of a female white classmate who once told me something like: *"hey girl, you need to get rid of that body hair. It is so nasty and dirty. Don't you see that it makes you look like "an animal"? Remember you no longer live in the African jungle, you now live in America!*" These "racial slurs" were so hurtful and made me feel so dirty that I started wondering if I shouldn't get my body shaved.

Amidst my struggles to make sense of shaving as an expectation of my cultural adjustment process in the U.S., I approached other African women of my community and was surprised that most of them confessed that they started shaving their bodies upon their move to the U.S. due to social pressure. Describing depilation norm as a social pressure, Terry and Braun (2013) say:

> An individual's hair display and/or removal choices and practices sit at a complex intersection of sociocultural meanings, norms and expectations, media and other influences, 'personal' desires and tastes, the desires and tastes of others, such as a sexual partner (which may be assumed, or expressed), and the intersection of the 'private' with the 'public'. (p. 600)

Feeling the same kind of pressure and given the negative reactions I received particularly about my facial hair/chin (Chapkis, 1986), I finally decided to shave my body. So one day I bought the shaving cream my American classmates recommended and shaved all my body from face to toes. I must admit that it was such a laborious and painful process that I didn't enjoy it even a bit. Indeed, I hurt myself many times using the razor. The next day I showed up in school after shaving, I received so many surprising reactions from my American friends. Some of the comments I received are: *"look at your skin, so soft, so smooth, and so beautiful;" "Your skin is shining. Now you can show 'your beef' without shame;"* and *"With these beautiful smooth legs I bet you'll have all the guys around you."*

The days that followed, I struggled to accept my "new self." I was uncomfortable in my own body. I felt out of my skin. For instance, when I touched my chin it was so smooth that I felt like a stranger in my own body. I was no longer "the lady with a beard," or "the hairy woman" like people used to call me in the Congo. Besides, my body hair started growing again. Even more, I had some allergic reactions on my face: pimples all over my chin. I complained to my classmates and they told me to take it easy. This wasn't a big deal and that next time I should probably go for waxing to prevent the allergy. After further research, I realized that once one starts shaving her body, you have to make it a habit and besides waxing was more costly. I got really revolted. This all shaving thing was just not making any sense to me. I asked myself why people had to be forced to go through such a painful process just in the quest of beauty. Ultimately, I realized that I was forced to conform to something I didn't feel comfortable with.

Through this process of self-reflexivity, I came to realize that body hair removal was not a universal norm across cultures (Tiggemann & Lewis, 2004). In fact, Ferrante (1988) notes that "norms about the proper amount and distribution of facial and body hair are rooted in and reinforced by the major symbolic roles hair has played in Western societies" (p. 224). In other words, it is important to note that, "what constitutes superfluous hair varies substantially not only across cultures but also within the same culture under different social conditions or during different time periods" (Ferrante, 1988, p. 220). So, I told myself: "Gloria after all, you are Congolese not American. So, why do you care about shaving? Why do you care about what people things? If someone likes you, he/she should accept you the way you are. So, stop worrying yourself with shaving. Just be yourself, accept who you are, and assume yourself the way you are."

Whereas I used my agency as way to challenge the prescribed depilation norm in order to assume myself as a "Congolese hairy immigrant woman" in the U.S. American culture, my hairy body was still a controversial issue in my everyday life. Of particular interest to me is health settings, where I was seen as the passive body of the Third word in need of Western medical intervention (Sastry & Dutta, 2012). The tale below describes this othering process:

Dr. Z was an African-American woman in her late forties who has been serving as my OB-GYN for many years. However, that day when I got to the hospital for my women's exams, I found out that from the nurse that she wasn't available and I was assigned to someone else. Dr. Y was a white woman probably in her early fifties.

"Hi, I am Dr. Y. I am going to perform your women's exams," she said.

"Hi, Dr. Y. Nice to meet you," I responded with a shy smile.

"And where are you originally from," she asked.

"I'm from The Congo, in central Africa," I responded. This question was so annoying to me because it was always followed by some stupid exotic comments and that is what exactly happened.

"Oh, wow interesting. You are the first patient ever from Congo I had to deal with. So how is the medical service over there?" she asked.

Quite frankly I wasn't in the mood for this kind of conversation, but I did my best to keep the conversation friendly. I provided her a brief synopsis of my gynecological medical background.

Then, she gave me the usual lecture of what women's exams were all about and why we had to do it. After she instructed me to lay on the bed so she can get started. As she was performing the exam, she suddenly stopped and said: "Wow, you're so hairy."

"It's hereditary. I got it from my mama. I also have a beard just like her," I said smiling innocently.

"Oh really?" she said with a disgusting tone of voice. Then, she added: "I need to have a close look at this" Then she started examining my body from head to toe.

"Why?" I asked her.

"Hum, hum …. This might be serious case of POCS," she replied.

"What is going on? Is everything okay? I don't get it." I asked her.

Then, she gave me a long lecture on POCS and all its symptoms, emphasizing: irregular menstrual cycle and infertility as the most common ones. I had no clue of what she was talking about. I told her:

"I don't think my hairy body has anything to do with what you said. I am naturally hairy just like my mom and siblings. I was born this way. I don't have any issue with my menstrual cycle, same for my siblings/relatives. Besides, Dr. Z has never mentioned anything about it, so I don't get it."

"I hear you, but we still need to check this. We have to make sure that all is fine with you because PCOS is a serious medical condition that requires attention," She added.

Even if I was an immigrant, I was not completely new to the U.S. health system. This was not my first women's exams since my move to the U.S. and Dr. Z has never mentioned anything about my hairy body. So, what was she implying? I could sense that something was weird with her examination. I started to get nervous.

"I don't think I am sick, I am fine. And besides, my mother and all siblings all have healthy babies. As for me, I don't intend to be a mother. It's not a matter of infertility because even back home my gynecologist assured me that all was okay with me. It is a matter of personal choice."

"Oh honey, don't be selfish. You have to give back to humanity. You're in your thirties and your clock is already ticking. So it is important to check if everything is okay." She said smiling.

Meanwhile she continued her examination of my hairy body with a set of inappropriate comments such as "too much hair here," "too much hair there," "the hair is so thick and coarse."

Dutta (2008) asserts that "the subaltern voice is marked by its absence, by not having been noticed" (p. 30). No matter what I did or say, it seemed to me that the woman wasn't ready to listen to me. Obviously, in the eyes of a White doctor, I was the subaltern whose voice didn't matter (Dutta & Basu, 2018). Even more, she did not even take into consideration the medical opinions of my other two OB-GYNs (Dr. X from the Congo and Dr. Z in the U.S.). I wonder if their opinions did not matter to her perhaps because they were both Blacks? Whereas one belonged to the Third world (Dr. X from the Congo) and the other lived in the Western world

(Dr. Z in the U.S.), I wonder if they both probably were perceived as "incompetent" because of the colonial legacy of white supremacy?

Dr. Y excused herself and stepped out the room: "I'll be right back," she said.

Then she came back after a few minutes with the nurse and another young white woman that she introduced to me as an intern. Why did she invite these people in the room without my consent I told myself? I wonder if this wasn't a violation of my privacy as a patient. Maybe I was probably biased and/or I overreacted and took it too personal. However, given my past experience in health encounters, I struggled to draw the line between what was medically allowed to be done/asked about or not on my "Black Congolese immigrant body." I also knew based on some recent medical visits that I have been subject to "extra attention" because of my ethnic and national identity. Sometimes, I was shocked by health care providers' level of ignorance about my country and/or Africa. For instance, when I showed proof of immunization record from my home country, I was asked if they were accurate. A nurse even told me that she didn't know that in Africa they also provided people health services for vaccines against tuberculosis. She probably didn't know that it was a requirement from the U.S. system for most, if not any international student, to do a set of medical exams including getting different types of vaccines before entering the U.S. territory.

The three white women gathered around me and engaged in a long conversation. So, there I was laying on the bed naked surrounded by three white women who were examining my hairy body and making all kind of medical assumptions about it. No one even bothered to ask my opinion at least. I felt like "an object of some sort ... or even an object of study" (Richards, 2008, p. 1717) "under Western eyes" (Mohanty, 2002, p. 499). As a Black female Congolese immigrant, I felt dehumanized: I was an object of study deprived of my agency and a mere recipient of the expertise of White doctors, who believed that they had the right to make all kind of decisions about my body/health without taking into consideration my opinion as if I had nothing important to say (Richards, 2008). I left Dr. Y's office with a lab work for a bunch of blood tests.

A couple of weeks after, I received a phone call from the hospital to follow up on my case. Dr. Z wasn't still back in town. So, I had to meet with Dr. Y again. I was so nervous the day of our appointment. When I first received the phone call, I was so scared that my women's exams may be came back abnormal. However, when I met with Dr. Y it was all about discussing the results of the blood tests about "my hairy body." She informed me that I had a hormone imbalance, and particularly a high level of testosterone. I told her that this wasn't new information to me because I was aware of it since I was in the Congo. So, I explained to her that my doctor told me about it already back home and reassured me that it was nothing to worry about. However, she dismissed all my explanation and insisted that I consult a specialist for further exams because she was worrying about my "medical condition." Additionally, she prescribed pills for hormone treatment and recommended me to a sex therapist because she said I needed therapy to learn how to deal/handle "my high libido" as a result of my "medical condition."

According to Dutta (2015), Western medicine today is driven by "the imagery of the passive Third World subject, depicted as a receptacle of traditional traits, and as the target of top-down interventions of development, rooted in West (read U.S.)-centric conceptualizations of linear economic trajectories to modernization" (p. 123). Describing this top-down model of intervention, Dutta and Basu (2008) denounce how it only "emphasizes the transmission of beliefs, information, and knowledge via one-way health messages from the core sectors of the globe to the subaltern spaces in the periphery, based on the assumption of the [Western] expert position of the sender of the message" (p. 560). For instance, Sastry and Dutta's (2012) study on the social construction of discourses about HIV/AIDS within the U.S. President's Emergency Plan for AIDS revealed that "the United States is portrayed as the altruistic savior, lifting the burden of the soul [while] the spaces of Sub-Saharan Africa, Asia, and the Caribbean emerge as the sites and targets of intervention" (p. 526). Likewise, the story provided above demonstrates that Dr. Y positioned herself as the "Western expert" whose missionary zeal was to save me the hairy Black Congolese woman from the Third world from "my medical condition."

Calling attention on the impact of the Western politics of intervention, Dutta (2007) reminds us that "the othering that drives the conceptualization and implementation of health communication interventions does violence to the culture by fixing it in terms of static characteristics as perceived and defined by the intervener" (p. 316). Similarly, although I insisted that I didn't need hormonal therapy, Dr. Y believed that this medical treatment was the best because her overall medical diagnosis was inspired by a static Eurocentric model of checkboxes applied unanimously to all patients regardless of their cultural and/or ethnic background (Dutta & Jamil, 2013). From a CCA postcolonial stance, such health encounter demonstrates how points of dominance are created through the dichotomous categories of "primitive" and "modern" within the healthcare system (Dutta, 2008). Likewise, as revealed by my lived experience I was "the sick primitive subaltern" and she was "the modern White Western doctor." In her eyes of a White health care provider, neither my cultural background, nor my voice or agency mattered in all the decisions she made about my own body. Consequently, I would argue that she used her power as a dominant actor of the U.S. healthcare system to maintain her control over and/or medically colonize my body (Dutta, 2008).

I left the hospital very disturbed and revolted that day. I wondered if I had the option to decline Dr. Y's medical recommendations. I kept asking myself what would be the consequences of doing so. Describing the tension between free choice and agency, Roach Anlieu (2006) writes:

> However, the concept of free choice in the context of medicalization is constrained by the power of medical advice, and the perceived risks of non-compliance. The risks of not following medical advice may implicate individual women as accountable for any outcome perceived to be socially undesirable. The choice to comply does give individual women some sense of agency while not disrupting dominant cultural expectations. (p. 363–364)

In a similar way, I must confess that as a subaltern, I struggle to make a decision regarding Dr. Y's recommendations because a colonial voice inside me was reminding me that I could pay the cost of neglecting medical recommendation coming from a "White American Doctor" (Dutta, 2008). However, Dutta (2008) also acknowledges that for subalterns, "agency taps into the ability of individuals and of their communities to be active participants in determining health agenda and in formulating solutions to a variety of health problems, as these are perceived by the community" (p. 7). Relying on my agency, I decided to consult other people for more clarity. Therefore, I intentionally ignored all the friendly reminders I received from the hospital concerning Dr. Y's recommendations until the return of my OB-GYN Dr. Z. I found out from my conversation with Dr. Z, my U.S. OB-GYN, and a phone call with Dr. X, my OB-GYN back home, that a medical perception of my "Black Congolese hairy body" as sick/ill was probably due to the fact that U.S. health care providers were not used to dealing with "hairy bodies" like mine. This explained maybe why Dr. Y made a big deal out of it. Equally important, both OB-GYNs reassured me once again that there was nothing medically alarming about my hairy body and made it clear that hormonal therapy was an option in case I really wanted to balance my level of testosterone.

Through the process of self-reflexivity, I came to realize that the medicalization of my body was more of cultural issue just because my "Black Congolese hairy body" was the disturbing and unexpected body of the "other" located outside of the spheres of American womanhood/femininity as defined by the U.S. health care system. I firmly believed that I wasn't sick, I was just a Black Congolese hairy woman who struggles with stereotypes and microaggressions because of her natural physical appearance. CCA stipulates that for the subaltern, "resistance is enacted in the act of returning the gaze" (Dutta, 2007, p. 323). In a similar way, I used a Congolese cultural background as an "oppositional gaze" (hooks, 2000) against the "Western gaze" in order "to talk back" (hooks, 1989) to the medical colonization of my hairy body. I decided to boycott Dr. Y's medical diagnosis and recommendations. I refused to consult a specialist as well as to follow the hormonal pills treatment and pursue sex therapy. In fact, for the subaltern, micro-level practices encompass "day-to-day acts of resistance" (Pawlowski, 2011, p. 27) among which the "refusal to take certain preventive measures as prescribed by the dominant paradigm" (Dutta, 2008, p. 14). Additionally, I asked my OB-GYN Dr. Z to inform Dr. Y on my behalf about my decision. I told her something like: *"tell Dr. Y that as I repeatedly mentioned to her 'I am not sick, I am fine.' I am just a Black Congolese hairy woman and she is not used to my kind of body."* Whereas, I felt empowered to use my agency in challenging the cultural meaning medically assigned to my hairy body, I wonder if this was a learning opportunity for Dr. Y to rethink how the dominant Eurocentric view shapes her medical expertise while dealing with immigrants people.

One long-term effect of the medical perception of my body as "ill" or "abnormal" is that whenever I go to the hospital for medical consultations I always feel like I owe medical providers some kind of explanation about the "excessive hair growth." While facing suspicious looks and/or stares on my naked hairy body, my magic formula is always: "I'm hairy, but I'm not sick. I am fine."

A Closing Tale

It was one of these beautiful sunny mornings. I had just woken up and as part of my morning ritual I glanced over my phone to check the daily conversation I have with my siblings back home on social media. The conversation revolved around everyday family issues. However, one thing in particular caught my attention on that day: a picture of my youngest sister's face with some weird white-ish cream all over her face. I tried to understand what this was all about, but I couldn't until I decided to track the conversation thread. I found the following lines:

"Hi all, hope you're all okay. Guess what? Our new boss at work who is a European White man has asked me to shave my facial hair. When I got to work this morning, I received a warning letter stating that I have to shave my chin ASAP otherwise I'll get fired."

I was speechless after reading these lines. I thought this was some kind of joke but it wasn't. It was indeed real because when I asked my sister if she was joking she just sent me another picture of her face completely shaved. As I looked at her hairless face, I felt like dealing with a stranger. She was no longer the same person to me. She wasn't my hairy twin sister anymore as people used to tease the two of us back home. Every single hair of her face was gone: chin, sideburns, and mustache. I felt so sad because knowing how much she was in love with her hairy body and praised it as one of her beauty assets, I could only image that this must have been a very painful experience for her. However, I was powerless, I couldn't help her. I didn't know what to do. I was away. I could only show my support to her from afar. Our conversation sounded like:

"I'm sorry that you have to go through this," I told her.

"It's okay, big sister. I'll be fine. You know how much I love my beard and sideburns, but I had no choice. I had to do it to keep my job." She replied.

After listening to these statements I was so revolted. So, I told myself it is true then that the universality of body hair removal "has been increasingly normative for appearance to play a role in decision to hire and promote women" (Toerien & Wilkinson, 2003, p. 338). I couldn't believe that this was also happening in the Congo. As a feminist, this reminded me again of one of these sexist policies imposed upon women's bodies to look a certain way. In fact, "the underlying message is the same: what a woman looks like is more important than the work she does" (Toerien & Wilkinson, 2003, p. 338). Thus, I told my sister:

"I see, but why didn't you resist? This man has no right to impose you how you should carry yourself or your body, this is not fair. What does this all shaving thing has to do with your job? You can sue him! Why is he disciplining your body like that?" I said.

"OMG, I can see that you're dreaming Gloria. This is the Congo. It is not the U.S. What kind of power do I have to say no to what a white man has decided? So just you know, I'm not the only one in the case. I have a female colleague who was recently suspended because she ignored the boss' warning about the same issue. As for me, I didn't want to end up like her. I need this job to survive." She told me.

My sister just called me out on my privilege. I live in a place where I can still openly claim to be a feminist and use my body as well as my voice to say no to some of the sexist practices imposed upon me. She was right. I was so unaware of my privilege that I failed to recognize the differences between the cultural contexts that shape our lived experiences as women with hairy bodies. I was using a Western lens to make sense of my sister's lived experience within the context of Congolese culture. How could I have forgotten that, unlike me, my sister was still living in a country where women's rights was not a priority and in many ways women still suffered different forms of oppression due to the political system, customs/traditions, etc. (Culture of the Democratic Republic of Congo, n.d.; Wango, 2010)? So how could she seek justice?

Although I may argue that the Congolese culture isn't a fertile terrain to seek justice for such issue, I am also revolted by the impact of white supremacy in my sister's experience.

What struck me the most in her sad experience is that her oppressor was not Congolese, but a white European man. Although my sister's boss was the only "white body" of the company, he was still the "powerful" body, mind, and spirit that dominated over all because he was obviously the incarnation of the "White Messiah" performing his/her missionary zeal. There lies similarity in our lived experiences as two black hairy Congolese women living at different places across the globe, yet carrying the colonial legacy of White Western norms of what a black "beautiful" and "healthy" female body should be/looked like in accordance with the "White master's" expectations. Our colonized Congolese Black female hairy bodies are seen as "dirty," "sick," and "unhealthy" in the eyes of these white Colonizers.

Concluding Thoughts

As noted by Koehn (2006), in the actual context of globalization, "many health outcomes are shaped by transnational interactions among care providers and care recipients who meet in settings where nationality/ethnic match is not an option" (p. 2). Therefore, in contrast to the traditional assumption that immigrants will adapt to the existing health system of the host country (Bollini, 1993), I agree with health scholars that the U.S. should develop culturally appropriate health services peculiar to the needs of immigrants (Bollini, 1993; Bollini & Siem, 1995; Dutta & Jamil, 2013; Kandula, Kersey, & Lurie, 2004; Koehn, 2006). In order to do so, Bollini and Siem (1995) cautions that "it is necessary to avoid the traditional approach, which sees the foreigner as passive and ignorant and the Western foreigner health professional as active and objective" (p. 826). For example, instead of evaluating immigrants' health experiences based on a checkboxes list designed from Eurocentric model as demonstrated in this autoethnographic piece, it is incumbent that health providers receive proper training about the social and cultural context shaping the service provided to their patients (Bollini, 1993; Bollini & Siem, 1995; Dutta & Jamil, 2013; Kandula et al., 2004; Koehn, 2006).

Health scholars claim that professionals of health often describe their patient's health issues/experiences through their own professional lenses failing to take into consideration how a patient's personal and sociocultural beliefs may impact their understanding/interpretation of their own related health condition (Dutta, 2008; Richards, 2008). Consequently, "the voice that is heard most often in medical narratives of various sorts is the voice of the distant expert, and this voice can be quite pernicious" (Richards, 2008, p. 1720). For instance, as demonstrated throughout this piece, western medical experts' reports/portrayals of Third world people/subaltern subjects are often filled with negative stereotypes, othering, and objectification while their voices are dismissed (Sastry & Dutta, 212). In contrast, Richards (2008) believes that the patient's voice should be privileged because the expert of lived experience of a given disease/illness is not the clinician/doctor, but the person/patient. Pursuing his argument, he claims that "one way of resisting [medical] objectification by others is by writing about oneself" (p. 1720) in order to reconstitute one's identity. Similarly, in this piece, I used autoethnograpy to tell the "previously untold, often oppressively silenced, story" (Chang, 2016, p. 446) of the medicalization of my hairy Congolese body to challenge the narrow Eurocentric view of what is medically defined as "a healthy body" and socially/culturally considered as "acceptable/appropriate femininity."

This paper expands on how research on the CCA can be applied to the lived experiences of immigrants other than Asian and/or of Asian descent living in the

U.S., and particularly African immigrants. In doing so, an important contribution of this study is to fill the gap on scholarship on African culture in the field of communication, and particularly mainstream health communication as well as critical intercultural communication scholarship. Scholars (Miller, 2005; Miller, Kizito, & Ngula, 2010) assert that whereas there is research on Africa in health communication, the scholarship produced reinforce the pervasive image of Africa as a poor continent in need of Eurocentric/Western interventions such as public health campaigns to combat prevalent diseases including but not limited to HIV/AIDS, malaria, and more. Miller (2005) decries this exoticism as the result of the lack of voices of African scholars that are often dismissed/unheard because Western scholars look at Africa as the "other in need of being spoken for, a 'them' that 'we' we need to explain" (p. 226). Although this study is limited to my own lived experience, a layered account of such experience through authoethnographic personal narrative/storytelling is a powerful way to lift up marginalized African voices because it allows me to" speak for myself" in order to break silence on the othering process African people are often subject to by Western people who tend to "speak for us" while conducting research on Africa. Thus, I believe that this study can serve as a springboard to promote more scholarship on CCA and African immigrants' lived experiences in diasporic/transnational context.

References

Basow, S. A. (1991). The hairless ideal: Women and their body hair. *Psychology of Women Quarterly*, *15*, 83–96.

Basow, S. A., & Braman, A. C. (1998). Women and body hair: Social perceptions and attitudes. *Psychology of Women Quarterly*, *22*, 637–645.

Basow, S. A., & Willis, J. (2001). Perceptions of body hair on white women: Effects of labeling. *Psychological Reports*, *89*, 571–576.

Bollini, P. (1993). Health for immigrants and refugees in the 1990s. A comparative study in seven receiving countries. *Innovation: The European Journal of Social Science Research*, *6*, 101–110.

Bollini, P., & Siem, H. (1995). No real progress towards equity: Health of migrants and ethnic minorities on the eve of the year 2000. *Social Science & Medicine*, *41*, 819–828.

Boylorn, R. M., & Orbe, M. P. (2014). Critical autoethnography as method choice. In R. M. Boylorn & M. P. Orbe (Eds.), *Critical autoethnography: Intersecting cultural identities in everyday life* (pp. 13–26). Walnut Creek, CA: Left Coast Press.

Chai, C.-L. (2009). Culture as enabler. *Science and Public,* 36(1), 76–77.

Chang, H. (2016). Autoethnography in Health Research: Growing Pains? *Qualitative Health Research*, *26*(4), 443–451.

Chapkis, W. (1986). *Beauty secrets: Women and the subversion of identity*. New York: Routledge.

Culture of the Democratic Republic of Congo. (n.d.). Retrieved on April 5, 2010 from http://www.everyculture.com/Bo-Co/Democratic-Republic-of-the-Congo.html

Dutta, M. J. (2007). Communicating about culture and health: Theorizing culture-centered and cultural sensitivity approaches. *Communication Theory, 17*, 302–328.

Dutta, M. J. (2008). *Communicating health: A culture-centered approach.* Cambridge, UK: Polity Press.

Dutta, M. J. (2015). Decolonizing communication for social change: A culture-centered approach. *Communication Theory, 25*, 123–143.

Dutta, M. J., & Basu, B. (2008). Meanings of health: Interrogating structure and culture. *Health Communication, 23*, 560–572.

Dutta, M. J., & Basu, B. (2009). Sex workers and HIV/AIDS: Analyzing participatory culture-centered health communication strategies. *Human Communication Research, 35*, 86–114.

Dutta, M. J., & Basu, B. (2018). Subalternity, neoliberal seductions, and freedom: Decolonizing the global market of social change. *Cultural Studies ↔ Critical Methodologies, 18*(1), 80–93.

Dutta, M. J., & Jamil, R. (2013). Health at the margins of migration: Culture-centered co-constructions among Bangladeshi immigrants. *Health Communication, 28*, 170–182.

Dyer, R. (1997). *White.* London: Routledge.

Ellis, C., Adams, T. E., & Bochner, A. P. (2011). Autoethnography: An overview. *Forum: Qualitative Social Research, 12*(1), 1–13.

Fahs, B. (2011a). Breaking body hair boundaries: Classroom exercises for challenging social constructions of the body and sexuality. *Feminism and Psychology, 22*, 482–506.

Fahs, B. (2011b). Dreaded otherness: Heteronormative patrolling of women's body hair rebellions. *Gender and Society, 25*, 451–472.

Ferrante, J. (1988). Biomedical versus cultural constructions of abnormality: The case of idiopathic hirsutism in the United States. *Culture, Medicine and Psychiatry, 12*, 219–238.

Fox, R. (2010). Re-membering daddy: Autoethnographic reflections of my father and Alzheimer's disease. *Text and Performance Quarterly, 30*(1), 3–20.

Holman-Jones, S. (2008). Autoethnography: Making the personal political. In N. K. Denzin & Y. S. Lincoln (Eds.), *Collecting interpretive qualitative materials* (pp. 205–246). Thousand Oaks, CA: Sage.

Holman-Jones, S., Adams, T., & Ellis, C. (2013). Introduction: Coming to know autoethnography as more than a method. In S. Holman Jones, T. E. Adams, & C. Ellis,(Eds.), *Handbook of autoethnography* (pp. 17–47). Walnut Creek, CA: Left Coast Press.

Hope, C. (1982). Caucasian female body hair and American culture. *The Journal of American Culture, 5*, 93–99.

hooks, b. (1989). *Talking back: Thinking feminist, thinking back.* Boston, MA: South End Press.

hooks, b. (2000). The oppositional gaze: Black female spectators. In J. Belton (Ed.), *Movies and mass culture* (pp. 247–264). New Branswick, NJ: Rutgers University Press.

Kandula, N. R., Kersey, M., & Lurie, N. (2004). Assuring the health of immigrants: What the leading health indicators tell us. *Annual Review of Public Health, 25*, 357–376.

Kitzinger, C., & Willmott, J. (2002). 'The thief of womanhood': Women's experience of Polycystic Ovarian Syndrome. *Social Science and Medicine*, *54*, 349–361.

Koehn, P. H. (2006). Globalization, migration, health, and educational preparation for transnational medical encounters. *Globalization and Health*. Retrieved from http://www.globalizationandhealth.com/content/ 2/1/2

Lunde, O. (1984). A study of body hair density and distribution in normal women. *American Journal of Physical Anthropology*, *64*(2), 179–184.

Lunde, O., & Grøttum, P. (1984). Body hair growth in women: Normal or hirsute. *American Journal of Physical Anthropology*, *64*, 307–313.

Miller, A. N. (2005). Keeping up with cartography: A call to study African communication. In W. J. Starosta & G.-M. Chen (Eds.), *International and intercultural communication annual* (pp. 214–236). Washington, DC: National Communication Association.

Miller, A. N., Kizito, M. N., & Ngula, K. W. (2010). Research and publication by communication faculty in East Africa: A challenge to the global community of communication scholars. *Journal of International and Intercultural Communication*, *3*(4), 286–303.

Mohanty, C. T. (2002). "Under western eyes" revisited: Feminist solidarity through anticapitalist struggles. *Signs: Journal of Women in Culture and Society*, *28*(2), 499–535.

Pawlowski, D. R. (2011). Communicating health: A culture-centered approach by Mohan J. Dutta. *Communication Research Trends*, *30*(1), 26–28.

Pelias, R. J. (2007). Performance writing: The ethics of representation in form and body. In N. K. Denzin & M. Giardina (Eds.), *Ethical futures of qualitative research: Decolonizing the politics of knowledge* (pp. 181–196). Walnut Creek, CA: Left Coast Press.

Richards, R. (2008). Writing the othered self: Autoethnography and the problem of objectification in writing about illness and disability. *Qualitative Health Research*, *18*, 1717–1728.

Richardson, L. (2000). Writing: A method of Inquiry. In N. Denzin & Y. Lincoln (Eds.), *Handbook of qualitative research* (2nd ed., pp. 923–948). Thousand Oaks, Ca: Sage.

Roach Anlieu, S. (2006). Gendered bodies: Between conformity and autonomy. In K. Davis, M. Evans, & J. Lorber (Eds.), *Handbook of gender and women's studies* (pp. 358–375). Thousand Oaks, CA; Sage.

Sastry, S., & Dutta, M. J., (2012). Public health, global surveillance, and the "emerging disease" worldview: A postcolonial appraisal of PEPFAR. *Health Communication*, *27*, 519–532.

Shah, P. N. (1957). Human body hair—A quantitative study. *American Journal of Obstetrics and Gynaecology*, *73*, 1255–1265.

Simpson, N. (1986). Unwanted hair. *British Medical Journal*, *293*, 348–349.

Spieldenner, A. R. (2014). Statement of ownership: An autoethnography of living with HIV. *Journal of Men's Studies*, *22*(1), 12–27.

Spry, T. (2011). *Body, paper, stage: Writing and performing autoethnography*. Walnut Creek, CA: Left Coast Press.

Terry, G., & Braun, V. (2013). To let hair be, or to not let hair be? Gender and body hair removal practices in Aotearoa/New Zealand. *Body Image*, *10*, 599–606.

Tiggemann, M., & Hodgson, Z. (2008). The hairlessness norm extended: Reasons for and predictors of women's body hair removal at different body sites. *Sex Roles, 59*, 889–897.

Tiggemann, M., & Kenyon, S. J. (1998). The hairlessness norm: The removal of body hair in women. *Sex Roles, 39*(11/12), 873–885.

Tiggemann, M., & Lewis, C. (2004). Attitudes toward women's body hair: Relationship with disgust sensitivity. *Psychology of Women Quarterly, 28*, 381–387.

Toerien, M., & Wilkinson, S. (2003). Gender and body hair: Constructing the feminine woman. *Women's Studies International Forum, 26*(4), 333–344.

Toerien, M., & Wilkinson, S. (2004). Exploring the depilation norm: A qualitative questionnaire study of women's body hair removal. *Qualitative Research in Psychology, 1*, 69–92.

Toerien, M., Wilkinson, S., & Choi, Y. L. (2005). Body hair removal: The "mundane" production of normative femininity. *Sex Roles, 52*(5/6), 399–406.

Toyosaki, S., & Pensoneau-Conway, S. (2013). Autoethnography as a praxis of social justice: Three ontological contexts. In S. Holman Jones., T. E. Adams, & C. Ellis (Eds.), *Handbook of autoethnography* (pp. 557–575). Walnut Creek, CA: Left Coast Press.

Wango, J. (2010, March 28). Why Congo is the world's most dangerous place for women. The Observer. Retrieved on April 5, 2010 from http://www.guardian.co.uk./lifeandstyle/2010/mar28/congo-women-danger-war-judith-wango

CHAPTER SIX

People of Color Don't Get That: An Analytic Autoethnography of Living with Celiac Disease

BY TOMEKA M. ROBINSON

Introduction

"Looking at your extensive medical history and the series of colonoscopies performed, which is abnormal to have as many as you have had at your age, I don't see any record of a celiac disease test. Have you ever been tested for celiac disease?" "No, I haven't, but what's another test at this point?" This was the conversation I had with a new physician in Fall 2009 after suffering from yet another mysterious attack that left me writhing in pain on the floor. A colleague heard that I had to cancel all of my afternoon appointments and scheduled me an appointment with her doctor. She said "while he does not have the best bedside manner, he will order test after test until he figures out what is wrong." Little did I know at the time, accepting this appointment was one of the best decisions that I could have made.

Celiac disease (CD) is an autoimmune disease that occurs in genetically predisposed individuals and is precipitated by the ingestion of gluten-containing grains: wheat, barley, and rye (Fasano et al., 2003). CD is associated with a number of health issues including: malnutrition, osteoporosis, iron deficiency anemia, and increased mortality (Godfrey et al., 2010; Jafri et al., 2008; Murray et al., 2003). While CD is one of the most common immunemediated disorders, the disease remains widely underrecognized and underdiagnosed (Alaedini & Green, 2005). CD is diagnosed via a simple blood test, though a biopsy often follows. The prevalence of CD is on the rise worldwide; however, the incidence and prevalence of CD vary significantly across different geographical regions of the world (Kang, Kang, Green, Gwee, & Ho, 2013). Cases have been found throughout Europe and in countries populated by those of European descent such as South Africa, Australia, New Zealand, and South America (Brar, Lee, Lewis, Bhagat, & Green, 2006). The disease also appears to be common in North Africa, the Middle East, and Northern India (al-Tawaty & Elbargathy, 1998; al-Hassany, 1975; Lionetti, Favilli, Chiaravalloti, Ughi, & Maggiore, 1999; ; Puri, Garg, Monga, Tyagi, & Sarawat, 2004; Tatar et al., 2004; Sood, Midha, Sood, & Malhotra, 2003). Moreover, there have also been documented cases in Cuba and in West Indian children living in England (Hung, Philips, & Walker-Smith, 1995; Sagaro & Jimenez, 1981). While once considered very rare in the United States, it is now estimated to occur in about 1% of the US population (Fasano et al., 2003). While the disease is multigenetic, there is a requirement that an individual possess the HLA alleles that encode for DQ2 and/or DQ8 (Louka & Solid, 2003). The prevalence of this disease in minority populations in the US is virtually unknown, partly because HLA DQ2 and DQ8 are regarded primarily as Caucasian genetic traits (Brar et al., 2006). While CD is considered rare in individuals of central or west African descent, one blood screening study by Not et al. (1998) found that 1 in 250 African-Americans had positive endomysial antibodies, a frequency similar to that of the entire study group. To date there have been no systematic screening studies among African-Americans or non-white Hispanics for the disease or the frequency of the DQ2 and DQ8 genes. While the low reported prevalence of the disease may be due to a lower frequency of the genetic markers and/or dietary, environmental & socioeconomic disparities (Kondrashova et al., 2008), it may also be the consequence of other factors such as implicit bias and the complex history within the United States of forced and voluntary intermixing between those of European and African descent.

Implicit Bias in Medical Encounters

In the United States, people of color face disparities in access to health care, the quality of care received, and health outcomes (Epstein, Ayanian, Weissman, Chasan-Taber, & Epstein, 2000; Fiscella, Franks, Gold, & Clancy, 2000; Mayberry, Mili, & Ofili, 2000; Nosek, Greenwald, & Banaji, 2007; Sabin, Nosek, Greenwald, & Rivara, 2009). Scholars have also found that people of color are also generally less satisfied with their interactions with health care providers (Beckman & Frankel, 1984; Hall et al., 2015; Johnson, Roter, Powe, & Cooper, 2004). Even when access-related factors such as insurance and socioeconomic status are controlled, racial/ethnic disparities in healthcare still exist. Therefore, provider attitudes and behavior have become a target area for researchers studying health disparities (Hall et al., 2015; Smedley, Stith, & Nelson, 2003). Although explicit displays of racial discrimination in healthcare settings have been on the decline, implicit attitudes that may influence provider behavior and treatment choices persist. According to Hall et al. (2015)

> patients of color may be kept waiting longer for assessment or treatment than their White counterparts, or providers may spend more time with White patients than with patients of color. In addition, providers may vary in the extent to which they collaborate with patients in systematic though nondeliberate ways, in considering treatment options based on patients' characteristics. Subtle biases may be expressed in several ways: approaching patients with a dominant and condescending tone that decreases the likelihood that patients will feel heard and valued by their providers, failing to provide interpreters when needed, doing more or less thorough diagnostic work, recommending different treatment options for patients based on assumptions about their treatment adherence capabilities, and granting special privileges, such as allowing some families to visit patients after hours while limiting visitation for other families. (p. 61)

The variations in practitioner behaviors may be based on positive and negative attitudes toward different racial and ethnic groups and these attitudes are often unconscious, therefore, making it harder to acknowledge and control.

One study by Blair et al. (2013) found that of the 210 clinicians who completed the measures of ethnic/racial bias test administered, approximately two-thirds had implicit bias against Black patients (43% moderate to strong bias) and Latino patients (51% moderate to strong bias), while reporting very little explicit bias against either group.

Another study by Shavers et al. (2012) conducted a systematic literature review on the prevalence, perception of and effect of racial/ethnic discrimination and institutional racism within health care settings. To be included in their study, articles had to be published in English, focus on US health care providers, patients, or US health care settings, report quantitative or qualitative results of racial/ethnic discrimination, patient or provider perceptions of race/ethnicity-based discrimination within US health care settings, or discriminatory attitudes and beliefs of US patients or health care providers. In the 58 articles reviewed, the reported prevalence of race/ethnicity based discrimination was between 6.9–52.0% for African Americans, 4.2–13.4% for Latinos and 0.4–6.0% for Non-Hispanic Whites in nine of the studies. Ten studies also reported perceived discrimination in health care of between 8.0–8.9% for American Indian patients, 12.3% for Puerto Ricans in the US, and 7.5% for Southeast Asians, and between 3.0–9.1% for Asian/Pacific Islanders. Their results show that African Americans and Latinos more frequently report race/ethnicity-based discrimination during their health care encounters compared to Non-Hispanic Whites, as are minority women compared with minority men. Findings from the majority of the reviewed articles provide evidence of the prevalence of provider explicit and implicit biases.

Moreover, Hall et al. (2015) completed a systematic literature review of articles that collected data from participants who were health care providers or were in training to become health care providers, measured and reported results on implicit attitudes toward racial/ethnic groups, and were written in English. They excluded studies that only examined explicit bias, as well as studies that examined implicit bias that was not related to race or ethnicity. In the 15 studies reviewed, 14 studies found evidence of low to moderate levels of implicit bias against people of color among health care professionals. Four studies found that health care professionals associate Black Americans with being less cooperative, less compliant, and less responsible in a medical context. Four studies also reported evidence of moderate levels of implicit bias against Hispanic/Latino/Latina individuals and one study specifically reported that professional tended to associate Hispanic/Latino/Latina people with noncompliance and risky behavior.

Implicit bias can and does negatively affects the health care delivered to racial/ethnic minority patients. Therefore, this autoethnography will delve into my personal experiences with an awareness of the intersections of race/ethnicity and the diagnosis of CD. The intention of this paper is to address the issue of implicit bias and discuss how as health communication professionals we have a role in addressing underdiagnoses of people of color living with chronic diseases.

Background and Context

Documenting my medical journey was unsettling at points. I have spent most of my life going from physician to physician seeking some answers for my "mysterious illness." While I have always expressed symptoms of what I have come to understand as CD, it wasn't until 2009 that anyone had an answer to what was plaguing my body. Navigating this journey is what led to my interest in health communication and education in part. More specifically, I wanted to be able to teach others, especially other people of color (POC), how to advocate for themselves better during medical encounters. As a scholar that often uses intersectionality and Critical Race Theory (CRT) as theoretical frameworks in order to better understand health, throughout my narrative references to the dimensions of oppression and marginalization within medical encounters will be utilized.

Moreover, I am deeply rooted in self-reflexivity and as such will position myself as being an upper middle class, mixed-race woman, who has always had access to quality health insurance and could afford any and all treatment options.

Intersectionality was founded in Black Feminism as a way to account for the various facets of identity in concrete, material, and positional ways (Crenshaw, 1991). Intersectionality includes race, class, gender, and sexuality in order to interrogate the ways that people have access to power and privilege, as well as how this access informs perceptions and beliefs. Intersectionality is not a static feature, but rather is fluid and can be used to explore norms and power in relation to a wide range of identities, including health conditions.

CRT specifically addresses how power is enacted through the lens of race. The basic CRT model consists of five elements: (a) the centrality of race and racism and their intersectionality with other forms of subordination, (b) the challenge to dominant ideology, (c) the commitment to social justice, (d) the centrality of experiential knowledge, and (e) the transdisciplinary perspective (Solorzano, 1997; Solorzano & Yasso, 2000). CRT also uniquely relies on narratives to substantiate claims. According to DeCuir and Dixson (2004), "an essential tenant of Critical Race Theory is counter storytelling" (p. 27). Deconstructing and understanding narratives can be used "to reveal the circular, self-serving nature of particular legal doctrines or rules" (Delgado & Stefancic, 2012, p. xvii). While many scholars argue for universalism over individual narratives, CRT emphasizes the role of individual narratives to the sense-making process, as we understand context through narrative.

Methods

An analytic autoethnography served as the research design for this study. According to Ellis and Bochner (2000) autoethnographic research is a "study and procedure that connects the personal to the cultural" (p. 739). More explicitly, "authors use their own experiences in the culture reflexively to bend back on self and look more deeply at self-other interactions" (Ellis, 2004, p. 46). Analytic authoethnography, first proposed by Anderson (2006), takes it a step further as the researcher is engaged within the group, setting, or society as a full and dynamic member, but holds a visible identity as a mindful researcher and social actor inside the ethnographic content (Marechal, 2010).

Notes from the Journal: Pre-diagnosis

As a child, I was the gross kid that you never wanted to invite to your birthday party. I could never predict exactly when I would get sick, but I would often leave from the party with a stomach ache and would start vomiting at some point. When my symptoms would persist for several days, my mom would schedule appointment after appointment trying to find some answer. The doctors said everything from a slight allergy to chocolate to perhaps I was drinking too many fluids. No doctor ever performed an allergy test on me to even test these theories, but all were certain that there was nothing to really be concerned about. According to my parents, I also experienced frequent vomiting as a baby after feedings and they sought medical interventions only to be told to switch to a different formula each time. Over the course of my adolescent and teen years, I was given a host of medications including ulcer and acid reflex treatements and nothing did the trick. The older I got, the worse the symptoms got and the longer the symptoms would last.

I had two incapaciting episodes that resulted in emergency room visits and one in a three day hospitalization. The first episode was in spring 2005 when I was a senior in college in Louisiana. I found myself laying on my debate coaches' office floor in extreme pain and continuously vomiting. One of my teammates eventually took me to the ER when he got out of class. Upon arriving, I waited for several hours to be seen by the physician and was eventually told that I probably just had food poisoning. I was given some fluids and was released. The doctors in this ER didn't order any tests even when I asked if there was anything they could run to see if that was all it was. I had food poisoning before and this felt very different. They reiterated that I probably ate something bad on campus and that it would eventually pass. So I went home and remained in my bed consuming only chicken broth for several days, until I felt that I could resume my normal schedule.

The second episode was in Fall 2007 when I was a doctoral student in Texas. I went to an animal shelter with one of my friends to adopt a dog. I felt the familiar hot flash, but this time I felt like I was going to black out immediately. My friend caught me and helped me to the car. He offered to drive me directly to the ER, but I stubbornly refused because I was tired of paying for medical bills and never getting an actual answer. About an hour later, the vomiting and pain was much more excruciating than previous episodes, so I called my friend back and he drove me to the ER. When we arrived, I was left laying on the floor of the ER for over three hours before I was even triaged. When the ER doctor finally saw me, he thought that I might have appendicitis and ordered tests. After the initial test, the nurse asked whether I had ever had my appendix removed because they could not find it. "My appendix is very much so still in my body." "Oh" was the response. At this point, I realized that I didn't trust this doctor or the hospital, but they admitted me and recommended that I have a colonoscopy and an endoscopy. I explained to the nurse that I have already had a colonoscopy the year before at the hospital in the neighboring town, but they wanted to run another one just in case the previous doctor missed anything. These doctors also couldn't find anything and ruled that I had an un-diagnosable illness and eventually released me. They saw value in my continuing my pescatarian lifestyle, but didn't offer any other suggestions. At this point, I was resigned to just having to learn to deal with it and praying that when I had an episode I was in a place where I could find a cool, hard, surface to lay down until it passed.

When I was released from the hospital, I was covered in bruises, had lost 10 lbs, and was so weak that I took a few days off from classes. When I returned to my advisor's office, she looked at me and asked whether someone was harming me. I later learned that the bruising was a result of my extreme iron deficiency because my body was not properly processing food.

Notes from the Journal: The Diagnosis

In Fall 2009, I had another debilitating episode in my office. My colleague scheduled me an appointment that afternoon and offered to drive me to it. Not wanting to be a burden to anyone, I waited until I was in a condition to drive to the appointment and met with the doctor. It took several hours for me to gain enough strength to walk down the stairs to my car and drive to the doctor's office. I finally got to the office and met with the doctor. After the medical interview where I explained my medical history to the doctor, the doctor asked whether I had ever had a CD test. I responded, "No, but what's another test at this point?" He added this to the full panel of blood work and tests that he wanted run. This was the first time that I didn't feel rushed in explaining my extensive medical history and felt that the doctor was actually listening to my symptoms. After he finished listening, he called in his nurse to conduct the blood tests and while they drew so much blood that I was certain that I didn't have any blood remaining, I was also relieved that finally someone was running more tests. I prayed that finally someone would find an answer and thus a treatment option that would actually work.

I eventually got the results from the CD blood test back and it produced inconclusive results. So, my doctor recommended that I see a specialist and have a biopsy. The nurse recommended that I start reading some literature on CD and start thinking about whether I thought that I could be compliant with going completely gluten-free. I found it a little odd that she asked about my ability to be compliant, but I scheduled the appointment with the gastrointestinalogist and immediately began to do my research. My mom also began searching for information about how she could adjust some of our traditional Creole dishes to be gluten-free, which is not an easy feat since most Creole dishes are roux based.

About a month passed before I could get in to see the specialist. Immediately upon seeing me, this doctor said that he wasn't certain why the referring physician even ordered a CD test because this is not a common disease for African-Americans. I told him "did you miss on my chart that I am actually Creole, not African-American?" I tried to explain to him that Creole is a mixture of mixture of French, Spanish, African, and American Indian. He completely ignored me and said that I could still go forward with having yet another colonoscopy and endoscopy, but he wasn't sure that they would find anything. I scheduled the procedure, but the confidence I felt just a month prior about finally getting a diagnosis was gone. After the visit, I called my mom and she assured me that if I needed to adopt a gluten-free lifestyle that we would figure out how to do it together.

It took another few weeks before I could get on the schedule for the third colonoscophy, endoscopy and biospy, but at this point, I had pretty much already adjusted my diet to being gluten-free and I had already started to feel better. No one at this point told me that I should have continued to consume gluten at my normal rate because this might alter my results. When the results came back, they could not definitively confirm that I had CD because it had been almost a month since I had consumed any gluten, so they wrote on my chart "suspected CD" and said that I had enough intestinal damage to believe that I did in fact have CD. They also said this could explain my extreme iron and Vitamin D & K deficiency. I was given two options at this point: go back to consuming gluten for at least a month and then have another test to get absolute confirmation or continue to live my life gluten-free without an official diagnosis. I chose the later because I could not bring myself to going back to feeling sick after finally feeling better and the doctor agreed with this choice.

Notes from the Journal: Finding Community with other CD Patients

Learning to live with any chronic disease is an adjustment. CD requires adopting a completely gluten-free diet. In the early days of diagnosis, I spent a lot of time on websites and blogs looking for tips for how I could learn to eat gluten-free. My training as a health communicator and educator gave me some insight into how to eliminate the illogical and faulty advice given on some blogs, but there were still some areas that were not ground in scientific evidence because it simply hadn't been studied yet. In 2009, CD was still very rare in the United States and learning how to completely eliminate wheat, rye, and barley was perplexing to say the least. Gluten was in almost everything and the few gluten-free products on the shelves, especially in the rural Ohio area I was living, were either disgusting, expensive, and/or of poor quality. I would often schedule weekend trips two hours away to Columbus, just to go to a Whole Foods to buy groceries.

While searching the blogs I found that everyone was looking for answers and were sharing their narratives with each other. One of the most eye-opening things within these forums I discovered was that many POC, especially women of color, were told the exact same thing, we were not susceptible to this disease because we were not White. Some of the women shared how they decided to adopt a gluten-free lifestyle even without a formal diagnosis because they found some reprieve in symptoms. Others shared how they kept searching for a doctor who would finally take their symptoms seriously. This was mind-boggling because we know that race is a social construct and more importantly that many POC have some Caucasian lineage in the US. I shared my story with several of the women too. Each of us had a similar story. The doctors simply saw Black or Brown skin and ignored everything else we mentioned about our lineage and/or medical history.

I continued searching the blogs for recipes and advice on where to find the best gluten-free food options. For several months, I attempted to remain pescatarian while also being gluten-free, but I realized that this was a poor choice as my food journals revealed that I was often consuming less than 700 calories a day. So, I decided to start slowly introducing meat back into my diet, a choice my mother and the rest of my family celebrated.

Notes from the Journal: Present Day Survival

Years after my diagnosis, I believe that I have adjusted fairly well to living a gluten-free lifestyle. There are more options available in grocery stores as bigger companies have decided to cash in on this niche market. This has caused the quality to improve while simultaneously making things more affordable. Restaurants are also doing a much better job of labeling and providing gluten-free alternatives. However, any time I have a meal not prepared in my own kitchen, I run the risk of cross-containmantion and getting sick. This is something that has happened to me many times. I now know within about two hours whether I have consumed something that contained gluten and thus find a space to just wait out the symptoms. Though some people take activated charcoal when experiencing a Celiac attack, I choose to just wait until the attack passes because the activated charcoal makes me vomit even more. These attacks often leave me weak and unable to move for at least a day depending on the amount of cross-containmantion that has occurred.

My rigourous professional and personal travel schedule makes it impossible to avoid eating at restaurants. So, I do my best to pack snacks and I research restaurants that provide gluten-free options. I am very reliant on an app called GF Card that translates an explanation of my disease into 50 of the most common languages. I show the card to my servers and they are able to talk to the chef to try to make accommodations for me. This has proven to be a lifesaver in many countries where my understanding of the language is deficient. I also spend a lot of time on other apps like Yelp, reading reviews to see if anyone has had any issues with cross-containation at the restaurant. In most major cities in the world, this is easy to do, but in more rural areas or countries like Italy, where gluten is a staple, I am often left with the option to only eat rice or lettuce for several days at a time. I know this is not healthy and I am often not consuming enough calories, but the alternative of consuming gluten is much worse.

While I am not still as active on the blogs and forums, I still share my experiences and talk to others who have similar symptoms about searching for doctors that will actually listen to them. I teach my students that it is important to remember that the biomedical model is not the only model of health care and they should not be afraid to seek second, third, or even fourth opinions if a doctor does not take into account your experiences or rushes you along within the medical encounter. Too often we elevate physicians to a God-like status and trust their advice more than we trust our own guts. It is our health and we have to take control of it.

When sharing my narrative, I am also very aware of the amount of privilege that I have. I am able to afford gluten-free food, seek medical treatment when necessary, and the education and ability to research and find options that suit my needs. Even while living in a food desert, I had the means to travel to grocery stores further away and could afford the more expensive food. While the gluten-free food industry has certainly become more affordable, it is still not cheap and for people that are reliant on food assistance programs like SNAP, WIC, or food banks, it is not available at all. I could not imagine living with my chronic disease and not having the options that I have now.

Discussion

Several scholars document the narratives of black and Hispanic women who tell of experiences where medical providers equated black and brown skin with being poor, uneducated, noncompliant, and unworthy. Therefore, we have to confront the role that racism plays in health outcomes. It is my firm belief that the more we understand and engage in intercultural communication the better our overall health outcomes will be. People of color receive different medical care than others and differences seem rooted in distrust, lack of knowledge and health risk, lack of access to medical information and services, and stereotypes affecting patient-caregiver communication.

People of color are less likely to pursue medical attention because they distrust the medical establishment (Hall et al., 2015; Smedley, Stith, & Nelson, 2003). This distrust may cause people to underutilize health services and doubt the validity of medical advice (Beckman & Frankel, 1984; Johnson et al., 2004). Outside of the historical mistreatment that people of color have received within the medical settings in the US, members of racial and ethnic minority groups are also more likely to feel that their doctors fail to listen, show respect, and explain things clearly.

One way to combat these issues is by incorporating the Culture-Centered Approach introduced by Dutta (2008). The Culture-Centered Approach builds on the criticism of other traditional health models and privileges the narratives that emerge through conversations with members of marginalized communities. Central to the Culture-Centered Approach is the understanding that communicating about health involves the negotiation of shared meaning embedded in socially constructed identities, relationships, social norms, and structures.

By situating the study of health communication culturally, the Culture-Centered Approach suggests that the very articulation of problems, development of solutions, and choices of theoretical and methodological tools are embedded in culture. The cultural lens provides the script for indicating which aspects of the problem will be highlighted and which aspects will be backgrounded or omitted.

Conclusion

There are a myriad of reasons why addressing cultural diversity in health makes sense. It is imperative that all caregivers learn to check their biases and start partnering with their patients of color in order to reduce health disparities and underdiagnoses. This is where health communication scholars should come in. We know that collaborative communication between patients and caregivers lead to better outcomes. Health communication is more responsive to the needs of community members and local levels when it privileges the voices of cultural participants and actively listens to them.

We also need to incorporate more intercultural theory and praxis into our teaching and research. Racism and xenophobia can literally make people sick, therefore, as communication scholars it is our duty to share our knowledge. Engaging in intercultural communication can be a transformative experience, not only because we learn about different cultures, but also because it pushes us to learn about ourselves. More importantly, engaging in intercultural communication within health can literally be the difference between life and death.

References

Alaedini, A., & Green, P. H. (2005). Narrative review: Celiac disease: Understanding a complex autoimmune disorder, *Annals of Internal Medicine, 142*(4), 289–298.

al-Hassany, M. (1975). Coeliac disease in Iraqi children. *Journal of Tropical Pediatrics, Enviornment, & Children's Health, 21*(4), 178–179.

al-Tawaty, A. I., & Elbargathy, S. M. (1998). Coeliac disease in northeastern Libya. *Annals of Tropic Paedriatrics, 18*(1), 27–30.

Anderson, L. (2006). Analytic autoethnography. *Journal of Contemporary Ethnography, 35*, 373–395.

Beckman, H. B., & Frankel, R. M. (1984). The effect of physician behavior on the collection of data. *Annals of Internal Medicine, 101*(5), 692–696.

Blair, I., Havranek, E. P., Price, D. W., Hanratty, R., Fairclough, D. L., Farley, T., … Steiner, J. F. (2013). Assessment of biases among Latinos and African Americans among primary care providers and community members. *American Journal of Public Health, 103*(1), 92–98.

Brar, P., Lee, A. R., Lewis, S. K., Bhagat, G., & Green, P. H. R. (2006). Celiac disease in African-Americans. *Digestive Diseases and Sciences, 51*, 1012–1015.

Choung, R. S., Ditah, I. C., Nadeau, A. M., Rubio-Tapia, A., Marietta, E. V., Brantner, T. L., … Murray, J. (2015). Trends and racial/ethnic disparities in gluten-sensitive problems in the United States: Findings from the National Health and Nutrition Examination surveys from 1988–2012. *American Journal of Gastroenterlogy, 110*, 455–461.

Crenshaw, K. (1991). Mapping the margins: Intersectionality, identity politics, and violence against women of color. *Stanford Law Review, 43*(6), 1241–1299.

DeCuir, J., & Dixson, A. (2004). So when it comes out, they aren't that surprised that it is there: Using critical race theory of analysis of race and racism in education. *Educational Researcher, 33*(5), 26–31.

Delgado, R., & Stefancic, J. (2012). *Critical race theory: An introduction*. New York, NY: New York University Press.

Dutta, M. J. (2008). *Communicating health: A culture-centered approach*. Malden, MA: Polity.

Ellis, C. (2004). *The ethnographic I: A methodological novel about autoethnography*. Walnut Creek, CA: AltaMira Press.

Ellis, C., & Bochner, A. P. (2000). Autoethnography, personal narrative, reflexivity: Researcher as subject. In N. K. Denzin & Y. S. Lincoln (Eds.), *Handbook of qualitative research* (2nd ed., pp. 733–768). Thousand Oaks, CA: Sage.

Epstein, A. M., Ayanian, J. Z., Keogh, J. H., Noonan, S. J., Armistead, N., Cleary, P. D., … Conti, R. M. (2000). Racial disparites in access to renal transplantation-clinically appropriate or due to underuse or overuse?. *New England Journal of Medicine, 343*, 1537–1544.

Fasano, A., Benti, I., Geraduzzi, T., Not, T., Colletti, R. B., Drago, S., … Hill, I. D. (2003). Prevalence of celiac disease in at-risk and not-at-risk groups in the United States: A large multicenter study. *Archives of Internal Medicine, 163*, 286–292.

Fiscella, K., Franks, P., & Gold, M. R., Clancy, C. R. (2000). Inequality in quality: Addressing socioeconomic, racial, and ethnic disparities in health care. *JAMA, 283*(19), 2579–2584.

Godfrey, J. D., Brantner, T. L., Brinkikji, W., Christensen, K. N., Brogan, D. L., Van Dyke, C. T., … Murray, J. A. (2010). Morbidity and mortality among older individuals with undiagnosed celiac disease. *Journal of Gatroenterology, 139*, 763–769.

Hall, W., Chapman, M. V., Lee, J. M., Merino, Y. M., Thomas, T. W., Payne, K., … Coyne-Beasley, T. (2015). Implicit racial/ethnic bias among health care professionals and its influence on health care outcomes: A systematic review. *Americal Journal of Public Health, 105*(12), 60–76.

Hung, J. C., Phillips, A. D., & Walker-Smith, J. A. (1995). Coeliac disease in children of West Indian origin. *Archives of Disease in Childhood, 73*(2), 166–167.

Jafri, M. R., Nordstrom, C. W., Murray, J. A., Van Dyke, C. T., Dierkhising, R. A., Zinsmeister, A. R., & Melton, L. J. (2008). Long-term fracture risk in patients with celiac disease: A population-based study in Olmsted County, Minnesota. *Digestive Diseases and Sciences, 53*, 964–971.

Johnson, R. L., Roter, D., Powe, N. R., & Cooper, L. A. (2004). Patient race/ethnicity and quality of patient-physician communication during medical visits. *American Journal of Public Health, 94*(12), 2084–2090.

Kang, J. Y., Kang, A. H., Green, A., Gwee, K. A., & Ho, K. Y. (2013). Systematic review: Worldwide variation in the frequency of coeliac disease and changes over time. *Aliment Pharmacology Therapy, 38*, 226–245.

Kondrashova, A., Mustalahti, K., Kaukinen, K., Viskari, V., Volodicheva, A. M., Haapala, A. M., … Epivir Study Group. (2008). Lower economic status and inferior hygienic environment may protext against celiac disease. *Annals of Internal Medicine, 40*, 223–231.

Lionetti, P., Favilli, T., Chiaravalloti, G., Ughi, C., & Maggiore, G. (1999). Coeliac disease in Saharawi children in Algerian refugee camps. *Lancet, 353*(9159), 1189–1190.

Louka, A. S., & Solid, L. M. (2003). HLA in coeliac disease: Unraveling the complex genetics of a complex disorder. *Journal of Tissue Antigens, 61*(2), 105–117.

Mayberry, R. M., Mili, F., & Ofili, E. (2000). Racial and ethnic differences in access to medical care. *Medical Care Research Review, 57*, 108–145.

Marechal, G. (2010). Autoethnography. *Encyclopedia of Case Study Research, 2*, 43–45.

Murray, J. A., Van Dyke, C., Plevak, M. F., Dierkhising, R. A., Zinsmeister, A. R., & Melton, L. J. (2003). Trends in the identification and clinical features of celiac disease in a North American community. *Journal of Clinical Gasteroenterlogy & Hepatology, 1*(1), 19–27.

Nosek, B. A., Greenwald, A. G., & Banaji, M. R. (2007). The implicit association test at age 7: A methodological and conceptual review. In J. A. Bargh (Ed.), *Social psychology and the unconcious: The automatcity of higher mental processes* (pp. 265–292). New York, NY: Psychology Press.

Not, T., Horvath, K., Hill, I. D., Partanen, J., Hammed, A., Magazzu, G., & Fasano, A. (1998). Celiac disease risk in the USA: High prevalenace of antiendomysium antibodies in health blood donors. *Scandanavian Journal of Gatroenterology*, 33(5), 494–498.

Puri, A. S., Garg, S., Monga, R., Tyagi, P., & Sarawat, M. K. (2004). Spectrum of atypical celiac disease in North Indian children. *Journal of Indian Pediatrics*, *41*(8), 822–827.

Sabin, J. A., Nosek, B .A., Greenwald, A., & Rivara, F. P. (2009). Physicians' implicit and explicit attitudes about race by MD race, ethnicity and gender. *Journal of Health Care Poor Underserved*, *20*(3), 896–913.

Sagaro, E., & Jimenez, N. (1981). Family studies of coeliac disease in Cuba. *Archives of Disease in Children*, *56*(2), 132–133.

Shavers, V. L., Fagan, P., Jones, D., Klein, W., Boyington, J., Moten, C, & Rorie, E. (2012). The state of research on racial/ethnic discrimination in the receipt of health care. *American Journal of Public Health*, *102*(5), 953–966.

Smedley, B. D., Stith, A. Y., & Nelson, A. R. (2003). *Committee on Understanding and Eliminating Racial and Ethnic Disparities in Health Care.* Washington DC: National Academy Press.

Solorzano, D. (1997). Images and words that wound: Critical race theory, racial stereotyping, and teacher education. *Teacher Education Quarterly*, *24*, 5–19.

Solorzano, D., & Yasso, T. (2000). Toward a critical race theory of Chicana and Chicano education. In C. Tejeda, C. Martinez, & Z. Leonardo (Eds.), *Demarcating the border of Chicana(o)/Latina(o) education* (pp. 35–65). Cresskill, NJ: Hampton Press.

Sood, A., Midha, V., Sood, N., & Malhotra, V. (2003). Adult celiac disease in northern India. *Indian Journal of Gatroenterology*, *22*(4), 124–126.

Tatar, G., Elsurer, R., Simsek, H., Balaban, Y. H., Hascelik, G., Ozcebe, O. I., … Sokmensuer, C. (2004). Screening of tissue transglutaminase antibody in health blood donors for celiac diease screeing in the Turkish population. *Journal of Digestic Diseases and Sciences*, *49*(9), 1479–1484.

PART 3:

Engaging Communities: Communal Complexity, Identity Politics, and Advocacy

CHAPTER SEVEN

HIV Drugs [Are] Like My Birth Control Pill: Lived Narratives of Black and Latino MSM in an Urban American Context

BY AMBAR BASU, PATRICK J. DILLON, SHAUNAK SASTRY, AND NIVETHITHA KETHEESWARAN

The Centers for Disease Control and Prevention (CDC, 2018a) reports that, despite making up approximately 2% of the United States' population, gay and bisexual men accounted for over 70% of new HIV infections in 2014. Recent surveillance data further indicate that within the general population of men who have sex with men (MSM), African American and Latino MSM continue to be disproportionately impacted by HIV; among those newly diagnosed as HIV-positive in 2015, approximately 39% were African American and over 26% were Latino (CDC, 2018a). Despite the inordinate rates of new infections within these populations, large numbers of HIV-positive minority MSM do not receive appropriate HIV-related medical care. The CDC (2018b) notes, for example, that among HIV-positive African American MSM diagnosed "in 2013 or earlier, 71% received HIV medical care in 2014, 54% received continuous HIV care, and 52% had a suppressed viral load" (para. 5).

Given the elevated incidence of HIV among minority MSM in the United States, scholars and government agencies have called for continued intervention efforts aimed at reducing HIV risk behaviors within these populations while linking those living with HIV to appropriate long-term medical care. In recent years, there has been increasing recognition that such efforts must address the cultural, social, and contextual factors that influence HIV-related behaviors among minority MSM (Basu, Dillon, Romero-Daza, 2016; CDC, 2018b; Dillon & Basu,

2014). The CDC has funded a number of programs that are specifically designed to reach minority MSM over the past decade; for example, their *Project PrIDE* initiative currently supports 12 local health departments engaged in implementing pre-exposure prophylaxis (PrEP) and Data to Care (i.e., using data to identify HIV-diagnosed persons not in care, and to link, engage, or re-engage them in HIV medical care) demonstration projects for gay and bisexual men of color (CDC, 2018b). While such programs have been initiated, there is little doubt about the need for continued efforts to develop and implement interventions that account for cultural and contextual risk factors that are unique to African American and Latino MSM, which—as we have argued elsewhere—"depend[s] in part on scholarship that focuses on patterns of communicating about HIV/AIDS within these populations" (Basu et al., 2016, p. 1367). There is, however, limited scholarship in (health) communication and related disciplines that addresses this important issue. We respond to calls to initiate such research in this chapter by reporting the findings of a qualitative study focused on documenting the HIV-related lived experiences of African American and Latino MSM living in a large city in the southeastern United States.

This chapter is organized into four main sections. The first section summarizes current literature focusing on HIV/AIDS-related communication among African American and Latino MSM. The next section describes the methods we used to collect and analyze narratives from a sample of minority MSM. The third section presents our interpretations of study participants' stories—focusing, in particular, on how cultural and contextual factors impact communication patterns pertaining to HIV/AIDS. The final section identifies the practical and theoretical implications of this work.

Literature Review

Risk Groups

The term "men who have sex with men" (MSM) emerged in 1992 out of necessity to recognize that when men engage in sex with other men, it is not necessarily a monolithic experience that can be captured under umbrella terms for sexual orientation like "gay" or "bisexual," or by terms for gender identification such as "female," "male," "transgender," or "queer." The more inclusive terminology of "MSM" therefore includes experiences such as heterosexually-identified men who engage in sex with men, bisexual men, male sex workers with any kind of orientation, and many more identifications across cultures (Beyrer et al., 2012). While HIV remains a global issue that affects the population at large, MSM have even higher rates of HIV due to several risk factors—including high frequency and number of partners, unprotected receptive anal intercourse, and injection drug use (Beyrer et al., 2012). In their study of global experiences of black MSM with HIV, Millett et al. (2012) identify criminalization, sexual identity, and financial factors as prevalent risk factors. While risk factors may differ based on region, the high rate of HIV and AIDS among MSM is still a pervasive global phenomenon, and a well-documented trend in the context of the United States as well.

In the United States, the incidence of infection among MSM increased 8% annually since 2001 (Beyrer et al., 2012). At greater risk in this population are minority MSM, because ethnic and racial minorities have less access to antiretroviral treatment, meaning that they likely have lesser chances of viral suppression (Beyrer et al., 2012). Millett et al. (2012) writes that in the USA, the chance of HIV infection is "72 times higher in black MSM than in general populations" (p. 412). These claims are similar to those of Beyrer et al. (2012), who note that black MSM have less access to antiretroviral treatment, and add that black MSM are "less likely to adhere to combination antiretroviral therapy than are MSM of other ethnic origins" (Millett et al., 2012, p. 415). As noted earlier, CDC figures point to a disproportionate incidence of new and continuing HIV and AIDS cases among minority MSM. The CDC states that nearly 83% of estimated new HIV diagnoses were among MSM aged 13 and older. Of those men, according to the CDC, 39% were African American and 24% were Latino. Further, according to the CDC website, from 2010 to 2014, HIV diagnoses increased disproportionately among Latino MSM—13% compared to a drop of 6% among White MSM and a drop of 2% among Black MSM. German et al. (2011) trace a rising incidence of HIV among black MSM by noting that black men made up 15% of AIDS cases in bisexual and gay men in 1989, and by 2007 black MSM accounted for approximately 25% of the total AIDS cases and 35% of cases within the MSM population itself. Several authors offer recommendations as to how to address these intersecting risks.

Some advocate continuing to expand current outreach and education programs to reach minority MSM (Koblin et al., 2000); others, such as, Sifakis et al. (2010) explain that preventative intervention should be "broad-based, culturally-appropriate and must take advantage of every opportunity in educational and clinical settings to promote HIV testing and facilitate knowledge of HIV serostatus" (p. 910). Dillon and Basu (2014) conclude that experiences of stigma largely impeded HIV prevention and enhanced HIV risk—a conclusion supported by Wilson et al.'s (2015) findings in their systematic review of 70 articles. Basu et al. (2016) state that intervention efforts to decrease HIV rates within the African American and Latino MSM populations have been criticized for their lack of cultural and contextual appropriateness.

Critical Intercultural Health Communication and the Culture-Centered Approach

Recent research in health communication highlights the importance of understanding and accommodating participants' culture and localocentric narratives in any initiative aimed at improving health and living conditions of marginalized communities (see Basu et al., 2016). Critical intercultural health communication, and the culture-centered approach to health communication (CCA), present intertwined theoretical frameworks that elucidate how such meaning-making/communication occurs in intercultural spaces situated at the margins of civil society (Dutta, 2008). Critical intercultural communication deals with questioning "issues of power, context, socio-economic relations and historical/structural forces as constituting and shaping culture and intercultural communication encounters, relationships, and contexts" (Halualani & Nakayama, 2010, p. 1). Further, issues of power and voice are critical when intercultural communication occurs at the margins of society, that is, between the dominant class and a marginalized community. According to Halualani and Nakayama (2010), critical intercultural communication studies is best suited to pay close attention to how discourse, history, economic and market conditions, geopolitics, global-local institutions and ideologies regulate processes of meaning-making/communication among and between cultural groups. In the context of health, and particularly when marginalized cultures are involved, critical intercultural perspectives aid in deciphering how discourses on health at the margins are left out of the mainstream society's health discourse. For instance, Basu (2010) notes how narratives on health and HIV/AIDS in marginalized sex worker communities are hardly ever recognized in the ways mainstream health policies and campaigns instruct the sex workers to work towards prevention and surveillance.

The Culture-Centered Approach centers these voices from the margins in dominant constructions of health. In the CCA, culture is conceptualized as a space of sense-making, struggle, and transformation, and such a conceptualization offers a lens to foreground alternative rationalities and marginalized narratives on health and living. These narratives, often of resistance, reframing, and localized vocalizations, highlight cultural artifacts and rules of negotiation that likely appear strange and paradoxical to the mainstream culture. This creates a space for re-inscribing narrations of the margins often voided in the mainstream's articulation of how health is and should be performed (Basu, 2017).

This chapter reports findings of a qualitative study aimed at understanding localized cultural and contextual vocalizations that speak to how MSM of color communicate about health and HIV/AIDS. Dillon and Basu (2014) argue that localocentric vocalizations of health and HIV/AIDS, as they materialize from within minority MSM cultural contexts, are crucial to understanding and addressing HIV/AIDS risk within these populations. Responding to this call, this manuscript brings together concepts in critical intercultural health communication and the CCA to report interpretation of data collected through face-to-face, qualitative, in-depth interviews with 17 Black and Latino MSM in an urban setting in the U.S. The broad research question that guided this study is: How do minority MSM construct meanings of health and HIV/AIDS?

Methods

Study Context and Participants

Our participants included 17 self-identified African American (n = 11) and Latino (n = 6) MSM who reside in a large city located in central Florida. There are an estimated 135,986 Florida residents living with HIV/AIDS—the third highest HIV prevalence in the United States (Florida Department of Health [FDOH], 2016a). As of 2016, 82,936 of those residents are male, 76% of whom were infected through male-to-male sexual contact; 28% of these men identify as African American and 28% identify as Latino (FDOH, 2016a). In addition to the large number of residents living with HIV/AIDS, Florida has, in recent years, also reported the highest HIV incidence rate in the United States (FDOH, 2016a). In 2016, 4,955 Florida residents were newly diagnosed with HIV—including 2,989 MSM (FDOH, 2016). 1,241 of newly diagnosed MSM were Latino while 883 were African American.

Given the well-documented difficulties associated with recruiting racial/ethnic minorities, particularly MSM of color, to participate in health research (see e.g., Abernethy etal., 2005; Bempong, Ramamurthi, McCuller, Williams, & Harawa, 2014; Yancey, Ortega, & Kumanyika, 2006), we established partnerships with a paid consultant and a local HIV/AIDS prevention organization to help us identify potential participants. The consultant, a HIV/AIDS peer educator and Latino MSM, also took part in the study and helped to refine our interview guide. After recruiting an initial sample, we continued identifying participants using a snowball sampling technique (Lindlof, 1995), in which participants provided our contact information to others who met the inclusion criteria and were interested in taking part in the study. Although we did not specifically inquire about the participants' HIV status, nine of the participants disclosed that they were HIV-positive.

Data Collection and Analysis

Data collection involved face-to-face, in-depth qualitative interviews with each participant. We conducted interviews using a semi-structured format (Frankfort-Nachmias & Nachmias, 1996), meaning that we introduced general topics and guided the discussion by asking specific questions while using spontaneous probes to address issues raised by the participants. We chose this semi-structured format because it allowed us to focus the conversation on HIV/AIDS while providing the flexibility for participants to discuss the topic in ways that were consistent with their experiences (see Lindlof & Taylor, 2011).

Study participation was voluntary and participants provided written consent prior to being interviewed. Participants were also compensated $30 for their time. The interviews ranged from 27 minutes to an hour and 15 minutes, with an average time of approximately 43 minutes. We recorded the interviews using a digital recording device and transcribed each interview verbatim. The transcripts totaled just over 187 pages of single-spaced text.

Our data analysis procedures were informed by constructivist grounded theory (Charmaz, 2000; Dutta, 2012). We analyzed the data using a process informed by Morse's (1994) four-stage qualitative analysis procedures: comprehending, synthesizing, theorizing, and recontextualizing. During the comprehending stage, the first two authors transcribed interviews as they were completed and met biweekly to discuss preliminary themes. The first author then began the synthesizing process by isolating discrete concepts within the preliminary themes that could be labeled and sorted. Through an intensive reading of the individual codings, the first author then clumped and reorganized the codings together until a tree of large-order and small-order themes emerged from the data. The conceptual categories were then checked and validated by the second and third authors. We then engaged in a process of theorizing. Morse (1994) describes theorizing as "he constant development and manipulation of malleable theoretical schemes until the 'best' theoretical scheme is developed" (p. 32). The final step of our analysis was to recontextualize the findings by identifying ways in which our theoretical explanations could prove useful within and beyond the study context.

Findings

In this section, we explain how a group of minority MSM in a southeastern city in the US link their conceptualization of health and HIV/AIDS with the role of the church, and with available HIV/AIDS cocktail drugs.

The Church and the Pastor: Necessary, Not Sufficient

Religious institutions have often been considered viable spaces for disseminating information related to health, particularly for communities that are difficult to reach via more conventional message channels or when the information is considered sensitive (see Abrams, 2000). A few of our research participants seemed to agree that the church can play a major role in addressing sensitive issues such as HIV/AIDS in the MSM community. Asked if he thought the church or other faith-based organization could try to do something to spread awareness about HIV or provide resources for health or HIV, one participant explained:

> … a situation like that would really be positive. I could really relate to that I could really go for that. I can really feel better knowing that okay this church or organization, this religious organization is getting together actually coming to reality on its not just a gay man's thing. It's something that is not our fault, you know? Um I don't know if a church can actually verify that this is not a gay man's fault. That this is not a disease developed to punish by God all homosexuals. If the church and these organizations can actually do these things then I can actually look like I would actually feel positive. I would actually know for a fact that okay hey things are gonna get better. So that would be a good idea.

Another participant agreed that religion was a "very big thing" in his (Latino) culture and that religion and religious leaders do "influence the way people think about behaviors." Another participant noted:

> [G]ay people are, are willing to go out there to do what they have to do to protect themselves. Knowledge is the key, if, yeah, I would go. If you know, exactly what it is then you know how to work around it and what to do, you would know how to handle it more better than if you were just ignorant and don't know nothing.

Most of our participants, however, regarded the church as a not-so-viable option in addressing HIV/AIDS issues in the minority gay community. One impediment, articulated most frequently, was the fact that most churches discriminate against homosexuals. A participant explained:

> And it's because someone, could have been a stoolpigeon, said that that's God's condemnation. So, you are forced to go to big momma's church of God and Christ every day or her Baptist church or her whatever or her Catholic church and the pastor gets up with all certainty and says, 'Fags are a bad thing.'

In fact, for another participant the church was a space of silence. "So, the church becomes this place where they don't … it's this whole mindset that if I don't talk about it then ...", he noted. A participant added that though there is extensive talk outside the churches that these places should be "accepting" of all people, it is only so, "outside." "In the church," he said, "they would not accept that [the church working with gay men] because it goes against what the Bible holds and what they believe in so dearly. No, they would not accept that at all." Another participant did not doubt that "the church cannot help" when it comes to acting as a nodal point of sharing information and helping to negotiate HIV/AIDS in the minority MSM community. "People don't talk too much about that, I [have been] going a couple time[s] to church and never hear people talking about HIV," another participant said.

There are other participants who pointed out that the messages circulating in the churches they knew about were not conducive to any type of dialogue or learning about how to address HIV/AIDS issues in the minority MSM community. One such participant explained:

> The church say this is the disease that is a punishment by God. You know so it messes with you. Not only physically but mentally. It makes it seem so some people go on this religious thing about punishment from God because you're gay. And you're not living right with the Lord and that's why you contracted this disease.

Another participant added:

> Once upon a time it was all about gay men disease cause we was doing cause they was gay, but know that other people have contracted it, heterosexual people are contracting it they blame and the reality is there is still people still blaming the gay man for this disease. It's a punishment by God to give to all gay men. And innocent women and innocent women and straight men got caught up in the rapture, you know what I'm saying. It's unfair to be labeled like that.

In other words, the church is considered in a not-so-favorable light by several participants, both Latino and African-American. While there is some agreement that the church can indeed serve as a site for spread of HIV/AIDS-related messages, generally the church is constituted by participants as the center of a discourse that stigmatizes them for their sexual identity. Hence they view the church as incapable of acting as a positive pivot in the community when it comes to creating an inclusive space for sharing information and initiating dialogue on risky sexual practices, health, HIV/AIDS and related issues.

The leaders of the churches also bear the brunt of the criticism from several of our study participants. A participant said this about a pastor:

> One of the biggest mega churches in the country, one of the pastors (inaudible) that he was going to be the next Billy Graham. You know, but now he is preaching diversity

> in his church. What did it take? Unfortunately, it was his son getting caught in a park in Atlanta exposing himself to an undercover officer. And as a father he must think, "why did my child go to such extremes?" Oh, because I preached that gay people are going to hell.

The diffusion of innovations model has often been centralized in health communication efforts when reaching out to hard-to-reach populations (Haider & Kreps, 2004). The model, used extensively across the globe, seeks to take health promotion messages to members of a community through its opinion leaders and decision-makers. The church and its leaders present a likely network for this model to play out in the case of minority MSM and HIV/AIDS. But, our minority research participants did not support this view. A participant explained that his attempts to get proposals to address HIV/AIDS issues in the minority MSM community passed in church councils repeatedly came to a naught. He said:

> Meanwhile while I am sitting on all these councils, it was something that we went through the churches to the pastors, to the deacons and we asked them to shoot it through their board and we were shot down unanimously. That's it; this is not going to be discussed in our church in our community.

Another participant reiterated the belief that churches will fail to act as spaces of HIV/AIDS information dissemination as long as the leadership of these institutions continue to stigmatize MSM. "Of course, but they don't come here. They don't come here," he noted. "I could have the biggest church in town by having all the gay folks in town and we'd just have a gay old time for Jesus. It does not happen because the stigma is that you can't be gay in churches," he added. Minority MSM come to churches, he noted, but they hide in the churches because the church does not subscribe to being a man who has sex with a man. One participant contended that his "gayness" stood in the way of him taking up leadership roles in his church. He noted, "Well I really can't um relate on that right now about the church because of the simple fact is that once upon a time when I was interested in taking a religious role I had tried to have come kind of affiliation with the church but the main thing the church was saying was that my gayness … that I couldn't come to church." Our research participants, both Latino and African-American, spoke about their own churches being discriminatory to them. Hence, for Latino MSM, it appears that the churches that served their respective Latino communities, did not subscribe to their sexuality. The same appears to be the case for our African-American participants. We could possibly argue that in our conversations with the participants, racial identity was sort of a constant and did not moderate the experience of these men with their respective churches as much as their sexuality did. We could also infer here that health campaigns that use religious institutions and leaders to target marginalized populations, might need to be recalibrated when it comes to communicating with minority MSM and their HIV risk relevance. In our discussions with our research participants, we were led to believe that the church and its leaders offer a space that is a necessary but not a sufficient condition for promotion efforts to address HIV/AIDS issues among minority MSM. A similar line of reasoning can be applied to using messages that primarily call for screening and clinical follow up in campaigns addressing HIV/AIDS among minority MSM.

False Truth: HIV Drugs Are Like Birth Control

Messages directed toward getting at-risk HIV populations to adopt positive health behavior—such as prevention through safe sex, screening, accessing medical services and maintaining medication—has been and continues to be a mainstay of HIV/AIDS campaigns globally. In the United States, a scrutiny of ongoing campaigns initiated by or supported by the CDC (see https://www.cdc.gov/hiv/group/msm/index.html) shows that an overwhelming number of them advocate talking to relational partners and or screening for HIV tests. Our participant narratives however lead us to ask: How well do messages aimed at screening, testing, medicating for HIV/AIDS work with minority MSM?

One of our participants said his siblings were not surprised that he is HIV-positive. He noted: "My brother and sister he has come to accept it. Um he accepts it but then when I finally told them that I was HIV-positive they both said, 'Well it's no surprise. With you being gay, we knew automatically you were gonna get it.'" He went on to add that his siblings think HIV is a "gay man's disease," and they "said they knew that eventually I would get it." Another research participant explained how his family told him to get his "AIDS-carrying ass away from them." And this was before he was "HIV-positive." He was barred from visiting his grandson and was called an "AIDS infected faggot" even before the HIV diagnosis. Living with HIV, it appears, is talked about as being a corollary to being gay. A participant, clarified:

> It made me feel like that like it's so common or like how can I say it? Like it's expected or something. You are gonna have you gonna eventually die from AIDS. That's the most like common thing said like being gay in the community like where I was raised or whatever. You gonna die from AIDS.

Living with HIV or AIDS because one is a minority MSM appears to be one discursive thread in the participant narratives. Another is the notion that living with HIV or AIDS is no more a death warrant. One participant explained:

> I mean it is scary, it's always gonna be scary, but as far as like when back in the days when you used to get and there was just nothing you could do about it. Now there's treatments for it. You know and now they've found people who live years with HIV and you know they were okay.

Another participant pointed to how the direct-to-consumer HIV/AIDS drug advertisements portray "healthy and vibrant" individuals. He asked: "Have you seen the recent medication ads? Have you seen any recent ads about HIV? Everybody's so health and vibrant, so beautiful." Such images normalize living with HIV and AIDS, leading to people living with the disease putting its negative side effects on the backburner. Yet another participant noted that he "feels really well lately" and that he is able to "just muddle through and keep it moving." A different participant added to this line of thinking. He said: "I just celebrated 17 years of being positive. So, um you know for me it's just something that I live with. Something that I deal with. You know it used to be my life for a long time and now it's just kinda like on thc backburner."

This perceived ease of living with HIV or AIDS, we argue, also leads to situations of easier disclosure about one's HIV/AIDS status, to families, and relational partners. For instance, a research participant in our study spoke about the practiced ritual in his household, of getting tested for HIV/AIDS and sharing the results with family. He explained:

> In my family … My mother, she drilled um the condoms before I even know what it was. She drilled it into our head, and once she found I was sexually active, she was taking me to go get tested. Even when I get tested, I make sure she gets the results, she knows I'm okay. And it is something we do talk about, you know.

Disclosing one's HIV/AIDS status is no more surprising in the minority MSM community, said one participant. "When I'm dating somebody or if I'm just meeting somebody right if I wanted to disclose, if I want to disclose to them before I have sex with them that I'm HIV-positive, it's not a surprise to a lot of people. It's like, 'Yeah I do too,'" he explained. Another research participant, added that "most people disclose their status" once he discloses his. He clarified:

> It's kind of hard for me to disclose my status, but once I do, I feel like a real big relief or whatever. It's just a lot of people I have disclosed my status to a lot of people that have disclosed theirs as well to me. So that's why I say it's like popular. It's not a surprise to people anymore when they hear it coming out of another gay man's mouth.

This apparent ease of living with HIV or AIDS, however, is a cause for concern, according to several of our research participants. One participant made this observation:

> [R]ealistically, folks think that they can take some pills and AIDS goes away. It doesn't go away! You just ... you manage it. But for some people their way of managing it is to pretend it does not exist. You know some people call their HIV and AIDS medicine their birth control.

Calling this phenomenon/situation a "false lull," a participant stated: "Yeah. And they don't have to deal with the numbers and the sicknesses and the running back and forth to the bathroom 20 times a day and they don't have deal with it and they don't know." A research participant narrated the story of his partner and his experience of living with regular HIV medications:

> And they don't know what it is like. When my partner had it, he had diarrhea every day of his life. But they think, they got new meds. And they don't know the details, and even when you are on medicine, baby you gotta get to work. And so he had to live with that. And he had to conquer that. And he had a rare strand. You know one in 1000 people get this rare strand because it's the HIV but worse. We're talking about that he had to go to Germany to find a topical that would help him deal with the sores.

These are HIV/AIDS narratives that go missing from the prevailing discourse on dealing with the disease through maintenance medications. Hence, communication from nodal agencies, such as the CDC, that call for regular clinical visits following screening and monitoring of intake of antiretroviral therapy medicines, might not be the solution to addressing HIV/AIDS issues among minority MSM. The research participant quoted above continued to explain:

> So people don't hear those stories. They don't realize that it's not just, well I just have to take some meds and think that it will just collaborate with their systems. They don't know that you can be screwed up until the doctors get it right.

Offering a similar argument, another research participant spoke about how difficult it was for his friend, "who transitioned all the way to AIDS," to live a "normal" life. There were some days, he noted, "where weeks at a time he's stuck in the house because he can't do anything." There is also the associated anxiety of not knowing what physical condition was a result of or was complicating the HIV infection, one research participant, noted, aboutliving with HIV. He added:

> Because of the fact that um so many people or even myself, to a certain extent, um although I try to not to attribute every little thing to the HIV, uh in the back of my mind I can't help but to wonder is this because I'm HIV-positive? Or will this affect my being HIV-positive?

A participant pointed out that the narratives presented by celebrities living with HIV/AIDS, such as Magic Johnson, are only "a part of the story." Magic

Johnson has been living with HIV since 1992 and our participant noted that even if Magic Johnson's wife proclaims that he is healthy and cured, that is not the case. "So people believe that they just need to go to his church. And his pastor can give holy oil to them so that they could be healed. He wasn't healed. It was just undetectable," the participant added.

A section of our research participants spoke about the fact this perception of "easily living with the condition" is more prevalent among younger minority MSM. More campaigns should target this population subgroup, they noted. One participant had this to say:

> A lot of people have become a little more relaxed and don't care and are not so crazy about getting information or protecting themselves. You find that a lot of these new kids who are just coming out of the closet and are just you know coming to terms with their own sexuality are so busy thinking that HIV/AIDS is a disease of the 90s. They're thinking that HIV and AIDS is something that happened in my father's time, not in my day.

Similar sentiments were expressed by another research participant. He felt that the "younger generation is not being well-educated about HIV and AIDS by choice because they find it too boring a disease to get interested in." Adding that this "younger generation" did not even bother to get screened, this participant pointed to providing incentives, such as money, to encourage regular screening.

Another participant agreed. He said that "right now the only thing that I think will attract the young crowd is something that by giving them something tangible that they can walk away with. Okay?" But then, he added, the minute they hear the name HIV and AIDS even related to the event "they're not gonna come."

In such a scenario, messages that aim to address HIV and AIDS issues among minority MSM youth should aim to disseminate "real stories," one research participant said. "Well the message should be that it's real. It's out there, and you can get it. It can happen to anyone. And that you should really protect yourself," he explained. Peer education is critical in this context, he added. Another participant stated:

> A young gay man, he should hear that. He should really hear that … I'm saying like another someone who is actually who actually has it isn't afraid to disclose that information and that is young reaching out to another young person who does not have it would be the best way to their attention. Peer education … That would … that would really open their eyes. Like, 'Wow, he's 21 too and he has it. He caught it at 18.'

In the following section of our paper, we tie the participant narratives we presented here to the theoretical assumption of our work and to address our research question. We also try to explain what these narratives mean for scholars and practitioners trying to address HIV/AIDS issues among Latino and African American MSM.

Discussion and Conclusion

Sontag (1989) writes that the modern HIV/AIDS discourse confers an identity to a risk group by creating a community and an experience that isolates and exposes the group to harassment and persecution. This creates an us-versus-them situation, particularly with poor and minority people living with HIV/AIDS being discoursed as the infected, vis-a-vis a general population that is framed as not-infected. Sontag contends that this discourse is created and sustained by mainstream biomedical 'experts', and that this discourse privileges certain types of meanings, preventive behaviors, and lived experiences associated with living with HIV/AIDS. In other words, the biomedical discourse on HIV/AIDS does not account for those narratives that emerge from the lived experiences of cultures at the margins living with HIV/AIDS.

Calling to attention this void, and drawing from the CCA's imperative to centralize localized vocalizations of minority MSM in an intercultural health communication context, our project points to novel and significant information about the HIV/AIDS-related experiences of African American and Latino MSM. Participants' narratives suggest that such experiences exist within a complex web of contextual, cultural, and structural factors, and identify several ways in which such factors are linked to difficulties in managing (the threat of) HIV/AIDS.

For instance, participants present a complex relationship with the church and its leaders. Long considered a viable medium and platform to connect to its members on health issues, particularly those issues that are sensitive and hard to discuss openly (Lumpkins, Greiner, Daley, Mabachi, & Neuhaus, 2011), the church and its leaders are a strict no-no for several of our participants who note the discrimination and shame they face from the church for being gay and susceptible to HIV/AIDS as a result of their sexual practices. Sontag (1989) writes that the HIV epidemic has been historically framed as one that results from deviance—moral laxity and socially/sexually non-permissive behavior The church appears to toe this discursive line.

In their meta-synthesis of journal articles dealing with minority MSM and HIV/AIDS, Dillon and Basu (2014) point to studies that confirm the importance of the church in the lives of minority MSM, but that the church also adds to the stigma associated with men having sex with men. Lumpkins et al. (2011) explain that African American clergy see themselves as health promoters and believe that their using the pulpit to endorse health information and health behaviors will indeed influence health behavior among underserved and minority communities. However, our participants are clear in their articulation that the church's discursive practices on being gay and on HIV/AIDS needs to be rethought to have any positive impact on the lives of minority MSM. This dual or divided relationship with the church and its leaders is similar to what Basu (2011) terms subaltern autonomous rationality, an alternative rationality on health and living vocalized in subaltern/marginalized classes that exists with, and often, in opposition to, the dominant discourse on health. For scholars and practitioners working to address HIV/AIDS among minority MSM, this could mean re-situating the 'target' of their campaigns—from minority MSM to the church and its leaders. A discursively-reorganized church will not only effectively reach minority MSM, it might also foster a revised rhetoric on being gay and HIV/AIDS in black and Latino communities.

In the context of our project, this marginalized autonomous/alternative rationality perhaps ought to accommodate what is not quite evident in the participants' narratives as well. This might include an interrogation of how identity positions beyond sexuality, such as race and class, affect relationships between minority MSM and the church and its leaders. It appears our research participants allude to the fact that the churches they visit provide services mostly to members of their respective communities. Hence, it is not clear how their racialized subject positions interject their relationships with these churches, given that the community being serviced in likely racially homogenous. However, it is likely that these racialized subject locations intersect with their class subjectivities to create divergent lived experiences. Cesaire (1972) talks about the insidious interlinkages of class and gender in the sustenance of racial oppressions. In several instances, our research participants spoke about being drained and emaciated from living with HIV/AIDS, which then could position their already "deviant" bodies as incapable of being productive members of prevailing socioeconomic systems. This might, in turn, mean the existence of multiple axes of marginalization for them—in terms of racial and class (in terms of living with HIV/AIDS) subjectivities. How minority MSM perceive and story health, illness, and HIV/AIDS amid these axes of marginalization could be one pertinent extension of this project. Participant narratives in this project also highlight an alternative vocalization on managing HIV/AIDS. Several research participants challenge the current biomedical storyline that HIV/AIDS leads to emaciation and ultimately, to death (see Sontag, 1989). The cocktail of antiretroviral therapy (ART) drugs changes the discursive canvas on HIV/AIDS to one from compulsory decay and mortality to one of sustainable management of health free of decay and quick death. This theorization is crucial because it means that time-tested fear-based campaign strategies that focus on the need to save oneself from physical and mental withering and death associated with HIV/AIDS might not work anymore. Instead, as our participants note, health promoters might want to focus future campaign efforts on the myths associated with easy management of HIV/AIDS using ART. Living with ART (and HIV/AIDS) is not as comfortable as it is often made out to be, according to several research participants. Campaign messages, chiefly those directed at the "younger generation" that is more at risk, must address perceptions such as living with HIV/AIDS medication is like popping one's blood pressure pills or "birth control."

The availability and promotion of HIV pre-exposure prophylaxis (PrEP), particularly targeted to MSM, complicates this discursive shift from "fearing" HIV/AIDS to "managing" and, possibly, not contracting HIV/AIDS even with hitherto accepted unsafe health practices, such as unsafe sex, substance abuse, sharing needles, etc. Spieldenner (2016) explains that such a discursive shift might necessitate a move away from promoting individual behavior change such as abstinence-only initiatives, condom use, HIV testing, condom negotiation, needle exchange, HIV disclosure, and sexual and drug-using risk reduction. In such a shifting biomedical and cultural scenario, localized vocalizations that emerge from minority MSM communities become critical to addressing the inequitable burden of HIV/AIDS in these minority communities.

References

Abernethy, A. D., Magat, M. M., Houston, T. R., Arnold, H. L., Bjorck, J. P., & Gorsuch, R. L. (2005). Recruiting African American men for cancer screening studies: applying a culturally based model. *Health Education & Behavior*, *32*(4), 441–451. doi: 10.1177/1090198104272253

Abrams, M. (2000). "Jesus will fix it after awhile": Meanings and health. *Social Science and Medicine*, *50*(1), 89–105.

Basu, A. (2010). Communicating health as an impossibility: Sex work, HIV/AIDS, and the dance of hope and hopelessness. *Southern Communication Journal*, *75*(4), 413–432. doi: 10.1080/1041794x.2010.504452

Basu, A. (2011). HIV/AIDS and subaltern autonomous rationality: A call to re-center health communication in marginalized sex worker spaces. *Communication Monographs*, *78*(3), 391–408. doi: 10.1080/03637751.2011.589457

Basu, A. (2017). Reba and her insurgent prose: Sex work, HIV/AIDS and subaltern narratives. *Qualitative Health Research*, *27*(10),1507–1517. doi: 10.1177/1049732316675589

Basu, A., Dillon, P. J., & Romero-Daza, N. (2016). Understanding culture and its influence on HIV/AIDS-related communication among minority men who have sex with men. *Health Communication*, *31*(11), 1367–1374. doi: 10.1080/10410236.2015.1072884

Bempong, G. A., Ramamurthi, H. C., McCuller, J., Williams, J. K., & Harawa, N. T. (2014).Recruiting black men who have sex with men and women (BMSMW) in an urban setting for HIV prevention research. *Journal of AIDS & Clinical Research*, *6*(1), 408. doi: 10.4172/2155-6113.1000408

Beyrer, C., Baral, S. D., van Griensven, F., Goodreau, S. M., Chariyalertsak, S., Wirtz, A. L., & Brookmeyer, R. (2012). Global epidemiology of HIV infection in men who have sex with men. *The Lancet*, *380*, 367–377. http://dx.doi.org/10.1016/S0140-6736(12)60821-6

CDC. (2018a). HIV among gay and bisexual men. Retrieved from https://www.cdc.gov/hiv/group/msm/index.html

CDC. (2018b). HIV care outcomes among blacks with diagnosed HIV—United States, 2014. Retrieved from https://www.cdc.gov/mmwr/volumes/66/wr/mm6604a2.htm

Cesaire, A. (1972). *Discourses on colonialism*. NY: Monthly Review Press

Charmaz, K. (2000). Grounded theory: Objectivist and constructivist methods. In N. K. Denzin & Y. S. Lincoln (Eds.), *Handbook of qualitative research* (pp. 509–536). Thousand Oaks, CA: Sage.

Dillon, P. J., & Basu, A. (2014). HIV/AIDS and minority men who have sex with men: A meta-ethnographic synthesis of qualitative research. *Health Communication*, *29*(2), 182–192. doi: 10.1080/10410236.2012.732911

Dutta, M. (2008). *Communicating health: A culture-centered approach*. Polity, Cambridge: UK.

Dutta, M. J. (2012). Hunger as health: Culture-centered interrogations of alternative rationalities of health. *Communication Monographs*, *79*(3), 366–384. doi: 10.1080/03637751.2012.697632

Florida Department of Health. (2016a). Epidemiology of persons living with HIV disease (PLWHAs) in Florida, 2014. Retrieved from http://www.floridahealth.gov/diseases-and-conditions/aids/surveillance/_documents/fact-sheet/Mens_Factsheet.pdf

Florida Department of Health. (2016b). Epidemiology of HIV among men who have sex with men (MSM) in Florida, reported through 2016. Retrieved from http://www.floridahealth.gov/diseases-and-conditions/aids/surveillance/epi-slide-sets.html

Frankfort-Nachmias, C., & Nachmias, D. (1996). *Research methods in the social sciences* (5th ed.). New York: St. Martin's Press.

German, D., Sifakis, F., Maulsby, C., Towe, V. L., Flynn, C. P., Latkin, C. A., … Holtgrave, D. R. (2011). Persistently high prevalence and unrecognized HIV infection among men who have sex with men in Baltimore: The BESURE study. *JAIDS Journal of Acquired Immune Deficiency Syndromes*, *57*, 77–87. http://dx.doi.org/10.1097/QAI.0b013e318211b41e

Haider, M., & Kreps, G. L. (2004). Forty years of diffusion of innovations: Utility and value in public health. *Journal of Health Communication*, *9*(Sup1), 3–11. doi: 10.1080/10810730490271430

Halualani, R. T., & Nakayama, T. K. (2010). Critical intercultural communications: At a crossroads. In R. T. Halualani & T. K. Nakayama (Eds.), *The handbook of critical intercultural communication* (p. 1). United Kingdom: Wiley.

Koblin, B. A., Torian, L. V., Guilin, V., Ren, L., MacKellar, D. A., & Valleroy, L. A. (2000). High prevalence of HIV infection among young men who have sex with men in New York City. *AIDS*, 1793–1800.

Lindlof, T. (1995). *Qualitative communication research methods.* Thousand Oaks, CA: Sage.

Lindlof, T. R., & Taylor, B. C. (2011). *Qualitative communication research methods* (3rd ed.). Thousand Oaks, CA: Sage.

Lumpkins, C. Y., Greiner, K. A., Daley, C., Mabachi, N. M., & Neuhaus, K. (2011). Promoting healthy behavior from the pulpit: Clergy share their perspectives on effective health communication in the African American church. Journal of *Religion and Health*, *52*, 1093–1107.

Millett, G. A., Jeffries, W. L., IV, Peterson, J. L.,Malebranche, D. J., Lane, T., Flores, S. A., … Heilig, C. M. (2012). Common roots: A contextual review of HIV epidemics in Black men who have sex with men across the African diaspora. *The Lancet*, *380*, 411–423. http://dx.doi.org/10.1016/S0140-6736(12)60722-3

Morse, J. M. (1994). "Emerging from the data": The cognitive processes of analysis in qualitative inquiry. In J. M. Morse (Ed.), *Critical issues in qualitative research methods* (pp. 23–43). Thousand Oaks, CA: Sage.

Sifakis, F., Hylton, J. B., Flynn, C., Solomon, L., MacKellar, D. A., Valleroy, L. A., & Celentano, D. D. (2010). Prevalence of HIV infection and prior HIV testing among young men who have sex with men. The Baltimore Young Men's Survey. *AIDS and Behavior*, *14*, 904–912. http://dx.doi.org/10.1007/s10461-007-9317-5

Sontag, S. (1989). *AIDS and its metaphors.* New York: Doubleday

Spieldenner, A. (2016). PrEP whores and HIV prevention: The queer communication of HIV Pre-Exposure Prophylaxis (PrEP). *Journal of Homosexuality*, *63*(12), 1685–1697, doi: 10.1080/00918369.2016.1158012

Wilson, P. A., Valera, P., Martos, A. J., Wittlin, N. M., Muñoz-Laboy, M. A., & Parker, R. G. (2015). Contributions of qualitative research in informing HIV/AIDS interventions targeting black MSM in the United States. *The Journal of Sex Research*, *53*(6), 642–654. doi: 10.1080/00224499.2015.1016139

Yancey, A. K., Ortega, A. N., & Kumanyika, S. K. (2006). Effective recruitment and retention of minority research participants. *Annual Review of Public Health*, *27*, 1–28. doi: 10.1146/annurev.publhealth.27.021405.102113

CHAPTER EIGHT

Social Media as a Transformative Force in Intercultural Health Communications: A Case Study of the BADASS Army

BY SPRING COOPER AND P. CHRISTOPHER PALMEDO

Social media, originally intended to improve communication between existing networks of friends (Van Dijck, 2013), is now transforming intercultural health communications in ways unanticipated a decade ago. Theoretical foundations of intercultural communications are being re-defined as social media dramatically and swiftly reshape how people self-identify, communicate, and associate within and among communities no longer bounded by political borders or geographic distance. With this change comes a theoretical juncture in intercultural health communications, enabling scholars in various social science fields to identify new possibilities for scholarly engagement (Hall, 1996). Theoretical frameworks, re-shaped through social media, are now being examined from different perspectives. Face-negotiation theory (Ting-Toomey, 1988a), for example, frames the "face" of self-image around conceptualizations of such emotions as shame, honor, social recognition and influence, and considers these emotions within high- and low-context societies. Social media is providing this area of scholarship with countless new topics of inquiry. Shaming and harassment—both of which have profound effects on health—are occurring in new ways and with different levels of intensity since the widespread adaptation of social media among adolescents and young adults (Van Royen, Poels, Vandebosch, & Adam, 2017). Social media enables important applicability to communication accommodation theory (Giles, Coupland, & Coupland, 1991), which looks at how identity navigates through communication partners, and now faces major theoretical modifications through the use of social media. This theoretical framework, which is concerned with how intergroup and interpersonal factors form boundaries between self and others and between different groups, can easily be linked to Facebook and WhatsApp groups, Instagram pages and Snapchat relationships. As the world adapts to new forms of relationships through social media, intercultural communications theories can facilitate insights to the problems and opportunities social media affords individuals, families, and communities.

Virtual Cultural Identities

During the hyper globalization that occurred at the turn of this century, people and societies' group identification ebbed and flowed through place-based communities, ethnicities and nation-states. Through industrialization and the commodification of culture (Harvey, 2002; Jones, 2009), the affinity groups identified by de Toqueville (1835) as flourishing in the United States in the early 19th century grew into numerous associations organized around like-minded interests. Until the emergence of social media, members in these affinity groups, including advocacy groups, fan groups and archivists, mostly formed relationships through one-way transmittals of communication via print media, email and face-to-face correspondence. The rise of social media radically changed that. In part because of their intended structure as a community builder (Van Dijk, 2013) and its technological structure as accessible to people all over the world, social media made it much easier for people to re-form their own cultural identities away from their own nuclear family, proximate friend groups and placed-based community and toward virtual communities unbounded by place or time zone. The mere fact that many of these communities are continuously and perpetually functioning around the clock imbues these communities with an intensity not seen before the use of social media (Xu, Bhargava, Nowak, & Zhu, 2012).

Today social media allows fan groups and other affinity-based associations to archive material as in the past, but also to create it as well. Social media allows nonprofessional archivists and activists to democratize cultural memory, and to mobilize political action (De Kosnik, 2016). In the realm of health communications, social media has facilitated new and often powerful communities formed around various categories of health information and advocacy. One example is among cancer patients and survivors, where now receive and share information in unprecedented ways. Social media, by extension, has facilitated new communities to be formed around these experiences, providing patients and advocates with information related to clinical outcomes, public health and political advocacy. Varieties of new cultural nuances are being found among and between groups, such as the differences found between communities organically formed and those intentionally created for a specific goal or intervention (Falisi et al., 2017).

Through emerging technical capabilities such as artificial intelligence, machine learning and data mining, and the nature of social media as a public source of detailed information, new public health capabilities are now being seen. Examples of this, which include epidemiological and surveillance capabilities present new implications for intercultural communication. Demographic extraction techniques and computational linguistics reveal that that new linguistic patterns are being created through these social media channels formed around health communications (and mediated by gender, race, income, and ethnicity, for example) (Beretta, Maccagnola, Cribbin, & Messina, 2015; Burger, Henderson, Kim, & Zarrella, 2011; Xu et al., 2016).

In terms of health impact, social media holds both promise and reason for concern. Evidence has shown that social media use by online communities can lead to improved cancer outcomes (Attai et al., 2015). At the same time, misinformation proliferated through online communities has been found to result in adverse health outcomes (Fernández-Luque, & Bau, 2015). One of the most powerful effects of the cultural forces of social media on public health can be found in vaccine hesitancy (Dubé, Vivion, & MacDonald, 2015; Goldstein, MacDonald, & Guirguis, 2015; Yaqub, Castle-Clarke, Sevdalis, & Chataway, 2014). Today, very powerful tribes (Godin, 2008) are being formed to spread information about concerns with childhood immunization or to disrupt the distribution of human papillomavirus (HPV) vaccination. One example of this can be found in Japan, considered a "high context culture," per Ting-Toomey (1988). In that country, social media enabled new communities to form internationally around hesitancy toward the HPV vaccine. Fueled by existing virtual communities formed in the United States and around the world, and compounded by unverified media reports of vaccine side effects, the Japanese Ministry of Health withdrew its recommendation for HPV vaccination in 2013, leading to the withdrawal of HPV vaccines from the Japanese health insurance program. As a result, HPV vaccine rates fell from around 70% to less than 1% of the population (Sipp, Frazer, & Rasko, 2018).

Social media allows conversations that once were held occasionally en masse and otherwise among small groups, to now be held continuously and among entire affinity communities. This allows people to be immersed in their communities, drawing them in more intensely and actively, and shielding them from countervailing opinions. Along with cancer treatment and vaccine hesitancy, social media is also transforming how newly formed communities re-shape important health issues such as provider utilization and referrals, alternative treatments and therapies, nutrition patterns and exercise behaviors. Social media has provided each of these of these domains with opportunities to improve health (through new evidence-based information) and also to devolve advances in health (through false information).

Social Media and Intercultural Health

Routes of Impact

The defined lines of geographic communities have become less important in the world of social media. The new communities that arise through social media may have some original basis in a geographic location, but the community-created shared values are what drive the social media presence and outreach. These communities are formed around the sharing of experiences and can be grown through hashtags and searches, allowing new people to find the groups. In some cases these communities have blossomed in physical locations where the opinions or ideas expressed within the online community would not have previously been tolerated in the "in real life" location.

Ziebland and Wyke (2012) have identified seven domains in which health may be impacted by social media, either positively or negatively: (1) finding information, (2) feeling supported, (3) maintaining relationships with others, (4) experiencing health services, (5) learning to relate the story, (6) visualizing disease, and (7) affecting behavior. While social media's health effects on all of these domains is important we will further explore the domain of relationships here, with the intention of understanding the community nature of these online groups and movements.

When we think about community as a health predictor or association, we should examine the academic construct "social capital," which is made up of social networks, norms of reciprocity or social support, and social trust (Ferlander, 2007; Putnam, 1993). Different forms of social capital may affect health in different ways. The social network is the basis for social capital, with participation in the network being a central behavior, while the norms and trust characterize it. The more durable networks contain more actual or potential resources within them (Bourdieu, 1985).

The norms of reciprocity or social support are composed of emotional, instrumental, informational support, and companionship (Cohen & Wills, 1985). The different types of support all contribute to the strength of social capital for each individual within a community. Another characteristic that defines someone's social capital is the type and strength of their ties to other individuals. The types of ties include bonding, bridging, and linking, any of which can be strong or weak in strength: bonding ties are ties with people of similar social characteristics; bridging ties are ties with people of differing social characteristics, and linking ties are ties with colleagues in differing levels of hierarchies. All of the types and strengths of ties have different purposes within one's social capital (Ferlander, 2007; Putnam, 1993).

Online communities have shown several positive networking impacts. For example, in a review of the research concerning Generation Y's use of social media, it was concluded that social media provides the function of formation and maintenance of social capital (Bolton et al., 2013). Online identities can nurture positive relationships and increase psychosocial well-being. However, there is also evidence to show that increased online involvement may serve to isolate individuals from the support they may be able to find in their geographical location (Ziebland & Wyke, 2012).

Both intentional online interventions and organic grassroots campaigns have the capacity to shift social capital and affect intercultural health. In a systematic review of systematic reviews of social media uses in public health, the following benefits were identified: increased community support, greater social connectedness, health management, health promotion, Internet support groups, knowledge acquisition, learning opportunities, and social interaction (Giustini, Ali, Fraser, & Kamel Boulos, 2018). Conditions that social media is used to manage include: depression, diabetes, mental health, sexual health, HIV and AIDS prevention, medication adherence, immunization and vaccination, obesity and weight management, cancer, cardiovascular disease, influenza, travel medicine, traumatic brain injury, infectious diseases, and non-communicable diseases (Giustini et al., 2018).

Here, we will examine one organically grown online group as a case study: The BADASS Army. We utilize a case study here to illustrate a concrete example of the theoretical concepts we have been discussing. The case study methodology involves inquiry into a specific phenomenon (Baxter & Jack, 2008); in this case, an online support/advocacy group.

Case Study: The BADASS Army

The BADASS Army is an organization that is "Battling Against Demeaning & Abusive Selfie Sharing," though it does much more than that. It was founded in August 2017 by Katelyn Bowden out of the need to support survivors of revenge porn and other forms of cyber sexual assault (CSA). To date, there are still not any easily found support networks for CSA survivors. Because the laws around CSA vary state to state, with several states having weak laws and a few states still have no laws against the crime of non-consensual sharing of images and videos, navigating one's rights after CSA is difficult. Moreover, there is a need for social support and recovery advice that is ideally located through social media: many CSA survivors cannot talk to family, friends, or geographically local support networks because of stigma and/or cultural expectations or laws (in some countries creating pornographic material is punishable by death).

The community operates through a private Facebook group page that an administrator provides access to. Once the administrator determines that the person requesting access is a survivor, they are granted access to the online community.

Katelyn Bowden began to build the community through contacts she met through her personal advocacy journey, and actively reached out to individuals she read about or heard about in the media. With her mother as her inspiration, who contacted the police, the FBI, and their senator when Katelyn found a non-consensually shared nude image of herself on the internet, Katelyn wanted to create an army of survivors that were fighting back. Getting people to join the movement wasn't hard, but helping them feel safe is. Many cyber sexual assault survivors are skeptical of messages or offers to help from strangers on the internet, since many of them have received upwards of thousands of unsolicited messages and offers to "help" find their nude images (which are often accompanied by threats to further spread the images if their offers aren't graciously accepted). Katelyn's vetting of members has contributed to the feeling of safety that survivors feel in her online group.

One of Katelyn's visions for her group, besides that of supporting other survivors, is starting to shift the attitudes and language around images that are non-consensually posted so that some of the stigma associated with them is removed. Instead of calling it "cyber sexual assault" or "revenge porn," she calls it simply "image abuse." Her perspective is that by changing what we call this problem, we can shift some of society's attitudes toward it.

For example, most of the rhetoric around revenge porn still places blame on the people who have been victimized, creating the idea that they had a choice in the outcome (Burns, in Nally & Smith, eds., 2015). This reinforces the belief that victims are somehow to blame, and prevents them from coming forward to report the crime (Evans, 2018). Non-consensual pornography dehumanizes and objectifies its subjects, and often empathy is difficult to garner, as many people, even if they reframe the victim's role into a "what if it was me?" frame, think they would never date someone who would expose them in that way (Donohue, 2017). However, taking a feminist re-approach with the "me" frame allows the problem to be conceptualized as one of sexual aggression, which provides space for criminalization (Donohue, 2017). The author states: "The difficult, necessary work before us is to imagine reform that animates inherent dignity and worth concepts that are non-positional, but universal and unalienable" (Donohue, 2017, p. 306). The re-imagination Ms. Bowden is creating is a step in this direction.

As the organization grows, fundamental strategic directions for the BADASS Army will be strongly influenced by the experiences and recommendations of the members themselves. This single case illustrates a problem (image abuse) caused by social media, leading to an online community formed to address the problem and to provide for support to people affected by the problem. The future of the group will depend on the collective action (group support, advocacy, policy change, etc.) of current and future members of the group. Intercultural communications theory, in turn, will adopt and evolve as groups like these form, grow, and lead us through our increasingly networked world in the 21st century.

References

Attai, D. J., Cowher, M. S., Al-Hamadani, M., Schoger, J. M., Staley, A. C., & Landercasper, J. (2015). Twitter social media is an effective tool for breast cancer patient education and support: Patient-reported outcomes by survey. *Journal of Medical Internet Research, 17*(7), e188.

Baxter, P., & Jack, S. (2008). Qualitative case study methodology: Study design and implementation for novice researchers. *The Qualitative Report, 13*(4), 544–559. Retrieved from https://nsuworks.nova.edu/tqr/vol13/iss4/2

Beretta, V., Maccagnola, D., Cribbin, T., & Messina, E. (2015). An interactive method for inferring demographic attributes in Twitter. *26th ACM Conference on Hypertext and Social Media*, 2015 September 1–4, Guzelyurt, Northern Cyprus, pp. 113–122.

Bolton, R.,Parasuraman, A.,Hoefnagels, A.,Migchels, N.,Kabadayi, S., Gruber, T., … Solnet, D. (2013). Understanding Generation Y and their use of social media: a review and research agenda. *Journal of Service Management, 24*(3), 245–267. https://doi.org/10.1108/09564231311326987

Bourdieu, P. (1985). The forms of capital. In J. G. Richardson (Ed.), *Handbook for theory and research for the sociology of education* (pp. 241–58). New York: Greenwood.

Burger, J., Henderson, J., Kim, G., & Zarrella, G. (2011). Discriminating gender on Twitter. The Association for Computational Linguistics 2011 Conference on Empirical Methods in Natural Language Processing; 2011 July 27–29; Edinburgh, United Kingdom. Association for Computational Linguistics; 2011. pp. 1301–1309.

Burns, A. (2015). In full view: Involuntary porn and the postfeminist rhetoric of choice. In Nally, C. & Smith, A. (Eds.), *Twenty-first century feminism*. London: Palgrave Macmillan.

Cohen, S., & Wills, T. A. (1985). Stress, social support, and the buffering hypothesis. *Psychological Bulletin*, *98*, 310–57.

De Kosnik, A. (2016). *Rogue archives: Digital cultural memory and media fandom*. Cambridge, MA: MIT Press.

De Toqueville, A. (1835). *Democracy in America*. New York: A Mentor Book from New American Library.

Donohue, C. P. (2017). A feminist framing of non-consensual pornography, 17 U. Md. L.J. Race Relig. *Gender & Class*, *247*. Available at: http://digitalcommons.law.umaryland.edu/rrgc/vol17/iss2/4

Dubé, E., Vivion, M., & MacDonald, N. E. (2015). Vaccine hesitancy, vaccine refusal and the anti-vaccine movement: Influence, impact and implications. *Expert Review of Vaccines*, *14*(1), 99–117.

Evans, J. (2018). Revenge porn victims not coming forward due to stigma around name of offense, police say. *ABC News*, 2 AUu. Available online at: https://www.abc.net.au/news/2018-08-03/revenge-porn-victims-not-coming-forward-due-to-stigma/10067570 (accessed 1 October 2019).

Falisi, A. L., Wiseman, K. P., Gaysynsky, A., Scheideler, J. K., Ramin, D. A., & Chou, W. Y. S. (2017). Social media for breast cancer survivors: A literature review. *Journal of Cancer Survivorship*, *11*(6), 808–821.

Ferlander, S. (2007). The importance of different forms of social capital for health. *Acta Sociologica*, *50*(2), 115–128. doi: 10.1177/0001699307077654

Fernández-Luque, L., & Bau, T. (2015). Health and social media: Perfect storm of information. *Healthcare Informatics Research*, *21*(2), 67–73.

Giles, H., Coupland, N., & Coupland, J. (1991). Accommodation theory: Communication, context, and consequence. In H. Giles, J. Coupland, & N. Coupland (Eds.), *Studies in emotion and social interaction. Contexts of accommodation: Developments in applied sociolinguistics* (pp. 1–68). New York, NY: Cambridge University Press; Paris, France: Editions de la Maison des Sciences de l'Homme.

Giustini, D., Ali, S. M., Fraser, M., & Kamel Boulos, M. N. (2018). Effective uses of social media in public health and medicine: A systematic review of systematic reviews. *Online Journal of Public Health Informatics*, *10*(2), e215. doi: 10.5210/ojphi.v10i2.8270

Godin, S. (2008). *Tribes: We need you to lead us*. New York: Penguin.

Goldstein, S., MacDonald, N. E., & Guirguis, S. (2015). Health communication and vaccine hesitancy. *Vaccine*, *33*(34), 4212–4214.

Hall, S. (1996). Cultural studies and its theoretical legacies. In K.-H. Chen and D. Morley (Eds.), *Stuart Hall: Critical Dialogues in Cultural Studies* (pp. 262–275), London and New York: Routledge.

Harvey, D. (2002). The art of rent: Globalisation, monopoly and the commodification of culture. *Socialist Register*, *38*(38), 93–110.

Jones, E. L. (2009). *Cultures merging: A historical and economic critique of culture*. Princeton, NJ: Princeton University Press.

Putnam, R. D. (1993). The prosperous community. The American Prospect, *4*(13), 35–42.
Sipp, D., Frazer, I. H., & Rasko, J. E. (2018). No vacillation on HPV vaccination. *Cell*, *172*(6), 1163–1167.
Ting-Toomey, S. (1988a). A face negotiation theory. In Y. Kim and W. Gudykunst (Eds.), *Theories in Intercultural Communication* (pp. 47–92). Newbury Park, CA: Sage.
Ting-Toomey, S. (1988b). Rhetorical sensitivity style in three cultures: France, Japan, and the United States. *Communication Studies*, *39*(1), 28–36.
Van Dijck, J. (2013). *The culture of connectivity: A critical history of social media*. Oxford, UK: Oxford University Press.
Van Royen, K., Poels, K., Vandebosch, H., & Adam, P. (2017). "Thinking before posting?" Reducing cyber harassment on social networking sites through a reflective message. *Computers in Human Behavior*, *66*,345–352.
Xu, J. M., Bhargava, A., Nowak, R., & Zhu, X. (2012, September). Socioscope: Spatio-temporal signal recovery from social media. In *Joint European Conference on Machine Learning and Knowledge Discovery in Databases* (pp. 644–659). Berlin, Heidelberg: Springer.
Xu, S., Markson, C., Costello, K. L., Xing, C. Y., Demissie, K., & Llanos, A. A. (2016). Leveraging social media to promote public health knowledge: Example of cancer awareness via Twitter. *JMIR Public Health and Surveillance*, *2*(1), e17.
Yaqub, O., Castle-Clarke, S., Sevdalis, N., & Chataway, J. (2014). Attitudes to vaccination: a critical review. *Social Science & Medicine*, *112*, 1–11.
Ziebland, S., & Wyke, S. (2012). Health and illness in a connected world: How might sharing experiences on the Internet affect people's health? *Milbank Quarterly*, *90*(2), 219–249. doi: 10.1111/j.1468-0009.2012.00662.x

CHAPTER NINE

Mexican-American Women, Prenatal Testing, and Definitions of Fetal Health: Challenging Social Perceptions of What Is "Healthy"

BY LEANDRA HINOJOSA HERNÁNDEZ

"Health" is a socially constructed concept and embodied experience that is defined in different ways by different cultural groups, particularly when cultural beliefs, attitudes, and preferences intersect with one's gender, relational status, and racial and ethnic identities. Definitions of health take on particular significance in prenatal testing contexts, where the ethical responsibility of prenatal life or death often falls on the shoulders of the mother involved (Lowy, 2017). To more clearly understand the ways in which culture, gender, and ethnic identity converge in an embodied maternal responsibility context, this chapter analyzes how two communities of Mexican-American women make sense of definitions of fetal health through prenatal testing procedures and experiences. In this chapter, I will (1) discuss the broader implications of these communities' culturally discursive constructions of health and (2) discuss the role of intercultural communication strategies that can assist healthcare providers in being more culturally competent communicators in ethically delicate situations such as prenatal testing.

Although research has explored Mexican American women's prenatal and postnatal depression (Marcus, Flynn, Blow, & Barry, 2003; Martinez-Schallmoser, Telleen, & Macmullen, 2003), postpartum fetal and maternal weight (Thornton et al., 2006), and other maternal and fetal health outcomes, one importantly related and understudied topic is that of Mexican American women's perceptions of fetal health as it relates to prenatal testing and screening. Does stress about fetal health routinized and highly scientized reproductive technologies are deserving of their role in women's lived pregnancy realities, particularly the amniocentesis because of its role in influencing a woman's decision to keep or terminate a pregnancy.

Decision-Making Processes

Considering the ethical and moral implications of prenatal testing and decisions that must be made after positive diagnoses (as they are so toxically labeled),[1] informed and shared decision-making (SDM) about prenatal testing has gained attention in health practice and health policy spheres. However, before one can understand informed and shared decision-making within this context, it is necessary to first describe the tenets of informed and SDM.

Informed and SDM is a communicative task and process that draws upon notions of informed consent and informed choice, which has been defined by Charles, Gafni, and Whelan (1997) as "disclosure of treatment alternatives rather than merely informed consent" (p. 681). Charles et al. (1997) note that SDM has four main characteristics: (1) it involves at least two participants (the patient and the physician), (2) both parties take steps to participate in the decision-making process, (3) information sharing is a prerequisite to SDM, and (4) a treatment decision is made upon which both parties agree (pp. 685–688). Charles, Gafni, and Whelan (1999) elaborate upon this characterization by noting that in a SDM approach, each person needs to be willing to engage in the process by both exchanging information *and* expressing treatment preferences, and that it should occur in a safe environment where the patient feels comfortable in exploring information and expressing opinions, ideas, and preferences. Ideally, if a patient and his/her physician engage in effective SDM, the high-quality decision should be one that, according to Epstein and Street (2007), is based on both the patient's values and understanding of the evidence and rationale for the decision. Thus, taken together, SDM is a process and social event between the patient and her provider that is characterized by trust, rapport, and active involvement and disclosure on behalf of all parties involved (Politi & Street, 2011).

However, SDM can become a complicated process when it involves the relationship between healthcare providers and pregnant women and the high-risk decision of undergoing prenatal testing. Bylund and Imes (2005) note that when considering SDM, it is important to consider the context within which the decision is being made. They argue that the medical context strongly impacts the nature and quality of the interaction, and the prenatal testing context is certainly an ethically- and morally-charged process that is characterized by high levels of stress, information seeking, information processing, and deliberation. Furthermore,

Emery (2001) argues that SDM from a genetic counseling and testing perspective is "a different breed of informed decision-making" that complicates informed choice and SDM because (1) genetic test results have broader implications than non-genetic test results and may be perceived differently; (2) carrier status might be difficult for parents to conceptualize, particularly from a gender role perspective (which typically views males as strong, perfect, and masculine, and females as weak, imperfect, and damaged); (3) genetic testing decisions are often multiple and sequential and are made at various levels that affect individuals and their families; and (4) most information is based on uncertainties and probabilities (p. 81). Thus, SDM about undergoing prenatal testing is a particularly delicate and tension-ridden encounter, and the process may not occur smoothly.

Women's Experiences with Prenatal Decision-Making

Women's experiences with reproductive technologies, particularly the amniocentesis procedures, have broadly been well documented. Katz Rothman's (1998) foundational research, for example, explored how the amniocentesis procedure radically altered women's pregnancy experiences, as well as American cultural values associated with motherhood and disability. Building upon Katz Rothman's (1998) work, Rapp (2004) also explored the meaning of the amniocentesis procedure for American women and utilized an intersectional approach by interviewing Caucasian, black, and Latina women from a variety of class positions and educational backgrounds. Women might accept prenatal testing because it is perceived to provide beneficial information or reject prenatal diagnostic screenings because of doubts of the tests' reliability, anxieties about genetic conditions and fetal health, and differences of opinion between spouses (Muller & Cameron, 2015). Hispanic/Latina women, in particular, have lower levels of first trimester prenatal care compared to non-Hispanic women, especially when pregnant for the first time (Selchau et al., 2017). However, when specifically concerning prenatal testing and the amniocentesis procedure, Browner and colleagues (1999, 2000, 2003) found that Mexican-origin women's willingness to accept the amniocentesis procedure was affected by several intertwined factors, including biomedical knowledge, lay knowledge, trust issues, translation issues, and relationships with providers.

Browner and Preloran, two significant scholars who have analyzed how Mexican women perceive and utilize prenatal testing, found that a majority of Mexican-origin women accept the amniocentesis procedure (Browner, Preloran, & Cox, 1999; Markens et al., 2003). There is a significant relationship between their positive perceptions of doctors' recommendations and their acceptance of the procedure (Browner et al., 1999), and they often believe that a negative test result would provide reassurance (Browner et al., 1999). However, those who refuse are skeptical of physicians and prefer to trust experiential knowledge sources (Markens et al., 2003). Moreover, "less acculturated Mexican women" are more likely to reject the test (Browner & Press, 1995) because they sometimes find the amniocentesis "frightening" (Browner et al., 1999).

From a relational perspective, Mexican-origin women they typically make the decision to refuse or accept the test alone, although spouses occasionally contribute (Browner & Preloran 1999; Browner et al., 1999). Research by Markens et al. (2003) illustrated the gendered dynamics of prenatal testing for Mexican women: "Most men in our study accompanied their partners to the genetic consultation, and of these, an egalitarian view of marriage and parenting was often espoused by both partners" (p. 473). For other participants, husbands were often not able to attend medical appointments because of economic unfeasibility, husbands often felt that prenatal testing was part of the "woman's domain" of authority and decision-making, and (in a small sample) husbands attended medical appointments to exert authority and provide "male approval" of screenings and procedures.

Moreover, in terms of other cultural beliefs and preferences, research suggests that religion has garnered conflicting results about its role in Mexican-American women's perceptions of and decisions regarding prenatal testing. Although one might hypothesize that Mexican-American women would be overwhelmingly Catholic and would decline prenatal testing and amniocentesis at higher rates than non-Mexican women, the small research that has explored this dimension has found that the role of religion is very flexible. Seth et al. (2011) evaluated the role of religion and spirituality as it relates to Latina women's prenatal diagnosis decisions and found that religious/spiritual beliefs were indeed important and provided comfort to the women as they dealt with the process, yet the risk of procedure-related complications played a more concrete role in the decision-making process than their beliefs did. Similarly, Atkin, Ahmed, Hewison, and Green (2008) found that women's decisions to undergo prenatal testing were generally related to their attitudes toward abortion and were mediated by religious and faith beliefs. While religion was an important variable in this study, what was most important was the woman's faith—"faith beliefs emerged as flexible, negotiable, and contingent: a resource, which could be used creatively to support and legitimate a person's decision" (Atkin et al., 2008, p. 29).

Finally, from a race/ethnicity perspective, Hispanic/Latina patients are less knowledgeable about genetic testing than their white counterparts and often have many misperceptions about the genetic testing process and what genetic testing actually assesses (Griffiths & Kupperman, 2008; Penchaszadeh & Punales-Morejon, 1998; Singer, Antonucci, and Van Hoewyk, 2004; Suther & Kiros, 2009).

Griffiths and Kupperman (2008) examined rural Latinas' understanding of prenatal testing and risks and found that they were overwhelmingly supportive of prenatal care because it assesses the fetus' health, *but* they had many misperceptions about prenatal testing, including the fact that a normal screening result automatically guarantees a fetus' good health.

Similarly, Penchaszadeh and Punales-Morejon (1998) surveyed 100 Latino patients prior to genetic testing and found: (1) two-thirds believed incorrectly that prenatal testing could detect all genetic diseases and mental retardation and that it could predict the overall health of the fetus; (2) less than 40% knew what prenatal testing actually screens for; (3) 31% reported undergoing prenatal testing at their physicians' insistence; (4) 63% refused prenatal testing because of fear of miscarriage; and (5) 30% stated that abortion would not be an option because of moral and religious beliefs. This lack of information and acquisition of incorrect information has the potential to negatively affect SDM because women might be making potentially life-changing decisions on a faulty information base.

Methods

In order to assess Mexican-American women's perceptions of prenatal testing and their social construction of fetal health, qualitative methods were utilized to explore participants' perceptions of the role of family members, health-related information, physicians, and religion in the prenatal testing decision-making process. Qualitative research allows for the exploration of human understanding, lived experience, and the nuances and negotiations that people experience in their everyday lives as they navigate the healthcare system and make important decisions about their health. It can also help unpack the processes surrounding healthcare communication and explore what "really" is going on (Britten, 2011, p. 388). Moreover, qualitative research is a useful tool for understanding societal issues that arise from cultural contexts (Covarrubias, 2002; Kreuter & McClure, 2004; Tracy, 2013). Issues experienced pertaining to ethnicity, gender, race, and sexual orientation can be understood, critiqued, and transformed through contextual studies that examine how these demographic categories are negotiated, ever-changing, and communicatively constituted (Tracy, 2013).

In order to understand participants' emergent and collaborative social realities, I conducted semi-structured, in-depth interviews with participants, which provided space for analysis of participants' views of reality (Reinharz, 1992) and pre-existing statistics and generalizations about Mexican-American women's perceptions of decision-making with spouses and clinicians about prenatal testing and amniocentesis. Moreover, in-depth interviews allowed me to explore the language used by participants to describe their experiences, garner their stories and explanations, and perhaps lead to new interview questions and phenomena that were not previously considered (Lindlof & Taylor, 2017).

After receiving IRB approval, I interviewed first-, second- and third-generation Mexican-American women between the ages of 30–45 who had at least one pregnancy and live in Houston or San Diego because I wanted to explore Hispanic/Latino within-group variation and analyze their reproductive experiences.[2] I specifically chose this population because much research has already explored how immigrant Mexican women experience their pregnancies and deal with the tensions of negotiating birth practices in Mexico and losing family ties, family traditions, and family support while making prenatal testing-related decisions and giving birth here in the U.S. (Galvez, 2011; Gutierrez, 2008). Little research has explored second- and third-generation Mexican-American women's negotiations of reconciling and making sense of their birth practices, beliefs, and traditions back in Mexico, particularly within a prenatal care/amniocentesis context, and the birth practices, beliefs, and customs they have experienced and perhaps adopted as they have lived here in the U.S. Given that the Hispanic/Latino population is growing here in the U.S., at almost 58 million individuals (Flores, 2017), and that this population is projected to soon become the majority in the next few decades, knowledge of Mexican-American women's experiences of making decisions with spouses and clinicians can help inform future genetic counseling and cultural competence curricula, as well as improve future healthcare encounters surrounding this complex decision-making process.

Thirty Mexican-American women were interviewed: 15 in Houston, and 15 in San Diego. I utilized the snowball sample recruitment method (Noy, 2008), meaning key informants in each city assisted with participant recruitment by suggesting friends, family members, and co-workers. Participants suggested women in their social networks as well, and I was able to conduct all of the interviews in each city within a one-month time span. Interviews with participants lasted on average one hour and were mostly conducted at local coffee shops.

After interviews concluded, I conducted a thematic analysis to explore the various themes, categories, and codes that emerged from the data and from my participants' experiences. According to Boyatzis (1998), thematic analysis is, in its most basic sense, a way of seeing. More specifically, Braun and Clarke (2006) claim it is "a method for identifying, analyzing and reporting patterns (themes) within data" (p. 79). Thus, I created categories and a coding scheme based on patterns, similarities, and notable exceptions in the data (Lindlof & Taylor 2017). I first identified categories pertaining to religiosity, identity, and SDM, which were then collapsed into themes and their corresponding categories.

Themes

The three primary themes that emerged relating to the participants' overwhelming rejection of the amniocentesis procedure were: (1) an unnecessary prenatal test, (2) intention to keep the pregnancy, and (3) no need for amniocentesis-related test results.

The Amniocentesis: An Unnecessary Prenatal Test

The most telling finding about Mexican-American women's relationship to the amniocentesis procedure is that they did not want it or see a need for it. Out of 30 participants, only *one* underwent the amniocentesis procedure because of a significant medical issue during one of her pregnancies that highly influenced her to accept the amniocentesis so that she could "prepare for her baby's future." Other than that, the remaining 29 participants refused the amniocentesis procedure during their pregnancies for a variety of reasons, and their religious, spiritual, and cultural values intertwined with their medical beliefs as reasons to reject the procedure.

"It Just Wasn't Necessary": No Reason for the Procedure

The first reason that the participants rejected the amniocentesis procedure is that, at a base level, they did not think it was necessary. Only 4 participants had positive or ambiguous test results after their blood screening, and the remaining 26 participants had normal test results after their blood screening. In this context, the "normal" blood test results indicated to them that "they had nothing to worry about."

Isa, a 34-year-old mother of four from Houston, said the amniocentesis procedure "just wasn't necessary because all the screenings came out fine. I might have at least kind of thought about the option of doing it if there was a problem, but since my blood tests were normal, I didn't see a need for it." Similarly, Nayara, a 33-year-old mother of four from Houston, stated: "I didn't really see a need to go through with it because my blood test came back normal. I didn't really see a need to go through with the amnio. It wasn't a huge concern for me to do more tests." Mireia, a 44-year-old mother of two from Houston, also shared Isa and Nayara's sentiments: "I mean, we didn't do the amnio stuff. Had there been issues that they'd found, I don't know, maybe I would've considered it or maybe not. But since it didn't really get to that point with either of my pregnancies, I didn't see a need for it."

Similarly, other participants mentioned that they saw no need for the amniocentesis, and as conversations unfolded, they pointed to structural factors such as the healthcare system, lack of insurance, and healthcare providers that also shaped their rejection of the amniocentesis procedure. For example, Evelia, a 32-year-old mother of two from San Diego, discussed how she had to go to a community clinic for low-income women for her prenatal care because she was a stay-at-home mom without insurance. Describing the clinic as "small, cramped, and low on time and resources," Evelia noted that even though she would not have gone through the amniocentesis procedure anyway, the clinic might be one of the reasons why she was not offered the amniocentesis procedure in the first place: "Yeah, the other test came out okay. The doctor said I didn't need the amnio because the blood screening was negative and that I didn't need to go that route. It was like a 2-minute conversation. In and out the door he went." Marita, a 34-year-old mother of three, went to the same clinic as Evelia and mentioned that the doctors there did not offer the amniocentesis procedure to her:

> I didn't even know that the amnio was an option! It was my first child, I didn't do that much research, and at the clinic, no one really told me anything about it. The clinic was always so packed with so many women needing to be seen, and the doctor would come in for like 5 seconds and then leave. Afterward, when I found out what the amnio was, there was no way that I was going to go through with that test! It just wasn't necessary because my original blood scan came out okay. The doctor came in and said, "Your blood tests were negative" and that was it.

In addition to Evelia and Marita, Anita, a 32-year-old mother of one from San Diego, went to a local neighborhood clinic because she did not have insurance. Anita described her local clinic with the same terms that Marita and Evelia used:

> Yeah, it was just a mess. Not enough staff, too many patients. They didn't even offer the amnio, they didn't ask, nothing. I didn't even know it was something that could be necessary. I don't know if it's because it's one of those clinics where it's low-income and for low-income people, so they didn't offer much there. I wouldn't have gotten it done, but they didn't even offer it.

Thus, for some of the participants, the amniocentesis procedure was not a necessary prenatal test because the initial blood screenings were negative, meaning there was no indication of chromosomal or genetic abnormalities, and participants did not think it was necessary to undergo more testing. However, as conversations progressed and narratives were recounted, it became clear that a variety of structural factors contributed to the participants' perceptions that the amniocentesis was not necessary. A handful of San Diego participants did not have insurance and as such went to community clinics for their prenatal care. With the participants' descriptions of low resources, overbooked patients, and overworked physicians, as well as the participants being uninsured, it is possible that these conditions contributed to the physicians telling the participants they did not need the amniocentesis or not even offering the procedure at all. Although research has illustrated that Mexican immigrants have lower rates of health insurance, less access to healthcare than documented citizens, and poorer experiences with overall primary care (Bustamante et al., 2012; DeRose, Escarce, & Lurie, 2007; DuBard & Gizlice, 2008; Ortega et al., 2007), this theme illustrates that Mexican-American women who are citizens (first through third generation) experience similar health disparities, particularly in prenatal testing contexts.

"It Won't Change the Outcome": Intention to Keep the Pregnancy

In addition to rejecting the amniocentesis procedure because they thought it was more unnecessary testing, participants from both Houston and San Diego also rejected the amniocentesis because they had no intention to abort their baby, regardless of any potential chromosomal or genetic abnormalities. Almost every participant said in some form or fashion that the amniocentesis "wouldn't change the outcome" and that they had their mind made up since the beginning of their pregnancies. The participants were steadfast in their beliefs that they would not abort their baby (not their "fetus," which is a key distinction that will be discussed later) because their baby was "a gift from God" and because they did not feel like Down syndrome or any other chromosomal condition would make their baby unhealthy.

First and foremost, participants mentioned that the amniocentesis was not necessary because they would not abort their babies who were "gifts from God." Noelia, a 37-year-old mother of two from Houston, stated, "Whatever I get, I get. That's what the Lord is going to bless me with. We always live by that saying that God only gives you what you can handle, and my baby is a gift straight from the man upstairs!" Similar to Noelia, Yessica, a 33-year-old mother of two from Houston, situated her amniocentesis rejection within religious values: "I didn't do the amnio because I was going to take what I can get. Whatever comes in my life, I'm going to take it regardless. I always think, let what comes, come. If that's what God's going to give me, then that's what He's going to give me. It wasn't going to change the outcome. I would never abort my baby."

Ysabel, a 33-year-old mother of two from Houston, stated: "I didn't do the amnio because it wasn't going to change my way of thinking about having the baby. I didn't really want to go that route because if my baby has something, then he has something. It wasn't going to chance the outcome of my pregnancy or my love for my baby." Dulce, a 34-year-old mother of two from Houston, also situated her rejection of the amniocentesis within her religious values: "I mean, I prayed about it and hoped to God that my baby would be okay, but it's just like what they say, I guess. Mexican-American women, we have a big faith. Whatever God gives us, that's what it is! It's meant to be, you know? He's giving it to me for a reason. That's why I didn't do the amnio. I was going to keep my baby regardless." Thus, the influence of the participants' religious and spiritual beliefs was an important component of their decision to reject the amniocentesis procedure.

In addition to the Houston participants, San Diego participants also shared this sentiment. Lara, a 32-year-old mother of two from San Diego, spoke of how her intentions to keep her pregnancy solidified her choice to reject the amniocentesis:

> I think for me at that point, it was more that the outcome of the test wasn't going to change anything. I think there's some people who want the test because they think more about the quality of life of the child and they want to have the option of to terminate or not to terminate. For me, it didn't really matter what the outcome of the test was going to be because I was going to keep my baby and love it anyways, so why have somebody prick me in the stomach?

Esperanza, a 36-year-old mother of two from San Diego, stated: "There was just no reason for it. I knew that whatever is going to come my way is going to come my way. The amnio test results wouldn't have changed my mind." Last, Beatriz, a 33-year-old mother of two from San Diego, encapsulated this theme when she noted: "I just didn't see the point in getting it done. It wouldn't have changed anything. It was just about me having my baby and that was it, you know? It's just that simple." Thus, participants overwhelmingly and repeatedly mentioned that the amniocentesis procedure was not necessary because they knew from the beginning of their pregnancies that they would not abort their babies, regardless of whatever conditions they might be born with. This conviction stemmed from their strong bond with the babies growing within them and their religious values, from which they believed that their babies were gifts from God that they needed to accept and love. Religiosity and spirituality play a significant role in Mexican/-American women's healthcare experiences: God is often seen as a "partner in healthcare" who plays an important role in decision-making processes (Jurkowski Kurlanska, & Ramos, 2010, p. 23). Moreover, from a fatalism perspective, spirituality and religiosity often lead to a lower locus of control whereby Mexican/-American women feel as if what happens to them is out of their control (Jurkowski et al., 2010), aspects of health and life are seen as coming directly from God (Musgrave et al., 2002), and conformity to God's will is often a guiding healthcare decision-making practice (Musgrave et al., 2002). In efforts to avoid essentialism, it is worth noting that participants viewed religion in an active manner whereby they evaluated their spiritual and religious beliefs in conjunction with their bonds with their babies, another important aspect of the decision-making process. In this context, a child was a blessing, regardless of a health anomaly or an illness that could be perceived as "unhealthy."

In addition to their religious and spiritual beliefs, participants also discursively constructed new definitions during their interviews of what it means for a baby to be healthy. Participants argued that they would not abort their babies because they would still be healthy, regardless of any birth defect. For example, Nayara, a 33-year-old mother of four from Houston, went back and forth about whether or not rejecting the amniocentesis during her fourth pregnancy was a bad choice. However, after praying about it, she felt confident about her decision: "I prayed every day—did I make the right choice? I realized eventually that I did, though. I still would've had her. It wouldn't have changed anything. As long as she was breathing, that's all that mattered to me. She still would've been healthy." This notion of the baby being healthy as long as s/he is breathing was also mentioned during Lourdes' description of why she did not want the amniocentesis procedure. Lourdes, a 32-year-old mother of four from Houston, said:

> I wasn't even concerned with the outcome, you know? If they said, like, if a red flag was raised, I would've told them, "Okay, as long as it didn't have to do with my baby biologically functioning or not existing or something, then why have [the amnio]?" As long as the baby is still breathing and the heart is still beating, then she'll be okay and she'll be healthy. As long as she's okay, then that's it.

In addition to Lourdes and Nayara, Dulce, a 34-year-old mother of two from Houston, situated her belief that babies with defects are still healthy within her lived experience of interacting with children who have Down syndrome: "I see a lot of Down syndrome kids that are talkative and normal. I also have a few friends with children who have Down syndrome, and you can't even tell that anything's wrong! They're perfectly healthy. I didn't really care about it. That's why I didn't do the amnio—it wasn't going to change the outcome." Yesenia, a 33-year-old mother of two from Houston, also mentioned her cousin with Down syndrome as a reason for believing that people with Down syndrome and other disabilities are still healthy:

> If she was happy and breathing, then she was healthy and that was it. I didn't do the amnio because I knew it wouldn't change a thing. My cousin has Down syndrome and

> is perfectly normal! He went through high school with no issues and was even prom king. If my baby had Down syndrome, then she had Down syndrome. She would still be another happy, joyous, and healthy addition to our lives. We would've had her regardless. It wouldn't have changed the way I love her.

Finally, Ysabel, a 33-year-old mother of two from Houston, also situated her belief that babies with defects are still healthy within her lived experience of being a mother to a first child with a disability: "I knew I didn't want the amnio from the very beginning. I was just going to go with it and hope for the best. There was no point—I wasn't going to NOT have my baby because of a disability. My first child has a disability and he's perfectly healthy."

Thus, participants overwhelmingly situated their rejection of the amniocentesis because they had no intentions of aborting their babies, and this was situated within a belief that a child with a genetic or chromosomal birth defect is still healthy. This belief stemmed from a variety of sociocultural and interpersonal influences, including their religious and spiritual beliefs and their experiences with other people who have Down syndrome. Since the participants already knew that they would not get an abortion, regardless of whatever genetic or chromosomal defect their children might have, then it was a logical next step that the participants saw no need for the amniocentesis test results.

"What Would I Do with the Information?" No Need for the Amniocentesis Test Results

Intertwined within interview discourses of pro-life, pro-disabilities, and religious values was the notion of information. Participants consistently noted during their interviews as they discussed their rejection of the amniocentesis that they did not know what they would do with the amniocentesis test results and thus realized that they did not need the amniocentesis. Participants weighed the pros and cons of the amniocentesis through deliberations about the utility of the genetic and chromosomal information that the amniocentesis test results could provide. Although this code shares many similarities with the two preceding codes, the key difference about this code is that the participants often construed the information that the amniocentesis could provide as a burden that they did not want. While some women would value this information as helpful for future planning purposes (i.e., preparation for a pregnancy termination or for a child with a disability), the participants explicitly noted that this information would be burdensome because (1) it would not change their mind about the outcome of their pregnancies and (2) because it would stress them out and ruin their pregnancy experiences, which many described as a time in their life that was supposed to be joyous and calm.

Flor, a 31-year-old mother of three from San Diego, said it best when she noted: "I didn't not want the test, I knew I wouldn't abort, so why would I even want that information in the first place?" Four participants *did* note that if their blood screenings came back positive, they might have considered the amniocentesis because they would have wanted the information so they could, as Mireia stated, "prepare for the future." The other 26 participants, however, argued that "the information" (the amniocentesis test results) was unnecessary.

For example, Elena, a 39-year-old mother of one from San Diego, expressed that her age was a worrisome factor during her pregnancy. She thought about the amniocentesis procedure for quite some time, yet finally decided against it, noting that the amniocentesis results would not affect her decision to keep her pregnancy:

> The more I thought about the amnio, I thought, "Well, is it *really* going to change what I'm going to do later? Is it going to change anything right now? What am I going to do with that information?" I figured there was nothing I could really do with the information since it wouldn't change my mind about whether to terminate the pregnancy or not. There was no point. There was no question about whether or not I was going to keep my baby, whatever the outcome might be.

Also concerned about her age, Noelia, a 37-year-old mother of two from Houston, was 36 when she gave birth to her second child. She contemplated the amniocentesis procedure, given that her doctor reminded her about how her age could contribute to birth defects. She eventually decided against the procedure after weighing the advantages and disadvantages of the amniocentesis and the information it could provide:

> You know, it's like nothing you can really prepare for when you're pregnant. You take it when it comes. What I've come to learn is what happens when you get tested and then it's positive? You stress out about it and you become depressed and then you have complications during your pregnancy because of the stress. Why do that to yourself? Why would you even want the information? I know people do it to prepare themselves, but what's there to prepare for? You have to prepare for a child no matter what. I just kept thinking to myself, "What am I going to do with the information? What's it for?" There's just no point.

Elena and Noelia both decided against the amniocentesis because they knew that the test results would not change their minds about keeping their pregnancies. While it might seem obvious that a woman might not want the amniocentesis if her initial blood screening was negative, 3 of the 4 participants who *did* have positive blood screenings still decided to reject the amniocentesis procedure for the same reason: they knew that they test results would not change their decision to keep their pregnancies.

Discussion

Overall, 29 of 30 participants refused to undergo an amniocentesis test, which challenges earlier research that found that Mexican-American women accept prenatal testing at comparable rates (Browner, 1999; Markens et al., 2003). The themes that emerged during the interviews created what the participants perceived as logical and straightforward thought processes for the amniocentesis rejection: the participants knew before the medical appointment that they would reject the amniocentesis because it would not change their intentions to keep their pregnancies, and because their varying religious and spiritual beliefs taught them to value life and their children's lives, regardless of the circumstances. These reasons are undoubtedly situated within a larger web of sociocultural factors, including their family relationships; their views of life, death, morality, and ethics; their support of disabled children and the possibility of having a disabled child; and their social construction of what is considered *healthy* in a prenatal testing context. This combination of sociocultural factors constructs what I am referring to as a "homegrown understanding"[3] of the participants' refusal of the amniocentesis procedure, which goes against some previous findings that oversimplify Mexican-American women's experiences with prenatal testing. In other words, Mexican-American women redefined "healthy," particularly in a reproductive prenatal testing context, at the intersections of their Mexican-American identity, gender identity, and religious/spiritual identity.

The first theme that emerged from interviews centered upon their perception of the amniocentesis procedure as a test that is unnecessary for two main reasons: the test would not change their intention to keep their pregnancies, and as such, there was no need for the information that the amniocentesis procedure could provide. Within this theme are many important discourses central to prenatal testing: the viability of the amniocentesis procedure; the role of health information within reproductive contexts; and ultimately, the relationships between and among prenatal testing, abortion rights, and disability rights. Although research suggests that Mexican women undergo the amniocentesis procedure at rates comparable to Caucasian women (Browner & Press, 1995; Hunt & de Voogd, 2005) and that they think amniocentesis results could make them feel more comfortable and reassured during their pregnancies (Browner, 1999), the participants in this study argued the exact opposite: that the test was unnecessary, the results were unnecessary, and the test seemed frightening and stressful.

A key factor that contributed to the participants' perception of the test being unnecessary was their conceptualization of what it means for a baby to be healthy. In every interview, participants consistently referred to their pregnancies as their "babies;" not a single participant referred to their pregnancy as "the fetus" or "my fetus." This is significant within the contexts of reproductive politics and prenatal testing because it radically altered the ways in which the participants viewed their entire pregnancies and created a very specific starting point from which they viewed prenatal testing. Participants noted that each time they underwent a blood test or an ultrasound, they were not testing or looking at a fetus or a "clump of cells"—they were very clear that they were looking at their babies, babies that they were excited about, babies that their extended family members were expecting, and babies that they had been planning for. In this context, a maternal-fetal cultural bond guided by what some participants referred to as a familial and cultural value provided a powerful decision-making impetus to reject the amniocentesis procedure. As Jesse et al.'s (2007) research illustrates, culture, faith, and spirituality impact women of color's pregnancies by providing guidance, support, strength, and the beliefs that pregnancies are blessings and rewards.

Related to this notion is what the participants viewed as "healthy," as most of them noted that their babies (not fetuses) would still be healthy if they had Down syndrome or spina bifida. A few of the participants had previous children with disabilities (autism and kidney issues), and other participants had family members or friends with Down syndrome. Participants relied on these experiential knowledge bases as they explained during interviews that children with genetic issues are still healthy, functioning individuals in society and as such, they noted that as long as their babies were breathing and moving, they were healthy. As Rapp (2004) has noted, the "choice" any woman makes to accept or refuse the test flows from "the way that both pregnancy and disability are embedded in personal and collective values and judgments within which her own life has developed" (p. 91). Although research suggests that women's positive attitudes toward disabilities in the context of prenatal testing might change once they receive positive prenatal test results (Press, Browner, Tran, Morton, & Le Master, 1998), this finding was not supported with the Mexican American women who participated in this analysis. There was no "provisional normalcy" with these participants: they supported the rights of disabled children to be born, and they would not abort their babies, regardless of any genetic issue. This decision was also powerfully impacted by the intersection of their ethnic identity, gender identity, and religious identity, as religious beliefs, spiritual beliefs, and the impact of family support and narrative medical information created a context that illustrated the lack of necessity for prenatal testing results and information.

In conclusion, the participants not only had a homegrown understanding of the amniocentesis that was influenced by their personal experiences, cultural beliefs, perceptions of risk, and relationships with family members, but it was also influenced by their interpretations of medical and scientific information. Many participants noted that they "had nothing to worry about" because of negative blood screenings or that they *were* worried because of positive blood screenings, and both indicate incorrect perceptions of what the blood tests actually screen for. Moreover, participants were also highly influenced by their family members' experiences with the amniocentesis procedure, particularly by their family members' false positive experiences. Although the amniocentesis procedure false positive rate is estimated to be 5% (Benn, 2002; Spencer, Spencer, Power, Dawson, & Nicolaides, 2003), participants perceived that the amniocentesis false positive rate is much higher. Due to all of these factors, participants chose the blood screenings and the ultrasounds instead of the amniocentesis. This decision-making process is evidence of what feminist scholars have referred to as "active engagement" with reproductive technologies. Instead of being compliant subjects within the medicalization of childbirth, women are increasingly becoming active participants within their reproductive healthcare as they evaluate medicalization, risk, complications, and the necessity of various prenatal tests (Fordyce & Maraesa, 2012). While the participants in this study did not necessarily reject biomedical reproductive care as an entire enterprise, they selected the tests that they perceived to be most valuable (Browner, 2012).

What emerged as one of the most interesting components of this segment of the interviews was that while participants rejected the amniocentesis procedure, they wholeheartedly accepted blood screenings and ultrasounds. This presents a bit of a contradiction, given that they adamantly opposed the amniocentesis procedure, yet the participants readily accepted blood screenings for four reasons: (1) they repeatedly mentioned that a negative blood screen result meant their children would be fine; (2) if anything was wrong with their child, they would find the anomaly during the ultrasounds; (3) they were under the assumption that the blood screenings and the ultrasounds were mandatory tests, whereas the amniocentesis was an optional procedure; and (4) the blood screenings and ultrasounds were less invasive and had lower associated risks. The amniocentesis, on the other hand, due to its ethnical implications, perceived complications, and invasive nature, was perceived as unnecessary and not always accurate. As Fordyce and Maraesa (2012) have noted, "women often exhibit particular strategies of engagement with available medical practices, using them creatively as well as actively to reflect on individual choice and in consideration of sociocultural constructs" (p. 7). In this study, participants were not "docile recipients of statistical risk categories," but rather "pragmatic actors" who made reproductive testing decisions based upon family values, religious beliefs, and personal and cultural interpretations of health and risk.

Notes

1. Positive diagnoses in prenatal testing contexts can be perceived as toxic because of the double nature of the term: on the one hand, the diagnosis in positive, indicating that a fetal abnormality could be present; on the other hand, this diagnosis is not always perceived as positive by family members involved who are then faced with a host of decision-making processes made necessary by the diagnosis.
2. Although I originally intended upon interviewing only second- and third-generation Mexican-American women, I realized in the midst of conducting interviews that accurately pinpointing participants' generational status proved to be a daunting task. Like me, many participants had parents with varying generational statuses, so I categorized their generational status according to their how they identified, not traditional definitions of first-, second-, and third-generation Mexican-American women.
3. In her book *Testing Women, Testing the Fetus: The Social Impact of Amniocentesis in America*, Rayna Rapp (2004) deployed the terms "homegrown epidemiology" and "homegrown statistics" to refer to the various ways in which minority women make sense of medical discourses about prenatal risk, as well as the ways in which they evaluate this information within their own "homegrown" understandings and constructions of prenatal risk as evidenced by their family members' experiences. A key example of this terminology is represented by Mireia when she stated, "Yeah, the doctors tell me that I'm in my 40s and at much higher risk. But so many of my aunts and cousins had babies at late ages and their babies were fine. I don't think I have anything to worry about."

References

Allyse, M., Sayres, L. C., Goodspeed, T., Michie, M., & Cho, M. K. (2015). "Don't want no risk and don't want no problems": Public understandings of the risks and benefits of noninvasive prenatal testing in the United States. *AJOB Empirical Bioethics*, *6*(1), 5–20.

American College of Obstetrics & Gynecology. (2014). *Frequently asked questions: Routine tests in pregnancy*. Retrieved from http://www.acog.org/~/media/For%20Patients/faq133.pdf?dmc=1&ts=20140220T1552062299

American Pregnancy Association. (2014). *Amniocentesis*. Retrieved from http://americanpregnancy.org/prenataltesting/amniocentesis.html

Atkin, K., Ahmed, S., Hewison, J., & Green, J. M. (2008). Decision-making and ante-natal screening for sickle cell and thalassaemia disorders: To what extent do faith and religious identity mediate choice? *Current Sociology*, *56*(1), 77–98.

Benn, P. A. (2002). Advances in prenatal screening for Down syndrome: II first trimester testing, integrated testing, and future directions. *Clinica Chimica Acta*, *324*(1–2), 1–11.

Boyatzis, R. E. (1998). *Transforming qualitative information: Thematic analysis and code development*. Thousand Oaks, CA: Sage Publications, Inc.

Britten, N. (2011). Qualitative research on health communication: What can it contribute? *Patient Education and Counseling*, *82*(3), 384–388.

Braun, V., & Clarke, V. (2006). Using thematic analysis in psychology. *Qualitative Research in Psychology*, *3*(2), 77–101.

Browner, C. H. (2000). Situating women's reproductive activities. *American Anthropologist*, *102*(4), 773–788.

Browner, C. H., & Preloran, H. M. (1999). Male partners' role in Latinas' amniocentesis decisions. *Journal of Genetic Counseling*, *8*(2), 85–108.

Browner, C. H., Preloran, H. M., Casado, M. C., Bass, H. N., & Walker, A. P. (2003). Genetic counseling gone awry: Miscommunication between prenatal genetic service providers and Mexican-origin clients. *Social Science & Medicine*, *56*(9), 1933–1946.

Browner, C. H., Preloran, H. M., & Cox, S. J. (1999). Ethnicity, bioethics, and prenatal diagnosis: The amniocentesis decisions of Mexican-origin women and their partners. *American Journal of Public Health*, *89*(11), 1658–1666.

Browner, C. H., & Press, N. A. (1995). The normalization of prenatal diagnostic screening. In F. D. Ginsburg & R. Rapp (Eds.), *Conceiving the new world order: The global politics of reproduction* (pp. 307–322). Berkeley: The University of California Press.

Bustamante, A. V., Fang, H., Garza, J., Carter-Pokras, O., Wallace, S. P., Rizzo, J. A., & Ortega, A. N. (2012). Variations in healthcare access and utilization among Mexican immigrants: The role of documentation status. *Journal of Immigrant and Minority Health*, *14*(1), 146–155.

Bylund, C. L., & Imes R. S. (2005). Communication and shared decision making in context: Choosing between reasonable options. In E. B. Ray (Ed.), *Health communication in practice: A case study approach* (pp. 69–80). Mahwah, NJ: Lawrence Erlbaum Associates, Inc.

Charles, C., Gafni, A., & Whelan, T. (1997). Shared decision-making in the medical encounter: What does it mean? (or it takes at least two to tango). *Social Science & Medicine*, *44*(5), 681–692.

Charles, C., Gafni, A., & Whelan, T. (1999). Decision-making in the physician–patient encounter: Revisiting the shared treatment decision-making model. *Social Science & Medicine*, *49*(5), 651–661.

Covarrubias, P. O. (2002). *Culture, communication, and cooperation: Interpersonal relations and pronominal address in a Mexican organization*. Lanham, MD: Rowman & Littlefield.

Derose, K. P., Escarce, J. J., & Lurie, N. (2007). Immigrants and health care: Sources of vulnerability. *Health Affairs*, *26*(5), 1258–1268.

DuBard, C. A., & Gizlice, Z. (2008). Language spoken and differences in health status, access to care, and receipt of preventive services among US Hispanics. *American Journal of Public Health*, *98*(11), 2021–2028.

Emery, J. (2001). Is informed choice in genetic testing a different breed of informed decision-making? A discussion paper. *Health Expectations*, *4*(2), 81–86.

Epstein, R., & Street, R. L. (2007). *Patient-centered communication in cancer care: Promoting healing and reducing suffering*. Bethesda, MD: National Cancer Institute, US Department of Health and Human Services, National Institutes of Health.

Flores, A. (2017). How the U.S. Hispanic population is changing. *Pew Research Center*. Retrieved from http://www.pewresearch.org/fact-tank/2017/09/18/how-the-u-s-hispanic-population-is-changing/

Florez, J. C. (2007). Knowledge is power. *JAMA, 298*(13), 1489–1490.

Fordyce, L., & Maraësa, A. (Eds.) (2012). *Risk, reproduction, and narratives of experience*. Nashville: Vanderbilt University Press.

Gálvez, A. (2011). *Patient citizens, immigrant mothers: Mexican women, public prenatal care, and the birth weight paradox*. New Jersey: Rutgers University Press.

Griffiths, C., & Kuppermann, M. (2008). Perceptions of prenatal testing for birth defects among rural Latinas. *Maternal and Child Health Journal, 12*(1), 34–42.

Gutiérrez, E. R. (2009). *Fertile matters: The politics of Mexican-origin women's reproduction*. Austin: University of Texas Press.

Hildt, E. (2002). Autonomy and freedom of choice in prenatal genetic diagnosis. *Medicine, Health Care and Philosophy, 5*(1), 65–72.

Hunt, L. M., & De Voogd, K. B. (2005). Clinical myths of the cultural "other": Implications for Latino patient care. *Academic Medicine, 80*(10), 918–924.

Hunt, L. M., de Voogd, K. B., & Castañeda, H. (2005). The routine and the traumatic in prenatal genetic diagnosis: Does clinical information inform patient decision-making? *Patient Education and Counseling, 56*(3), 302–312.

Elizabeth Jesse, D., Schoneboom, C., & Blanchard, A. (2007). The effect of faith or spirituality in pregnancy: A content analysis. *Journal of Holistic Nursing, 25*(3), 151–158.

Jurkowski, J. M., Kurlanska, C., & Ramos, B. M. (2010). Latino women's spiritual beliefs related to health. *American Journal of Health Promotion, 25*(1), 19–25.

Katz Rothman, B. (1994). *The tentative pregnancy: Amniocentesis and the sexual politics of motherhood*. London: Pandora.

Kreuter, M. W., & McClure, S. M. (2004). The role of culture in health communication. *Annual Review of Public Health, 25*, 439–455.

Lindlof, T. R., & Taylor, B. C. (2017). *Qualitative communication research methods*. Thousand Oaks, CA: Sage Publications.

Löwy, I. (2017). *Imperfect pregnancies: A history of birth defects and prenatal diagnosis*. Baltimore, MD: Johns Hopkins University Press.

Marcus, S. M., Flynn, H. A., Blow, F. C., & Barry, K. L. (2003). Depressive symptoms among pregnant women screened in obstetrics settings. *Journal of Women's Health, 12*(4), 373–380.

Markens, S., Browner, C. H., & Preloran, H. M. (2003). "I'm not the one they're sticking the needle into:" Latino couples, fetal diagnosis, and the discourse of reproductive rights. *Gender & Society, 17*(3), 462–481.

Markens, S., Browner, C. H., & Mabel Preloran, H. (2010). Interrogating the dynamics between power, knowledge and pregnant bodies in amniocentesis decision making. *Sociology of Health & Illness, 32*(1), 37–56.

Martinez-Schallmoser, L., Telleen, S., & Macmullen, N. J. (2003). The effect of social support and acculturation on postpartum depression in Mexican American women. *Journal of Transcultural Nursing, 14*(4), 329–338.

Muller, C., & Cameron, L. D. (2015). It's complicated–Factors predicting decisional conflict in prenatal diagnostic testing. *Health Expectations, 19*(2), 388–402.

Noy, C. (2008). Sampling knowledge: The hermeneutics of snowball sampling in qualitative research. *International Journal of Social Research Methodology, 11*(4), 327–344.

Ortega, A. N., Fang, H., Perez, V. H., Rizzo, J. A., Carter-Pokras, O., Wallace, S. P., & Gelberg, L. (2007). Health care access, use of services, and experiences among undocumented Mexicans and other Latinos. *Archives of Internal Medicine, 167*(21), 2354–2360.

Papantoniou, N. E., Daskalakis, G. J., Tziotis, J. G., Kitmirides, S. J., Mesogitis, S. A., & Antsaklis, A. J. (2001). Risk factors predisposing to fetal loss following a second trimester amniocentesis. *BJOG: An International Journal of Obstetrics & Gynaecology, 108*(10), 1053–1056.

Penchaszadeh, V., & Punales-Morejon, D. (1998). Genetic services to the Latino population in the United States. *Public Health Genomics, 1*(3), 134–141.

Press, N., Browner, C. H., Tran, D., Morton, C., & Le Master, B. (1998). Provisional normalcy and "perfect babies": pregnant women's attitudes toward disability in the context of prenatal testing. In S. Franklin & H. Ragone (Eds.), *Reproducing reproduction: Kinship, power and technological innovation* (pp. 46–65). Philadelphia: University of Pennsylvania Press.

Rapp, R. (1996). Power of "positive" diagnosis: Medical and maternal discourses on amniocentesis. In D. Bassin, M. Honey, & M. M. Kaplan (Eds.), *Representations of motherhood* (pp. 204–219). New Haven, CT: Yale University Press.

Rapp, R. (2004). *Testing women, testing the fetus: The social impact of amniocentesis in America.* Abingdon UK: Routledge.

Reinharz, S., & Davidman, L. (1992). *Feminist methods in social research.* London: Oxford University Press.

Rothman, B. K. (1998). *Genetic maps and human imaginations: The limits of science in understanding who we are.* New York, NY: WW Norton & Company.

Sadlecki, P., Grabiec, M., Walentowicz, P., & Walentowicz-Sadlecka, M. (2018). Why do patients decline amniocentesis? Analysis of factors influencing the decision to refuse invasive prenatal testing. *BMC Pregnancy and Childbirth, 18*(1), 174.

Selchau, K., Babuca, M., Bower, K., Castro, Y., Coakley, E., & Flores, A., … Shattuck, L. (2017). First trimester prenatal care initiation among Hispanic women along the US-Mexico border. *Maternal and Child Health Journal, 21*(1), 11–18.

Seth, S. G., Goka, T., Harbison, A., Hollier, L., Peterson, S., Ramondetta, L., & Noblin, S. J. (2011). Exploring the role of religiosity and spirituality in amniocentesis decision-making among Latinas. *Journal of Genetic Counseling, 20*(6), 660–673.

Singer, E., Antonucci, T., & Van Hoewyk, J. (2004). Racial and ethnic variations in knowledge and attitudes about genetic testing. *Genetic Testing, 8*(1), 31–43.

Spencer, K., Spencer, C. E., Power, M., Dawson, C., & Nicolaides, K. H. (2003). Screening for chromosomal abnormalities in the first trimester using ultrasound and maternal serum biochemistry in a one-stop clinic: A review of three years prospective experience. *BJOG: An International Journal of Obstetrics & Gynaecology, 110*(3), 281–286.

Stainton, T. (2003). Identity, difference and the ethical politics of prenatal testing. *Journal of Intellectual Disability Research, 47*(7), 533–539.

Suther, S., & Kiros, G. E. (2009). Barriers to the use of genetic testing: A study of racial and ethnic disparities. *Genetics in Medicine, 11*(9), 655.

Thornton, P. L., Kieffer, E. C., Salabarría-Peña, Y., Odoms-Young, A., Willis, S. K., Kim, H., & Salinas, M. A. (2006). Weight, diet, and physical activity-related beliefs and practices among pregnant and postpartum Latino women: The role of social support. *Maternal and Child Health Journal, 10*(1), 95–104.

Tracy, S. J. (2013). *Qualitative research methods: Collecting evidence, crafting analysis, communicating impact.* Hoboken, NJ: John Wiley & Sons.

PART 4

Engaging Borders: Intercultural Complexity, Identity Politics, and Advocacy

CHAPTER TEN

Health in the Margins: Cultural Borders in Contestation

BY MOHAN J. DUTTA AND SATVEER KAUR-GILL

The body performs health in complex and contested ways, shaped by cultural dynamics, understandings, and interpretations (Airhihenbuwa, 1995). Typically read through the dominant ideologies of health, the constitution of the healthful body is often biomedically driven, and situated within the materiality of structures (Dutta, 2008). The dominant systems of knowing and understanding health act as the borders of what can and cannot constitute health meanings; these borders simultaneously reify and reproduce the structures that constitute the terrains of social organizing. The healthful body is described through a singular lens of normative health understandings and behaviors. Migrant health is often understood through the lens of the host culture, ignoring social, cultural and political economy of migrant life; more specifically for migrants that are constructed for exclusion and temporariness within the borders of the host country. The margins represent these exclusions, where the omission of cultural voices renders impossible alternative readings of what can constitute health meanings (Dutta, 2012). Whose voices are erased from contributing to dominant health narratives? How are these voices erased from dominant health organizing? These critical questions are the starting point for generating alternative health knowledge that remains in the margins of health meanings.

We work through the context of Singapore, a global economy projected as a model of Asian development, sustainability, and digital transformation. Singapore, as a model of the "Asian turn," depicts the ways in which Asia emerges in the global neoliberal order and its imaginaries of the future. Singapore positions itself as a milieu of development in Asia with the "intellectual, material, and symbolic source of neoliberal Asian imagination projected on the global imaginary as the crossroads of the Asian turn" (Dutta & Kaur-Gill, 2018, p. 4068) and the imaginations of model migration and its exportation to the world (Dutta & Kaur-Gill, 2018). Yet, unskilled migrant work in Singapore continues to be a site of exploitation. Ripe conditions structurally embedded in the policies of hire and management, contribute to the exploitation of unskilled migrant workers, specifically migrant domestic workers and migrant construction workers that come from paupered spaces of South East Asia and South Asia. The flexible labor regulations in the hire of migrant workers, tied to the organizing of labor around transnational capitalistic ideas of unregulated labor have created conditions that pay workers poorly and accord little protection to their labor (Escobar, 2012). The neoliberal system of organizing labor in extensible ways, coupled with global migration have systematically created precarious conditions for laborers that partake in unskilled work (Escobar, 2003), impacting how workers come to discuss their health outcomes while acting as temporary migrants (Dutta & Kaur, 2016). In adopting the case study in Singapore, where a significant portion of migrant workers are unskilled workers and working in conditions of precarity, our ethnographic exploration of worker conditions and health are discussed in the context of how precarious work is fashioned through mechanisms of control, surveillance, and the state work of temporariness in their lived experiences as workers. Temporariness is connected with the kind of labor one is hired to perform. For foreign domestic workers (FDWs) and foreign construction workers (FCWs) in Singapore, the temporariness of labor "reflects liability to variation or the ability to be changed" (Boersma, 2018, p. 5). This state of temporariness as a lived experience for the marginalized migrant worker is a starting point in mapping out precarity in labor, impacting health vulnerabilities.

Migrant Labor

Labor mobility across geographic borders is not a contemporary phenomenon. Yet, the manifestation of work conditions for those that conduct work in informal economies such as domestic work (Anderson, 2000; Dutta et al., 2018) or work that is typically considered "dirty, dangerous, and difficult (3D)" such as construction work (Kaur, Tan, & Dutta, 2016), continue to emulate conditions that reflect indicators of both modern-day slavery and elements of human trafficking (Parreñas, 2001;

Yea, 2018). Workers from both these categories share common narratives. Dusk to dawn labor, conditions of indenture, isolation, and confinement, vulnerabilities to abuse, limited or marginal health and informational access are some of the many indicators of poor employment conditions, with indicators fitting into markers of modern-day enslavement and the trafficking of labor (Yea & Chok, 2018; Yeoh, Baey, Platt, & Wee, 2017). The construction of the unregulated market with limited state interference, coined as the neoliberal system of organizing labor (Saad-Filho & Johnston, 2005) is best a communicative inversion by states that ignore the problem of poor work conditions that are exacerbated precisely because of unregulated markets that maximally extract profits from workers, while limitedly providing for proper work conditions (Dutta, 2017b). Communicative inversions refer to how communicative acts of equality are displayed, when in fact it presents the very obverse of the material realities of the situation (Dutta, 2015). The exploitation of migrant workers in Singapore is reproduced through a plethora of communicative inversions carried out by the state. This chapter seeks to interrogate these communicative inversions of health that enable the marginalization of unskilled migrant workers in Singapore and disrupt these inversions through the activist insertion of migrant voices. Worker voices shared in this chapter have been changed to protect their identities.

The Singapore migration model privileges certain types of migrants known as expatriates while leaving unskilled migrants such as FDWs and FCWs to the fringes of Singapore society (Yeoh, 2006). They are regulated, surveilled and managed through temporary visa programs. Singapore also continues not to ratify with the Domestic Workers Convention, 2011 (No. 189), an international convention that protects the interest of domestic workers, outlining the conditions for decent employment in the field of domestic work (Paul, 2017). It is important to recognize that the exploitation of unskilled migrant workers begins structurally when they arrive and are immediately labeled as a particular type of migrant. This label both discursively and materially immediately relegates them to the margins of the local space (Dutta & Kaur, 2018). The labeling of the worker as an FCW or FDW has become a marker of marginalizing discourse, where the attribution of *maids* for FDWs (Yeoh & Huang, 1998) is often classed and raced. By nature of being identified as a *maid*, already complicates their struggle of negotiating space both public and private. Similarly, the use of the term *banglas* on FCWs in the local context is fashioned in derogatory ways, racializing construction work. The class prejudice, as well as the racial prejudice, is "clearly at work in shaping the spatial politics of exclusion in the city" (Yeoh et al., 2017, p. 645). A key aspect of the social shaping of workers lives as migrants in Singapore is in the hiring policies structured for its temporariness. Ong and Yeoh (2013) explain that discriminatory experiences of workers by locals "reflect a 'use-and-discard' sentiment among the general population who want foreign workers to do the work that citizens shun, but at the same time wish that these workers could be erased from the landscape" (p. 94).

In short, it is through these multiple erasures built into the system of hire that migrant worker voices remain absent in how dominant discourse comes to shape their lived experiences as workers in the nation-state. In recovering these absences, the ethnographic study sought to uncover the narratives of workers through dialogic openings that create opportunities for workers to recover these erasures through their own storied descriptions of what it means to embody the experience of a migrant worker in Singapore.

Narratives of Marginal Bodies

The narratives of Jamal, a construction worker, and Julie, a domestic worker articulate the lived experiences of feeling everyday enslavement in their lived experiences as migrant workers. Consider Jamal who arrives in Singapore from Bangladesh as a construction worker. He borrows a sum of money to travel to Singapore for work. Upon employment, he pays a significant sum of money back to the agents by whom he has been recruited. This system of being bonded, because of having to pay back debts for employment, leaves Jamal continually stressed. He, therefore, partakes in overtime work that pays him a slightly better wage, sometimes working 12 to 16-hour shifts on the job. A few months into his job stint, the hard labor takes a toll on his body and mind, but he continues working to pay the debt back in the next six months. On an unfortunate afternoon, he is injured in a construction accident, while conducting dangerous construction work. His employer sends him to a clinic that is informally known to send injured construction workers back to work quickly. This doctor then writes Jamal a two-day medical leave certificate and sends him back to work. Over time, his broken leg from the previous incident intensifies. He then seeks assistance from his employer to take him to the hospital. The employer refuses to do so. Jamal who speaks limited English is unable to locate the information he requires to seek proper assistance. Instead, the next day a gang of men that work for his employer surround him and threaten him. They ask him to pack his belongings and take him to the airport. The employer in sum sees no more value in keeping Jamal, cancels his contract, and sends him back home. To ensure that he does not report the injury or seek compensation for the injury, the worksite hires runners to threaten and intimidate him. They also ensure to take him to the airport so that he will not run away. This is not just Jamal's story, but Amir, Malik, and Feroz who have all faced similar situations when they had become injured on the job and were considered liabilities for their employers. Malik describes the ordeal of waiting for medical help when he was injured,

> when those fell on me, and then broke my leg immediately, even my boot was broken and turned upside down … No, I was lying on floor after accident, nobody cares, everyone is working, I was crying in pain …

When the interviewer probed further to understand how he moved forward with receiving medical help, Malik shared:

> Yes, then supervisors were also working, I told them send me to hospital, they don't respond, he told boss will come and send me to hospital, long time passed but boss didn't come, there were some workers from another company who were there, they told me to call police, call the ambulance, otherwise your legs situation will be worse, then they call ambulance from my mobile and I was sent to hospital.

It was only till intervention by workers from a separate company that were not precarious in this context because they belonged to a different company, were able to render help to Malik by using his mobile phone to call for medical services.

In not too different ways, Julie arrives in Singapore with a recruitment debt. These debts can range from approximately 1000 to 2000 USD, with monthly salaries that range from a mere 200 to 500 USD. Julie pays the agency monies without receiving any form of documentation. She elaborates,

> A lot of money. Actually I still have the receipt. The medical … is thirty five. Also for the … Before I live in Philippines also, I still give them another thousand. No receipt, no sign. I just give the money. Another thousand, it's worth three fifty Singapore dollars.

Julie describes the burden of debt on the domestic worker to partake in this labor. The mental stress caused by taking on debts begins even before Julie arrives to her place of work. When she arrives, she conducts domestic work in her place of employment but also lives there. Her employers work her from six in the morning to midnight, sometimes waking her up in the wee of hours of the night for meals, massages, or other requests. Julie has not received eight hours of rest since she arrived. During the day, she accidentally dozes off and is chided. Her employer pays her 10 USD on Sundays so that she is unable to take her off day. She also has no room to herself and sleeps in the kitchen on a thin wooden mat. She is only allowed to use her mobile phone during her rest times. The employment conditions are too difficult, and she asks her employers for an off day and higher pay. Two days later, she is asked to pack her things and is dropped off to the airport. The employer has cancelled her contract and blacklisted her with the Ministry of Manpower Singapore, claiming that she had stolen their items.

The stories of Jamal and Julie are not unfamiliar. During our ethnographic encounters with over 150 disenfranchised foreign domestic and construction workers, narratives of work conditions emulating precarity for the purposes of maximum profiteering are commonplace. It is within worker narratives that we locate health meanings as intimately tied to labor. There is a particularity to labor amplifying health vulnerabilities in the case of foreign workers in Singapore. Through culture-centered interrogations of health (Dutta & Jamil, 2013), we locate alternative rationalities in the articulation of health meanings by communities living at the margins of state borders, incorporated into the sites of state-capitalist reproduction as precarious labor, and simultaneously excluded from possibilities of articulation. The state renders these bodies invisible from dominant health ideologies, where invisibility here is constituted by the absence of communicative infrastructures, materially and symbolically. These material and symbolic erasures are tied to the technologies deployed by the state to discipline the subaltern body, to extract labor from it, and to erase it from opportunities of access to fundamental resources of health. Technologies such as cameras placed on worksites and surveillance instruments such as machine-based check-ins, on one hand, count the body of the migrant worker, and on the other hand, erase the voice that emerges from the body. The voiceless body of the migrant worker is thus produced through an array of techniques of technology, disciplining the worker and simultaneously producing the threat of being deported. Spaces where migrant workers spend their leisure times on their day off (Sunday) are flooded with lights and cameras, marked by high volumes of police presence to discipline migrant bodies. Narratives of alcohol consumption and rioting workers are deployed as justifications for control, simultaneously obfuscating the structural contexts of migrant work.

FCWs express health as feeling safe and the ability to access clean, fresh, and nutritious food at worksites, where physical labor is performed for an average of 12 hours a day, while FDWs construct health meanings as having access to their fundamental rights as human beings. As simply put by Eka, "… health for me is eating enough food, it is not really enough food, proper food, and then having enough sleep also." Health meanings constructed by FDWs include not being physical, verbally or mentally threatened, having access to their income, rest hours, health insurance and privacy (Dutta et al., 2017). However, these notions of health remain shadowed, while the state constructs health for migrants as a body that is disease free. By adopting health security as a measure of inclusion to its borders, the state determines what sorts of migrant bodies can perform in the economy that will not threaten or compromise productivity and efficiency. Thus, migrant health is read parochially by the state, measured using rigid guidelines on what sorts of healthful bodies are acceptable within its borders. The reading of health by the state for migrants include the clearance of four types of infectious diseases, for FCWs and FDWs that include tuberculosis, HIV, syphilis, and malaria (Ministry of Manpower, 2018a). For the state, migrant health is read through the organizing of health using a neoliberal model that determines what sorts of bodies are most productive and efficient, materially produced as vastly underpaid labor to be exploited by capitalist formations (Dutta, 2016). For FDWs the state's reading of a healthy domestic worker is one that does not fall pregnant during her time as a domestic worker in Singapore, surveillance through compulsory six-monthly medical examinations (Ministry of Manpower, 2018b). A pregnant FDW threatens how the state manages what kinds of economic citizens it accepts within its borders as permanent or temporary. Techniques of surveillance such as mandatory medical exams discipline the FDW body, ensuring that her body is compliant with the pregnancy regimens imposed by the state.

Our extended ethnographic work with low-skilled migrant workers through the framework of the culture-centered approach (CCA) that seeks to build migrant worker-driven activist and advocacy interventions serves to shift the meanings of health by anchoring worker voices. Drawing upon participant observations, in-depth interviews, and collaborations with advisory groups of migrant workers conducted over six years, we note that migrant bodies offer alternative rationalities of health that invert the dominant axioms of health understandings. The body emerges through the voices of migrant workers, articulated through the communicative infrastructures built through our ongoing academic-activist collaboration. The dominant axioms of understandings often limit and disable a structural critique of health and healing; these erasures by the structure are disrupted through embodied voices. The placing of the body in the discursive space emerges as an interruption of the material structures of migrant worker exploitation that fundamentally threaten migrant health. Through the presence of the body and its experiences, neoliberal discourses of migration and mobility are disrupted.

Voice, Body and Structural Transformation

Fundamentally, the starting point of the CCA is in centering voice. It takes a critical approach to how voice is incorporated into theory, practice, and research (Dutta, 2014). In working with vulnerable communities, the CCA recognizes the peripheral ways in which marginal voices remain erased from dominant agendas while at the same time voices form the basis of state's narration of engagement. In the case of foreign workers in Singapore, this is shaped by the immobilities and invisibilities of workers in the city-state (Yeoh & Huang, 2010; Yeoh et al., 2017). Despite, mobility for locating labor across geographic boundaries, workers face significant barriers in achieving mobility within the spaces where they conduct their labor. They are rendered to the margins of the space, socially, politically, economically. In the chapter, the stories of worker plights highlight the invisibilities and immobilities faced. These immobilities structurally limit workers from accessing health resources required. In centering worker voices, the limitations of structure, articulated agentically (voice), informs how the health marginalities and threats surface while conducting transnational labor. The key assumption on voice in the CCA is that it must be foregrounded for the purposes of challenging the taken for granted dominant assumptions, by probing into where the silences and erasures remain (Pal, 2014). Voice in the CCA is therefore theorized as a dialogic opportunity, with 'listening' acting as a central methodological tenet for detailing alternative imaginations of knowledge building vis a vis subaltern life. It is particularly interested in the project of recovering the erased subject, by centering the voice of those that remain unengaged by dominant systems. The centrality of voice is built into the methodological positions of the CCA that include ethnographic interviews, in-depth interviews, participant observations, focus groups, advisory board sessions, and empowerment focused workshops (Dutta & Kaur-Gill, 2018). The starting point of the project on foreign workers in Singapore centers on setting up methodological infrastructures that allow for voices of workers to remain central in the interventions. The narratives from the interviews shed salient light on the structural limitations of what it entails being a migrant worker, setting up the context for understanding precarious work. During the advisory board sessions, key issues on health as labor were thematized. During these sessions, the vulnerabilities of the worker body as systematically in a state of marginality remained consistent.

Voices of Precarity

Domestic workers in sharing the context of their fractured lives from poor employment situations described how health meanings were tied to having worker rights respected. This triggered workers to design a health intervention focusing on employers and the state to consider the fundamental rights of workers as requiring respect and dignity. The health of workers was constructed as having attention paid to labor rights by structural actors. For example, Julie who was overworked by her employers emphasized that health meant having eight hours of rest a day and having a proper private space to sleep. For Maria, health meant being paid for her work.

Mary had gone without pay for two entire years. She was illegally deployed by her employers to work both at their home and as a food deliverer, without ever receiving her pay. She describes the ordeal:

> 30 minutes, if you are fast. But I have so much to deliver, so many styropore (referring to the boxes in which one delivers food), you have to be fast. I bring so many of them: styro, plastics. My entire arms are full. Then I still have to go to Paramount. Especially when the bars start to open at night, oh my, it's so difficult. And there's always massive orders ... you don't even get to eat even if you're very hungry. Because there are so many orders, then we have to bring the plates too.

During the time spent with her, Mary's story had become national news for having worked without pay for such an extended period of time (Heng, 2014). She left without recovering a penny from her employers and was owed an approximate of 6500 USD. During her time at the non-governmental organization, where she was seeking redress for her plight, Mary suffered multiple health threats and emergencies. The precarity of health conditions of domestic workers is tied to the precarity of the labor. For Maria, had her basic rights been respected which entailed getting paid and on time, her health outcomes would remain relatively unthreatened.

In other narratives, feelings of entrapment, isolation, and physical abuse led to detrimental health vulnerabilities with some narratives involving extreme health risks when removing themselves from poor employment conditions. Ika, a domestic worker from the Philippines was never allowed to leave her employer's home. She was confined and made to work in a harsh environment that entailed getting hit by her employer every now and then. She was also provided very little food by her employers that led to her losing an extensive amount of weight in a short period of time. As the hunger pangs escalated, Ika retrieved a piece of fish from the refrigerator. Her employers found out and beat her brutally, including making her drink bleach. She could not tolerate the abuse any longer and decided to escape. She climbed out of the window from the high rise building she lived in. In the process, she fell and was badly injured. The trauma of the experience, along with all of the right violations done unto her by her employers had serious health outcomes. Despite surviving the fall, Ika continues to relive the trauma on the perils of her labor experience. For Ika, therefore, health meanings again centered on the need for her basic rights to access food, to not be physically abused, or confined. In stringing these narratives together, we hear domestic workers articulating health as a domestic worker as compromised by work conditions. Work conditions are the catalyst to vulnerable health.

The complex health vulnerabilities take form in the orchestration of labor as a domestic worker. June arrives in Singapore as a migrant domestic worker. By nature of her employment, she will only receive a temporary visa, subject to her contract. There are strict regulations to her employment by the state, ensuring that June will have to leave the country upon contract expiry. Her employer typically has the power to decide her leaving, even if her contract is for two years. Her employer also has the power to blacklist June with the Ministry of Manpower Singapore, limiting her entry back to Singapore again. Furthermore, June's health screening in Singapore before employment entails a pregnancy screening and a six-monthly medical assessment for the purposes of detecting sexually transmitted disease and to verify any impending pregnancy. Work permit and contract will be canceled if June fails the assessments. From their very arrival, migrant domestic workers like June are managed for the purposes of surveilling their bodies to ensure temporariness is constantly communicated to them during their stay. The intentions of surveilling are deeply rooted in the state's model on the type of migrants that can belong to its borders and those that cannot. In the early phases of the extended ethnographies conducted with domestic workers, we spoke to the caseworkers that assist distressed domestic workers. Bon, the caseworker had described a domestic worker that had failed the health assessments three times. She had already taken on a loan for the job and could not pass the test. Bon described,

> And another thing is that ... when the domestic worker they come here, they have to go for testing. When one of a domestic worker die, because he (referring to she) failed to pass the testing for three times, and that meant when she go back to Indonesia, she might have to pay the loan. Ar.. so, she cannot take it. She hanged herself in the agency.

Bon essentially describes the conditions of indenture structured in domestic work that can have severe repercussions on the lives and health of workers. Health precarities of workers are deeply interconnected with the hiring practices of the labor. Here, Bon describes how domestic workers already materially dispossessed are made to take up loans just to access work. In the Philippines for example, rife under-employment that cut across gender lines, push women to find work beyond local geographies (Paul, 2015). In order to find work overseas, domestic workers take on loans to be placed with an agency. Despite, taking on loans, work may not always be guaranteed or the temporariness of work as an FDW where they can be deported on the disposition of their employers pushes domestic workers to be in a constant state of health precarity. In the case of Bon's narrative of the FDW, the fear of debts to find domestic work became a significant health threat. Stories like these remain erased in the dominant health understandings of migrant health. Unskilled foreign workers in Singapore remain excluded, are social and politically disenfranchised, resulting in a lack of attention to their health needs. Labor policies for unskilled migrant workers structurally set the tone for exploitative labor conditions. In this chapter, we discuss the inclusions and exclusions of migrant bodies that are relegated to the peripheries of the state. In interrogating these divisions, a culture, structure, agency reading of migrant bodies in Singapore on health, brings to light migratory labor as an impediment in achieving good health. Health for unskilled migrant workers in Singapore is a contested space. With civil society actors internationally and nationally championing for better health and social rights of these workers (Yeoh & Annadhurai, 2008), the state continues to communicatively erase rights violations and exploitative conditions of workers.

FCWs faced their own sets of challenges in trying to reduce health vulnerabilities. A key health theme among FCWs related to managing worksite injuries in their health agendas. Consider Khan, a foreign construction worker earning less than 500 USD a month. He works at the construction site from seven in the morning. With limited material resources and poor wage structure, health access remains limited. Khan, therefore, normalizes the worksite injuries encountered. He shares:

> That's usual. Good health is the precondition of work ... In Singapore not any company give the opportunity for a good treatment. Just when there is someone got an accident then they had to manage the treatment. Even some worker got a little sick but they had to join work.

A key aspect of construction worker discourse is in normalizing worksite injury as being part of the risk when taking up the job. Khan, for example, shares that he knew that he could be severely injured as a construction worker in Singapore. He understands the risk, but material deprivation back home takes precedence and therefore, he cannot be risk-averse. He discusses many times that safety regulations at his worksite are incomprehensible as they are not in a language he understands. The manufacturing of communicative infrastructures on workplace safety was rendered inaccessible This had left him injured a few times. In Dutta (2017a), ethnographic interviews with FCWs in Singapore included life-threatening injuries including life and death situations, situating these life-threatening injuries amid the everyday deprivations back home. Storied descriptions of severe worksite injuries, such as workers being killed by a cement mixer or having parts of their body broken from construction accidents (Dutta, 2017b). Health for FCWs is therefore shaped by vulnerabilities being part of the everyday experience of a worker. The health dangers in the everyday life of a construction worker meant securing the health and wellness for their materially deprived families back home. Familial access to materiality was grounded in their health meanings. and at the same time shaping the need to participate in dangerous work.

In considering the narratives reproduced in this chapter on the health of migrants as belonging to a contested space, a structural reading of hire situates the ecology of exploitation encased in labor management by the state. From debt engagement to worksite risks, health precarities exists within the ecology of the labor. Migrant workers are exposed to a myriad of health risks that are built into the system, including conditions of accommodation, deprivation of food and fresh food as well as rest hours, worksite health precarities, both mental and physical, are all part of the contextual embodiment of being a migrant worker in the local space. Therefore, in transforming the context of health precarities in migrant work, the underlying structures that threaten health is a point of evaluation. Domestic worker centered health promotion interventions adopting a culture-centered frame, focused on telling stories about the hidden structures that create health immobilities for workers such as creating rights focused documentary titled "Respect Our Rights" scripted co-constructively with domestic workers. Integral to the development of the documentary was the centering of domestic worker voices. Rights focused discourse was framed in the intervention material that focused on getting structural actors to respect the basic rights of workers. These rights were in fact spelled out in their contractual clauses. When they faced violations in their place of employment, domestic workers wanted swift justice by state actors. During a post-interview with one of the participants of our ethnographic work, she summed up conceptually how the rights focused health intervention impacted her health understandings, "I want only justice for us … to say what their rights are, to defend this, respect our rights." Health is centered in communicatively protecting and safeguarding fundamental rights. Health is "I can say what is my right" shared by a participant after the culture-centered health intervention.

Based on this insight, our dominant abstractions of health are questioned, and new entry points are created for building an alternative understanding of migrant health. Anchoring the CCA as a basis for voice creates spaces for cultural scripts to detail health agendas for health promotion within community spaces (Dutta & Basnyat, 2008). Ideas of structural transformation are located within these cultural scripts. Structural transformation of migrant work and health are in the culture, structure, agency reading of the stories of migrant work and precarity. In doing so, centering voices becomes an act for disrupting the hegemonic imaginations of migrant labor as achieving better health and social outcomes and achieving mobility. The idea that globalization processes and neoliberal reforms generate even and equal health outcomes are disrupted when narratives of worker abuse are generated and become scripts for intervention and change. The assembly of mobility and movement within the ideology of the neoliberal landscape is communicated as emancipating the impoverished South. Dutta and Kaur-Gill (2018) position that the neoliberal landscape that champions migration, "obfuscates the structural disenfranchisements that constitute and necessitate movements of the poor among sites of precarity" (p. 4069). Sites of precarity are created by conditions of labor structured by neoliberal reforms and globalization processes, threatening the health of the raced, classed, and gendered migrant body that remains in contestation. By paying attention to lived experiences of those in the peripheries, the material realities of low-skilled migrants in Singapore are unpacked, where interpretations on the benefits of labor deregulation are in fact far from the material outcomes of being a labourer in this context. The deployment of such communicative inversions that sell the broader sense-making of neoliberalism as bringing about benefits of globalization for economic growth is disclosed. It is in the very state structuring of neoliberal policies as reflected in the storied descriptions of material realities by workers that reveal the vicious cycle of economic abuse faced by migrant workers.

References

Airhihenbuwa, C. O. (1995). *Health and culture: Beyond the western paradigm.* California, CA: Sage Publications

Anderson, B. (2000). *Doing the dirty work: The global politics of domestic labour.* London, UK: Zed Books.

Boersma, M. (2018). Filipina domestic workers in Hong Kong: Between permanence and temporariness in everyday life. *Current Sociology.* https://doi.org/10.1177/0011392118792928

Dutta, M. J. (2008). *Communicating health: A culture-centered approach.* Cambridge, UK: Polity.

Dutta, M. J. (2012). *Voices of resistance: Communication and social change.* Purdue University Press.

Dutta, M. J. (2014). A culture-centered approach to listening: Voices of social change. *International Journal of Listening, 28*(2), 67–81. doi: 10.1080/10904018.2014.876266

Dutta, M. J. (2015). *Neoliberal health organizing: Communication, meaning, and politics.* Walnut Creek, CA: Left Coast Press.

Dutta, M. J. (2016). *Neoliberal health organizing: Communication, meaning, and politics.* New York, United States: Routledge.

Dutta, M. J. (2017a). 3 negotiating health on dirty jobs. In *Culture, migration, and health communication in a global context.* New York, NY: Routledge. 45–59.

Dutta, M. J. (2017b). Migration and health in the construction industry: Culturally centering voices of Bangladeshi workers in Singapore. *International Journal of Environmental Research and Public Health, 14*(2), 132. doi: 10.3390/ijerph14020132

Dutta, M. J., & Basnyat, I. (2008). The case of the radio communication project in Nepal: A culture-centered rejoinder. *Health Education & Behavior, 35*(4), 459–460. doi: 10.1177/1090198106296009

Dutta, M. J., Comer, S., Teo, D., Luk, P., Lee, M., Zapata, D., … Kaur, S. (2017). Health meanings among foreign domestic workers in Singapore: A culture-centered approach. *Health Communication*, *33*(5), 1–10.

Dutta, M. J., Comer, S., Teo, D., Luk, P., Lee, M., Zapata, D., … & Kaur, S. (2018). Health meanings among foreign domestic workers in Singapore: A culture-centered approach. *Health Communication*, *33*(5), 643–652.

Dutta, M. J., & Jamil, R. (2013). Health at the margins of migration: Culture-Centered co-constructions among Bangladeshi immigrants. *Health Communication*, *28*(2), 170–182. https://doi.org/10.1080/10410236.2012.666956

Dutta, M., & Kaur, S. (2016). Communicating the culture-centered approach to health disparities. In J. Yamasaki, P. Geist-Martin, & B. Sharf (Eds.), *Storied health and illness: Communicating personal, cultural and political complexities*. Illinois: Waveland Press.

Dutta, M. J., & Kaur-Gill, S. (2018). Precarities of migrant work in Singapore: Migration, (im) mobility, and neoliberal Governmentality. *International Journal of Communication*, *12*(2018), 4066–4084. Retrieved from https://ijoc.org/index.php/ijoc/article/view/9664

Escobar, P. (2003). The new labor market: The effects of the neoliberal experiment in Chile. *Latin American Perspectives*, *30*(5), 70–78.

Escobar, A. (2012). *Encountering development: The making and unmaking of the third world*. Princeton, NJ: Princeton University Press.

Heng, L. (2014, July 23). Maid worked 17-hour-days for two years with no pay. Retrieved from https://www.tnp.sg/news/others/maid-worked-17-hour-days-two-years-no-pay

Kaur, S., Tan, N., & Dutta, M. J. (2016). Media, migration and politics: The coverage of the Little India riot in the Straits Times in Singapore. *Journal of Creative Communications*, *11*(1), 27–43. doi: 10.1177/0973258616630214

Ministry of Manpower. (2018a). *Medical examination for foreign worker*. Retreived from http://www.mom.gov.sg/passes-and-permits/work-permit-for-foreign-worker/sector-specificrules/medical-examination

Ministry of Manpower. (2018b). *Employer's guide: Foreign domestic worker*. Retrieved from http://www.mom.gov.sg/passes-and-permits/work-permit-for-foreigndomestic-worker/employers-guide

Ong, F. C., & Yeoh, B. S. (2013). The place of migrant workers in Singapore: Between state multiracialism and everyday (Un) cosmopolitanisms. In L. A.Eng, , F. L. Collins, & B. S. A. Yeoh (Eds.), *Migration and diversity in Asian contexts* (pp. 83–106). Singapore, SG: Institute of Southeast Asian Studies.

Pal, M. (2014). Solidarity with subaltern organizing: The Singur movement in India. *The Electronic Journal of Communication*, *24*(3–4). http://www.cios.org/EJCPUBLIC/024/3/024343.html

Parreñas, R. S. (2001). *Servants of globalization: Women, migration, and domestic work*. Stanford, CA: Stanford University Press.

Paul, A. M. (2015). Negotiating migration, performing gender. *Social Forces*, *94*(1), 271–293. doi: 10.1093/sf/sov049

Paul, A. M. (2017). *Multinational maids: Stepwise migration in a global labor market*. United Kingdom: Cambridge University Press.

Saad-Filho, A., & Johnston, D. (2005). *Neoliberalism: A critical reader*. Illinois: University of Chicago Press.

Yea, S. (2018). Helping from home: Singaporean youth volunteers with migrant-rights and human-trafficking NGOs in Singapore. *The Geographical Journal*, *184*(2), 169–178. doi: 10.1111/geoj.12221

Yea, S., & Chok, S. (2018). Unfreedom unbound: Developing a cumulative approach to understanding unfree labour in Singapore. *Work, Employment and Society*, *32*(5), 925–941. doi: 10.1177/0950017017738956

Yeoh, B. S. A., & Annadhurai, K. (2008). Civil society action and the creation of "transformative" spaces for migrant domestic workers in Singapore. *Women's Studies*, *37*(5), 548–569. doi: 10.1080/00497870802165550

Yeoh, B. S. A., Baey, G., Platt, M., & Wee, K. (2017). Bangladeshi construction workers and the politics of (im)mobility in Singapore. *City*, *21*(5), 641–649. doi: 10.1080/13604813.2017.1374786

Yeoh, B. S. A., & Huang, S. (1998). Negotiating public space: Strategies and styles of migrant female domestic workers in Singapore. *Urban Studies*, *35*(3), 583–602. doi: 10.1080/0042098984925

Yeoh, B. S. A., & Huang, S. (2010). Transnational domestic workers and the negotiation of mobility and work practices in Singapore's home-spaces. *Mobilities*, *5*(2), 219. doi: 10.1080/17450101003665036

Yeoh, B. S. (2006). Bifurcated labour: The unequal incorporation of transmigrants in Singapore. *Tijdschrift voor economische en sociale geografie*, *97*(1), 26–37.

CHAPTER ELEVEN

Transcending In/Visibility, Isolation, and Stigma: Trauma-Informed and Culture-Centric Mental Health

BY LARA LENGEL, ADAM SMIDI, AND NORA ABDUL-AZIZ

The Arabic word, *majnūn* [مجنون] is often attributed to the canonic love story of Qays and Layla. Originating in 5th century Persia, then reworked seven centuries later by Persian poet Nizami Ganjavi, the literary work traces Qays Ibn al-Mulawwah's unrelentless passion for Layla and his histrionic efforts to woo her, leading community members to call him *Majnūn* [madman] or crazy. Etymologically, *majnūn* relates *al-junun* [madness] and to the notion of possession or insanity; *jinna* is "possessed by a *jinn*" [demon]; *jen-zadegi* [possession by *jinns*, or demons] (Hassouneh & Kulwicki, 2009). *Majnūn* and *al-junūn* are terms that continue to be used in Muslim socities to indicate any kind of impairment of judgment or behavior disorder (Al-Issa, 2000a, 2000b); it can also be interpreted as "fool" (Hassouneh & Kulwicki, 2009).

Words Matter

Words matter. In subject matter fraught with stigma, words matter immensely. Given that continued use of *majnūn* and *al-junūn* from the medieval age to the present is just one example of many, the rhetoric of mental health across all cultures has contributed to a "millennia-long history of social exclusion and prejudices" (Rössler, 2016, p. 1250). In the monumental work, *Madness and Civilization: A*

History of Insanity in the Age of Reason, Foucault (1965) notes "Language is the first and last structure of madness, its constituent form; on language are based all the cycles in which madness articulates its nature" (p. 100). The rhetoric within the Foucauldian "first and last structure of madness" is also vast, including a copious lexicon, in the English language alone, of at least 250 words to describe persons with mental illness (Rose, Thornicroft, Pinfold, & Kassam, 2007), including, but certainly not limited to, "lunatics," "nutcases," "nutters," "psychos," and "whack jobs." Conversely, and perplexingly, the words "insane" and "crazy" are now so embedded in ableist discourse to mean anything from surprising to extreme, unbelievable, or absurd that the widespread use of these words not only offer lazy substitutes for more precise adjectives, but trivialize mental illness.

As words matter, so too, does communicating about mental health conditions in order to reduce the stigma associated with them. This is not a simple task. There is widespread critique of the five editions of the American Psychiatric Association's Diagnostic and Statistical Manual. There are ongoing debates on appropriate language. One term is "persons with mental illness," commonly used in the psychiatric and psychological fields (Granello & Gibbs, 2016), and by the World Health Organization, and the UN (United Nations High Commissioner for Human Rights, 2002, p. 1). However, critics (see, for instance, Charland, 2013; Hopkins & Battin, 2004; Murphy, 2013; Ratcliff, 2008) argue that term emphasizes a medicalization model through the inclusion of the word illness. Mental health advocates, such as the UK Mental Health Foundation (MHF) (n.d.), recommend terms such as "psychiatric survivors" to highlight that "some forms of psychiatric treatment can be considered abusive. They campaign for reforms to end the powers of psychiatry to compulsorily detain people and enforce treatment against their will" (para. 11). Words we prefer include, first, "persons with experience of mental and emotional distress" (MHF, n.d., para. 9), second, neuroatypical, a term acknowledging that many persons with experience of mental and emotional distress have IQs in the ranges of very superior intelligent and genius, and, third, "experts by/through experience," which, according to the Mental Health Foundation (n.d.), is a "more recently coined term used by the recovery movement to draw attention to expertise of people with mental health problems gained through personal experience, and their expertise about their own mental health" (para. 6). "Experts by/through experience" is particularly salient as it highlights a collaborative, "participative approach to treatment that acknowledges a person's ability to work in partnership with the mental health services and professionals towards their own recovery" (MHF, n.d., para. 6). Further, it acknowledges that such experts have often spent great time, energy and effort to gain expertise, self-reflexivity, and awareness about deeply misunderstood phenomena. We support language that situates mental and emotional distress as not a weakness, not a phenomenon to be feared, but rather an experience appropriate to the unhealthy, harmful, and traumatic conditions of the world, and that encourages people to seek support, talk about their pain, and feel less alone.

Awareness and Advocacy Matters

Attention to the discursive, cultural, and socio-political nuances of mental health, particularly in critical intercultural, health, or organizational communication studies, is sparse. Further, while there is large body of research on Muslim mental health (See, for instance, Arsha & Falconier, 2019; Byrne, Mustafa, & Miah, 2017; Hamsyah & Subandi, 2017; Keshavarzi & Haque, 2013; Rondelez, Bracke, Roets, Vandekinderen, & Bracke, 2018; Stuart & Ward, 2018), our exhaustive literature review, to date, attests that only one study emerges from the field of communication (Ahmad, Harrison, & Davies, 2008). We aim to fill this gap by focusing on Muslim faith-based health organizations' efforts to address the complex intersecting and marginalizing tendencies of mental illness, xenophobia, dis/misinformation-based anti-Muslim Othering, and the emotional trauma of Islamophobia.

The study builds on our broader research program (See Lengel & Holdsworth, 2015; Lengel & Smidi, 2019; Smidi & Lengel, 2017) on cultural and politico-religious discourses about Muslims, and on interfaith dialogue, organizational support, and community building to examine the health impact of incendiary and divisive rhetoric and the "manufacture of paranoia toward Islam" (George, 2016, p. 146) on Muslim American citizens, Arab American citizens, and Arabs and Muslims worldwide.[1] Given that religious Othering is, as Alexander and colleagues (2014) argue, a "most pressing intercultural urgency" (p. 38), we aim to gain insight into the ways in which religion-based nationalism and ethnocentrism perpetuate social, cultural, political inequality which, in turn, can exacerbate depression, anxiety, and other mental health concerns.

Critiquing Ableism Matters

Highlighting community-centered approaches to culture and health is central to our analysis. Community-centered approaches to mental health within faith communities, however, pose unique challenges, as many religious communities' leaders and organizational members maintain conflicting attitudes and beliefs about mental health, perceptions of the existence and treatability of mental illness, and how to address neuroatypical persons and persons with experience of mental and emotional distress (Caplan, 2019; Iheanacho, Stefanovics, & Ezeanolue, 2018). This is not surprising given that "public knowledge about mental disorders has received significantly less attention than physical diseases" (Neely-Fairbanks, Rojas-Guyler, Nabors, & Bamjo, 2018, p. 162).

In addition, the privilege of ability has resulted in a lack of understanding about mental illness and emotional distress. In response, the National Alliance on Mental Illness "encourages collaboration among the mental health community and other community-based organizations" to development and implement culturally relevant and community responsive mental healthcare services and programs (Greenstein, 2016, para. 2). In addition, collaboration across community organizations, healthcare organizations, and scholars is needed. Deanna Fassett (2013) makes the case for critical intercultural communication studies on dis/ability:

> While disability studies exists as a field in its own right, and while communication scholars may certainly benefit from these researchers' insights, critical intercultural communication scholars are, by their commitment to interrogating and better understanding the intersections of identity, power and culture as constituted in communication, well-positioned to engage in analysis of how we become (and come to see ourselves as) ability-privileged or disabled. (p. 461)

In our own efforts to become and come to see ourselves as ability-privileged or disabled, it is important to situate ourselves in this project. Our self-reflexivity, positionality, lived experience, and professional expertise inform our study. I (Lara) have been an advocate for mental illness awareness for years, but even more so since I lost my brother to death by suicide in 2012. As a result of this family trauma, I have been increasingly open to disclosing my own experiences with major depressive disorder, and the accompanying challenges of performing the "normalcy," efficiency, and efficacy required of modernity. I (Nora) am a Syrian-French-American pre-med undergraduate student who aims to specialize in surgery and serve in *Médecins Sans Frontières* in the Middle East and North Africa. I have witnessed the collective trauma in the Syrian diaspora and see the emotional toll it has taken on my community. I (Adam) am an advocate for and leader within the Muslim American community, involved in assisting newly settled Syrian refugees and their negotiation of social exclusions and the post-traumatic impact of the vast death and destruction they and their families have experienced in Syria and the U.S. I also serve as a volunteer and board member of numerous Muslim faith-based organizations, and have personally assisted many Muslim Americans in acquiring employment, transportation, and housing through collaboration within Arab and Muslim communities' professional network across the bi-state region which has been a safe refuge for Arab and Muslim immigrants for over a century. Together, we bring our own commitment to community, our specific scholarly areas of critical intercultural communication, organizational communication, and culturally sensitive healthcare to analyze the discourses and perceptions of mental illness, particularly as these discourses and perceptions intersect with identity, culture, and power.

This type of interdisciplinary collaboration across intercultural and organizational communication and medicine is crucial for knowledge and praxis. Fassett (2010) notes that "research in intercultural communication has been shaped by a general lack of attention to ability and disability as cultural" (p. 463). Psychiatric dis/ability as a cultural phenomenon has even less attention in communication and healthcare research. In his study on the production of the psychiatric subject, Roberts (2005) suggests mental illness "is not to be understood as some universal, a temporal and objective category" (p. 37). Rather, he draws from Foucault who historicizes the concept of mental illness as emerging at "a certain historical point within a particular culture and society, and 'politicises' that concept by showing how its emergence was inextricably bound to the political concerns, norms and values of that culture and society" (p. 37). For our analysis, we situate mental illness, generally, and the Muslim psychiatric subject, specifically, in the "current historically and politically constituted psychiatric discourses" (p. 37) emerging since 9/11 and, more recently, the increase of anti-Muslim and anti-immigrant sentiment in the U.S. since 2015.

In addition, we analyze the "truths" that emerge from the intersection of identity, culture, and power. Foucault (1977) argues that the "truth" of a cultural group is formed by "the ensemble of rules according to which the true and the false are separated and specific effects of power attached to the true" (p. 132). Here we can apply the "truth"/myth of danger to persons with mental illness and to Muslims. The perception that persons with mental illness are necessarily a danger to their communities is widely held historically and globally (See, for instance, Saleem & Anderson, 2013; Stuart, 2003).[2] In various global and cultural contexts, media framing of persons with mental illness grotesquely perpetuates the public perception that they are violent (McGinty, Webster, Jarlenski & Barry, 2014). For instance, in a study of violent attacks on German public figures by persons suffering from psychiatric disorders (Angermeyer & Matschinger, 1995), German citizens surveyed reported a significant increase in desire to maintain social distance from persons with mental illness immediately following reported acts of violence; such social distance never returned to previous levels. The attacks also increased public perception of persons with mental illness as dangerous, violent, and unpredictable.

Understanding Intersectional Oppression Matters

The widespread essentializing equating of Muslim with terrorist (See, for instance, Morey & Yaqin, 2011; Semati, 2011; Shaw, 2012; Sultan, 2016) makes critiquing the dominant cultural perceptions linking mental illness and violence of paramount importance to this analysis. So, too, is intersectionality, which can be described as how "various socially created categories interact in intersecting systems of oppression" (Turner, 2011, p. 345). The unique complexity of perceptions, challenges, and discrimination experienced by Muslims and other marginalized communities is illustrative of intersectional oppression, multiple systems of marginalization emerging from "formations of complex social inequalities" (p. 345).

The health disparities experienced by underserved and marginalized communities illuminate the "complexity of the intertwined influence of both individual social positioning and institutional stratification on health" (Gkiouleka, Huijts, Beckfield, & Bambra, 2018, p. 92). As evidenced throughout this volume, there are a number of underserved communities in healthcare, resulting from intersectional oppressions and structural socioeconomic and other forms of inequity and injustice. These communities, argue Padela, Killawi, Forman, DeMonner, and Heisler (2012), "receive a lower quality healthcare in part due to the inadequate assessment of, and cultural adaptations to meet, their culturally informed healthcare needs" (p. 708).

Given the struggles inherent in negotiating intersectional oppression, Arab Americans and Muslims in the U.S. "may be among those with the highest risk for stress related mental disorders" (Hassouneh & Kubwicki, 2009, p. 196). Further, given this risk, much more scholarship and praxis is needed to assess the impact of these intersectional oppressions, most notably Islamophobia, on the mental health of Arab Americans and Muslims. The lack of research is particularly remarkable given the vast increase of hate crimes and incidents of bias against Muslims in the United States, which, after increasing by 1,600% from 2000 to 2001, surged another 67% from 2014 to 2015, and has continued to rise since (Abu-Ras & Suarez, 2009; Disha, Cavendish, & King, 2011; ProPublica, 2017; Southern Poverty Law Center, 2017). Globally, the rise in hate crimes and bias incidents has increased substantially. For instance, between 2012 and 2015, there was a 253% increase in hate crimes targeting Muslims in Canada (Minsky, 2017).

Mis/Perceptions and Multiple Layers of Othering

> "The first thing they asked was if I was going to be violent."
>
> —Kadijah Faaria Aleema Islam (2017), a person living with Bipolar Disorder, while seeking entry to a Muslim shelter (para. 5).

Despite the widespread research confirming that persons with mental illness are far more likely to be victims than perpetrators of violence (See, for instance, Harvard

Health Publishing, 2011; Latalova, Kamaradova, & Prasko, 2014; Stuart, 2003), the misperceptions that mental illnesses necessarily leads to violence remains strong across both dominant and marginalized cultural communities.

The mis/perceptions and multiple layers of Othering manifest in the complex juxtaposition of violence/submission for Muslims, particularly for Muslim women. Along with Muslims being "among those with the highest risk for stress related mental disorders," Hassouneh and Kubwicki (2009) suggest "Arab-American Muslim women, in particular, have experienced high levels of post-911 trauma, acculturative stress, and stress related to perceived discrimination" (p. 196).

Denial and Isolation

> "I felt entirely alone … I prayed, fasted, performed my duties with enthusiasm and was still suffering."
>
> — Noura Rockwood (2013)

In a rare personal narrative about Bipolar Disorder and the isolation experienced after disclosing her illness those closest to her, Rockwood (2013), in the independent media organization, *The Islamic Monthly,* recalls:

> [After] I was finally able to confide in them that I had been diagnosed with depression[,] I expected my friends to wrap their arms around me and offer religious and worldly advice on how to feel better, supported and to never feel alone again. Instead, they withdrew from me, regarded me with suspicion, and told me just to pray more. I felt rejected, and blamed. Was it that God was angry with me? Did God love me at all, and this question was the source of my pain? This reaction caused a new framework to develop in my mind, one in which suffering was punishment, neglect and anger—something I somehow deserved. (para 4)

Further exacerbating isolation is the unwillingness of many highly religious Muslims to maintain a close relationship with, have their children interact with, or consider marrying a person with mental illness (Tabassum, Macaskill, & Ahmad, 2000), as well as the preference for psychiatric hospitals to be isolated and distant from communities (Al-Adawi et al., 2002; Coker, 2005).

Many very religious followers of not only of Islam, but other religions including Christianity, tend to resist understanding the complex range of origins of mental illness from chemical imbalances in one's brain to surviving trauma. In a study of American Muslims' perceptions of mental illness (Padela, Killawi, Forman, DeMonner, & Heisler, 2012), respondents stated Allah is "the ultimate doctor. He is the one that brought down the disease. He is the one that brought down the cure" and "healing is in the hand of God before everything" (p. 849).

The impact of denial within oneself and, usually more salient, within family and community (Jozaghi, Asadullah, & Azim Dahya, 2016) is exacerbated by stigma which leads to people not disclosing an emotional disorder or neuroatypical condition to family, friends, and community. The stigmatization renders mental illness invisible, hidden within families, or hidden within the individual suffering, who feels that s/he will receive no support if the suffering is disclosed. S/he suffers alone, and feels punished by God.

Stigmatization and Shame

> "… similar to other faith groups, the main challenge would be stigma associated with mental health … many people go without seeking counseling or any other support because of stigma."
>
> —Kameelah Rashad, Muslim Chaplain at the University of Pennsylvania on the challenges facing Muslim Americans (cited in Blumberg, 2015, paras. 5 & 6)

It distresses us to know that despite the preponderance of research addressing the stigma associated with mental health generally (See Anglin, Link, & Phelan, 2006; McGinty, Goldman, Pescosolido, & Barry, 2018) and, specifically, in Islam (See, for instance, Abdullah, & Brown, 2011; Abu-Ras & Abu-Bader, 2008; Abu-Ras, Gheith, & Cournos, 2008; Abdullah & Brown, 2011; Ali, Milstein, & Marzuk, 2005; Al-Krenawi & Graham, 2000; Gary, 2005; Hamdan, 2009; Phillips & Lauterbach, 2017; Trein, 2017), stigmatization surrounding mental illness continues to prevail. Many Muslims who suffer from anxiety, depression, and other mental illness often refrain from seeking help, out of fear they will be viewed as lacking in faith. The complex nature of stigmatization of mental illness in the Muslim community emerges from intersectional oppression, what researchers have termed "double stigma" to denote the layered nature of stigmatization both within and outside cultural groups, primarily emerging from religious and ethnocentric Othering (Ciftci, Jones, and Corrigan, 2012, p. 17). Stigma is also salient in the nomenclature of violence: Is the perpetrator of a mass shooting a "terrorist" or "lone wolf"? Whiteness allows for a "troubled youth" of Anglo-American heritage to commit a mass murder at his school; he is not labelled a "terrorist." White men and boys who commit mass murder in the U.S. are often identified as mentally ill, while any Middle Eastern or Islamic appearing individual is ascribed the identity of terrorist.

Although, as Bryant (2018) of the National Alliance on Mental Illness argues, one "can't 'pray away' a mental health condition," highly religious individuals and groups tend to mistrust mental health professionals and the disciplines of psychology and psychiatry (para. 9; See Aloud & Rathur, 2009; Breakey, 2001; Jozaghi, Asadullah, & Dayha, 2016; Pilkington, Msetfi, & Watson, 2012; Smietana, 2013). This is particularly the case among Evangelical Christians and African Americans, as well as in the Muslim community where some Imams and community leaders see the mental health profession as "anti-religious," fraught with "materialistic or reductionistic approaches to understanding the human condition," and undermining of Muslim beliefs (Breakey, 2001, p. 62). Highly religious Muslims believe mental illness is a punishment or test from God (Abu-Ras, Gheith, & Cournos, 2008; Padella et al., 2012; Rassoll, 2000). God decides who should have an illness; He is the only one who can provide a cure. This point of view is echoed by many religious followers who are unfamiliar with medical research of illnesses broadly, and the neurobiological nuances of mental illnesses specifically. In the mindset that only God can heal, they refuse, or may be entirely unaware of, available medication, therapy, and treatment.

The stigma associated with mental illness for most marginalized communities, Muslims included, is "the overwhelming hindrance to accessing services, due to the strong cultural prohibitions on exposing any personal or family matters to outsiders" (Youssef & Deane, 2006, p. 43). Nevertheless, it is important to note the diversity across Muslim communities. Urban, highly educated Muslims, particularly those living in the west, are less prone to stigma and shame. By contrast, for example, the majority of Muslim families in rural areas and in more remote locations such as Ethiopia have experienced stigma due to having a relative with a mental illness (Shibre et al., 2001). Given that mental illness is viewed by highly religious Muslims as a hazard to the social well-being of their communities, persons living with mental illness should be hidden, segregated from "normal" society, made invisible through isolation and silence within families and communities. Further, psychiatric facilities are often situated out of view, segregated from community centers. The stigma does, however, span urban and rural areas and cultural contexts. Given the widespread nature of stigma, some health organizations have centered in their missions on stigma reduction. For instance, the Muslim Wellness Foundation (2017) aims to reduce stigma surrounding mental disorders by providing education to Muslims through an "interdisciplinary, spiritually relevant, community based public health approach to wellness" (para. 1). The Foundation has noted a particular need among African American Muslims as, historically, the Black community has been reluctant to discuss mental illness. Lack of knowledge leads some members of this community to believe it is a sign of failure, could harm their career and relationships, and something about which to be ashamed. Mental Health America (2007) reported 63% of African Americans believe depression is a personal weakness, while 31% of consider depression a health condition. Religious leaders, often seen as a cultural bridge between healthcare providers and those seeking care, are often the initial responders to mental health concerns among Black cultural communities (Mantovani, Pizzolati, & Edge, 2017).

Collective and Community Trauma

Some of the most pressing trauma-inducing events facing marginalized communities—the discrimination against Arab Americans, Muslims, and Muslim-appearing persons since the tragic events of September 11, 2001, the devasting impact of gun violence that has most negatively impacted black and brown communities, the rise in police killings of unarmed African American men, and the detainment of undocumented Central American immigrants—all have the capacity to incite collective and community trauma.

Collective trauma, defined as "the impact of adversity on relationships in families, communities and societies at large. This includes natural and human-caused disasters as well as the cumulative effects of poverty, oppression, illness, and displacement" (Saul, 2014, p. 3). It is important to note that "Catastrophic events often open up or exacerbate previously existing fault lines of racism and other forms of discrimination, social and economic inequalities, and prior historical traumas" (p. 4). Such collective trauma, which has also been referred to as cultural or community trauma, results from psychosocial ramifications of intergenerational histories of trauma from chattel slavery, and its accompanying legacies, including but not limited to, 19th and 20th century lynchings to contemporary racial profiling (See Akbar, 1996; Alexander et al., 2004; Cross, 1998; Eyerman, 2001; Overstreet & Braun, 2000; Williams & Williams-Morris, 2000). The Muslim Wellness Foundation (2017) argues, "In a post-9/11, post-Ferguson Trump era, it is important to discuss the cultural and spiritual resilience which have strengthened Black Muslims through the centuries and the strategies/coping mechanisms that will serve the community as they face new threats to their collective well-being" (para. 7) (See, also, Tynes, Willis, Stewart & Hamilton, 2019; Weinstein, Wolin, & Rose, 2014).

The cumulative impact of collective or community trauma has been documented in the forced migration and continued oppression of Native American First Nations (Brave Heart, 1999; Brave Heart & DeBruyn, 1998; Jervis & AI-SUPERPFP Team, 2009), the Holocaust (Hirschberger, 2018; Lazar, Litvak-Hirsch, & Chaitin, 2008), and genocides and wartime sexual violence in Rwanda and Bosnia and Herzegovina (Klain, 1998; Lengel, 2018). Vital efforts to advance the conceptualization and treatment of community trauma has emerged from Bosnia and Herzegovina where, at the University Clinical Center at the University of Tuzla, work on community-wide post-traumatic stress in the Balkans, Libya, and Syria where civilians have been particularly impacted by armed conflict in densely populous urban areas.

Intergenerational, collective and community trauma has also been found. Given that more than 70 years have spanned since the systematic genocide of European Jewry, Roma/Sinti and other groups by the Nazis during World War II, the most robust analyses of intergenerational, community-wide trauma has centered around survivors of the Holocaust (See, for instance, Adelman, 1995; Bar-On, 1995; Davidson, 1980; Doucet & Rovers, 2010; Fromm, 2012; Gottschalk, 2003; Kellerman, 2001; Kidron, 2003; Shrira, Menashe, & Bensimon, 2019). The intergenerational traumatic impact of more recent genocides have also been analyzed. For instance, Hasanović, Pajeviić and Sinanonviić (2017) found, of the groups of children displaced by the Bosnian war, those who experienced the highest severity level of post-traumatic stress were the children who witnessed the massacre of the entire male population at Srebrenica. The researchers argue, "It is important that both military and political decision makers should bear in mind the potential mental health consequences of war, especially in urban areas. It is the responsibility of the medical profession to educate decision makers to consider the consequences of exposure of children to war trauma" (p. 24).

Trauma-Informed Interfaith and Community-Centered Support

Given the isolation that oppressed groups experiencing emotional or mental distress tend to experience, community support and efforts are vital. The unity of the Muslim people is represented in Islam by the concept of the *ummah* [community], which is a crucial virtue in Islam and central to Muslim identity. In chapter 3 verse 103 of the *Qu'ran*, God calls to believers to "hold firmly to the rope of God all together and do not become divided. And remember the favor of God upon you—when you were enemies and He brought your hearts together and you became, by His favor, brothers [and sisters]" (*Qu'ran* 3:103, Oxford World's Classics edition). Originating as a unifying classification to describe the community of the Muslim faithful in the Arabian Peninsula during the life of Muhammad, *ummah* in contemporary contexts represents the communal unity of all Muslims globally. In Islamic teachings on egalitarianism, all Muslims are equal, regardless of culture, nationality, ethnicity, or gender.[3] According to Islamic scripture, human differences between Muslims are natural, but the unity of God's word is equally supreme to all.

In order to achieve true unity in the *ummah*, loving for one's brother or sister exactly as one would love for oneself, and treating all equally regardless of ethnicity, nation, gender, cultural heritage, religion, or the status of their mental health upholds a unified *ummah*. The notion of ummah has recently been expanded and extended to an interfaith *ummah* in the face of horrific hate- and bias-centric mass murders at, first, the Tree of Life Synagogue in Pittsburgh on October 27, 2018, and, second, Masjid Al Nour and the Linwood Islamic Center in Christchurch, New Zealand on March 15, 2019. The mass murderer of worshippers at the Tree of Life Synagogue (cited in Dale, Lauer, & Breed, 2018) was overheard telling Pittsburgh police that "all these Jews need to die" (para. 3).

Immediately after the murder of 11 worshippers at Tree of Life, the deadliest attack on persons of Jewish heritage in U.S. history, through numerous faith-based organizations and crowdfunding campaigns, Muslims throughout the U.S. hosted vigils and raised over $1.4 million (USD) for survivors and family members of those murdered. In Pittsburgh, Muslims stood guard outside synagogues throughout the city and suburbs, attended mourning services, and walked alongside Jewish brothers and sisters who felt unsafe (Khan, 2019). In turn, after the worst mass murder in New Zealand's history by a self-identified white nationalist whose live-streamed shootings in Christchurch left 50 Muslim worshippers dead and scores more injured, Jewish communities immediately reciprocated by leading vigils for their Muslim brothers and sisters and raising funds for the New Zealand Attack Emergency Relief Fund. The Board of the Jewish Federation of Greater Pittsburgh took a leading role in the fund-raising efforts. Meryl Ainsman, Chair of the Board (cited in Khan, 2019), said "Unfortunately we are all too familiar with the devastating effect a mass shooting has on a faith community" (para. 4).

Even the most neurotypical person could be emotionally harmed by such a tragedy. Dr. Anthony Charuvastra (2017) of the Seleni Institute, a nonprofit organization whose mission is to "destigmatize and transform mental health and wellness by addressing real-life issues that challenge the emotional health of women, men, and their families", notes, "After national tragedies—such as the horrific shooting in Las Vegas, we all walk around in a world that is materially the same for the majority of us, but psychologically altered. There are still the same necessary routines: making breakfast, getting the kids to school, riding the train to work. Yet we go through them with a new awareness of our own vulnerability" (para. 1). Chauvratra (2017, October 2) reports, "In climates of fear, life is more difficult for everyone. Children have trouble playing, adults can find it hard to be loving, and workers are distracted by their anxieties. Fear is bad for body and soul. So, even though it may seem difficult, finding a way to feel safe is essential to living well and thriving" (para. 2).

In their study on the Mental Health Consequences of Mass Shootings, Lowe and Galea (2017) cite the growing body of research indicating that "exposure to assaultive violence, or learning that a close friend or loved one has faced such exposure, is associated with an increased incidence of a range of negative mental health outcomes, among them posttraumatic stress disorder (PTSD) and major depression" (p. 62; see, also, Fergus, Rabenhorst, Orcutt, & Valentiner, 2011; Hughes et al., 2011; Smith, Abeyta, Hughes, & Jones, 2014). Analyzing the impact of the Christchurch murders, Pardeep Singh Kaleka (2019), a former police officer and Licensed Therapist specializing in trauma-informed approaches to treat survivors of violence, notes "We now understand that communities can suffer similar symptomatology when not even directly affected by the violence themselves. Simply put, the threat of violence to marginalized in-group members can have severe consequences on quality of life concerns for those group members who identify or empathize with that group" (para. 15). Kaleka, whose father, Satwant Singh Kaleka, was killed in the August 5th, 2012 Sikh Temple of Wisconsin murders, co-founded the organization Serve 2 Unite with Arno Michaelis, a former white supremacist who instrumental in start a gang in the late 1980s that produced the Sikh Temple Wisconsin murderer. He argues, "Communal trauma has to be at the foundation of our public health model to ensure that systems have sufficient knowledge bases to inform their practices" (Kaleka, Michaelis, & Fisher, 2018, para. 16).

Community Trauma and Rising Hated

> "There was a river of blood coming out of the mosque, and that's a scene that you don't forget."
>
> — Paul Bennett, Christchurch New Zealand ambulance officer, fighting back tears as he described arriving at the Al Noor Mosque (cited in Fifield, 2019, para. 7)

> "None of us are doing OK right now."
>
> — Sara Mansour, two days after the mass murders in Christchurch (2019, para. 7)

Community or collective trauma can span within and across religious and ethnic communities. In fact, early on in the development of discipline of traumatology, Caruth (1995) suggested "trauma itself may provide the very link between cultures" (p. 11). In Christchurch, for instance, a city of fewer than

400,000 people, many first responders, like Paul Bennett, and educators have some kind of connection to the victims. Iona Holsted of the New Zealand Ministry of Education (cited in Fifield, 2019) noted that twenty schools and three early-childhood centers in Christchurch had direct connections to victims. She also stated "We have traumatic incident teams. They comprise people who are trained in understanding the impacts of trauma, and how behaviors change after trauma" (para. 11).

In their study, Contradicting Borderlessness: Tracing the Mediated Circuits of Ethnonationalist Belonging, Newsom and Lengel (in press) note, "While certainly the worst case of a hate and bias-centric mass murder, Christchurch is merely one example of the singling out of Muslims in the immigration 'crisis,' that has been increasingly at the center of the strategic narrative of Othering in Europe and the U.S. and, since March 15, Australia and New Zealand." In this narrative of Othering, specific groups are singled out by white ethno-nationalists, with racist and ethnocentric, inaccurate perceptions of the alleged cultural alienation, lawlessness, militancy, and, in the case of Muslims, an erroneous appraisals of their hyper-involvement in terrorism (Newsom & Lengel, in press). Media coverage further enflames this process, as these events related to the strategic narrative of Othering, particularly in center-right to extreme-right media organizations, are deemed "newsworthy" or, at least, able to increase ratings due to their emotionally-charged content (Newsom & Lengel, in press). Further, viral media spreads specifically targeted, niche audience-tailored coverage of so-called "hot button" topics and incidents through biased and polarized media. "Mediated processes, especially through interactive social and digital media platforms, both encourage the legitimization of polarized biases, and generate community-building among those espousing similar values, ethics, and concerns" (Newsom & Lengel, in press; see, also, Gat, 2017).

While the oxymoronic white transnationalist/nationalist community expands and extends its "religious racialization" (Schaefer, 2015, p. 128) efforts to dehumanize and demonize all they perceive to be "The Other," interfaith community building between Jewish and Muslim groups is central to both groups' well-being. Such interfaith community building is particularly relevant when considering community trauma (Fromm, 2012). With *ummah* at the center of their missions, an increasing number of nonprofit Muslim faith-based health organizations are advocating for destigmatizing mental illness and seeking help, enhanced community outreach, research, and education both within and outside the Muslim community. Elsewhere (Abdul-Aziz, 2019), we highlight efforts of Muslim faith-based health organizations worldwide addressing the stigma of mental illness in Muslim communities, the distressing in/visibility of Muslims particularly since

9/11, and the ongoing trauma of being blamed, erroneously, for the tragic events on that day (Lengel, in press).

Intercultural Healthcare Literacy Matters

In their study published in *Journal of Muslim Mental Health*, Khan and Ecklund (2012) argue, "Greater understanding of non-Muslims' affective response to Muslims might be useful information to guide efforts to reduce prejudice toward this group" (para. 5). We concur and we return to our positionalities as scholars. My [Adam's] family story includes coming to terms with my sister who experienced the effects of having to keep turmoil inside herself. When I (Adam) was younger and still living in my parents' home, one of my sisters was having a difficult time in her marriage and divorced her husband. My mother was devastated: "How will the community view my daughter now?" "Who will ever marry a divorced woman that has a son?" When my sister moved back to the family home it was very difficult for everyone to deal with all of the questions being asked. I do not recall anyone, including myself, asking my sister how *she* was feeling. Instead nothing was discussed, all kept secret. Over time, my sister bought into the narrative surrounding her, thinking perhaps the sadness she lived with *was* all her fault, and she was no longer good enough to be part of the community. At times she would be my loving sister, and at many other times I saw a much different side—an angry and depressed woman, convinced her own family and entire community around her viewed her as a second-class citizen.

At the time I didn't understand my sister's atypical behavior. Nor did my extended family and friends who felt sorry for her, and called her situation unfortunate. If she was physically ill our family would not have hesitated a second before seeking medical care, yet her mental struggles were kept quiet and secretive. One reason for this is that our community views mental illness as a sign of weakness in faith or a lack of appreciation in God (See Aghababaei & Tabik, 2013). Even my sister herself would not have the courage to come to terms with and openly admit her depression. She knew what the response around her would be: "Maybe you are not praying enough?" and "You should be thankful to God for everything you have." I remember my mother at one point being certain that an evil eye had been cast on her, and that she had been possessed by *jinn*–a supernatural being. Had my sister and family been given knowledge and understanding about mental health sooner, perhaps we would have better understood what she was going through and how to treat it. The first step is to normalize the idea of mental health in the Muslim community. Local Imams of mosques should receive mental health training sessions, and speak about it during the sermons. While many Muslims today would not imagine reaching out to their local Islamic center for help with mental struggles, they could potentially serve as a useful arena to bring religious leaders and mental health professionals to the same table. Medical professionals, too, must do their part. The study of medicine often leaves little to no room for spirituality, for belief in a higher healing power. If practitioners are not sensitive and culturally competent they can quickly lose patient rapport and trust.

Reflecting on my own spiritual growth, I [Adam] now see where religious and community leaders could play a central role in reducing stigma of mental illness. Almost every Friday of the last couple decades, at my community *masjid* [place of prayer], I attended *Yawm al-jum'ah* [Day of Assembly] for *ṣalāt* [prayer]; not once did I hear a *shaykh* [elderly religious leader] or *imam* give a *khutbah* [sermon] that even mentioned mental illness. Any time the topic was brought up among peers, we all assumed that it could only happen to people with weak *iman* [faith], as we had been taught that good, faith practicing, Allah loving Muslims could never experience such negative symptoms. While my experience has taught me that *iman*, *'aylah* [family], *ummah* [community], and other factors can certainly help support persons with mental illness, these central foci of Muslim life cannot guarantee mental health. My experience is not unique; Shaykh Dr. Yasir Qadhi (2018), who has studied Islamic scholarship at some of the most rigorous seminaries in the world, says "I studied many disciplines and read hundreds of works, never once was the subject of counseling even covered" (para. 6). He emphasizes "the average shaykh is not qualified to be a family counselor, or a marriage therapist, or a psychiatrist who can help you with OCD, depression, mental trauma, sexual abuse, substance abuse, or a host of other issues that they haven't been trained to deal with" (para. 8).

Religious leaders like Dr. Qadhi are beginning to shift the narrative surrounding mental illness—from stigmatized to a real health condition, no different than a physical illness that requires one to seek help from a trained healthcare professional. Their centrality in communities will have a robust impact to help community members to understand that no one needs to feel shame and isolation if they need help, and that seeking guidance from healthcare practitioners is not only appropriate but necessary. They can also encourage dialogue to enhance understanding within and across communities and, aligned with the Islamic concept of *khidmak-e-kkalq* [service to community/service to humanity], to encourage increased community service and outreach to help reduce the stigma, shame and isolation associated with mental illness.

Finally, as evidenced throughout this volume, more attention and effort is needed to reduce health disparities, more attention to the words practitioners and community members use to identity neuroatypical persons with experience of mental and emotional distress, and more effort to communicate about mental health in order to reduce bias, stigma, and shame. These concerns, in addition to religious Othering, are intercultural urgencies (Alexander et al., 2014) that require insight into the ways in which the intersectional nature of Othering perpetuates social, cultural, political inequality which, in turn, can exacerbate depression, anxiety, and other mental health concerns. Such intercultural urgencies reinforce the need to highlight health organizational, cultural, and spiritual efforts to support mental health of marginalized communities and to advocate engagement with increasingly diverse communities, and to foster culturally-specific, culturally-inclusive, and culturally-inspired approaches to benefit health and well-being.

Notes

1. We concur with Edwards (2014) who argues, "religion is poorly understood and often defined in imprecise or fallacious ways, resulting in inaccurate references to and representations" of both Islam and Muslims, and suggests "U.S. public discourse has often collapsed the religion and ethnicity through the logics of Orientalism" (para. 1) (See, also, Said, 1978).
2. It is important to note that the *Qu'ran*, being the written word of God in the Arabic language, cannot be definitively translated because doing so might lead to the loss of God's literal meaning. Since the bulk of Muslims are non-Arabs, the Arabic language is a unifying conveyor of Islamic teachings and prayers.
3. See Abdul-Aziz, Smidi & Lengel (forthcoming) for an analysis of Muslim mental health organizations including The Institute of Muslim Mental Health, Muslims Thrive, ICNA Relief, Muslims for Humanity, The Family and Youth Institute, and the Syrian Telemental Health Network.

References

Abdul-Aziz, N. (2019, February). Overcoming the stigma of mental illness in Muslim communities and increasing the need for cultural competence to address health inequities. Presented at the Fourth Annual Undergraduate Symposium on Diversity, Bowling Green State University, Bowling Green, Ohio, February 15, 2019.

Abdullah, T., & Brown, T. L. (2011). Mental illness stigma and ethnocultural beliefs, values, and norms: An integrative review. *Clinical Psychology Review*, *31*, 934–948.

Abu-Ras, W., Gheith, A., & Cournos, F. (2008). The imam's role in mental health promotion: A study at 22 mosques in New York City's Muslim Community. *Journal of Muslim Mental Health*, *3*, 155–176.

Abu-Ras, W. M., & Suarez, Z. E. (2009). Muslim men and women's perception of discrimination, hate crimes, and PTSD symptoms post 9/11. *Traumatology*, *15*, 48–63.

Academic Autistic Spectrum Partnership in Research and Education. (2015). AASPIRE's use of "person first language." Retrieved from http://aaspire.org/?p=about&c=language

Adelman, A. (1995). Traumatic memory and the intergenerational transmission of Holocaust narratives. *The Psychoanalytic Study of the Child*, *50*(1), 343–367.

Aghababaei, N., & Tabik, M. T. (2013). Gratitude and mental health: Differences between religious and general gratitude in a Muslim context. *Mental Health, Religion & Culture*, *16*(8), 761–766.

Ahmad, M. K., Harrison, J., & Davies, C. L. (2008). Cultural sensitivity in health promotion program: Islamic persuasive communication. Paper presented at the 6th International Conference on Communication and Mass Media, May 19–22, 2008, Athens, Greece.

Al-Adawi, S., Dorvlo, A. S., Al-Ismaily, S. S., Al-Ghafry, D. A., Al-Salmi, A., Burke, D. T., … Chand, S. P. (2002). Perception of and attitude towards mental illness in Oman. *The International Journal of Social Psychiatry*, *48*(4), 305–317.

Al-Issa, I. (2000a). Mental illness in medieval Islamic society. In I. Al-Issa (Ed.), *Al-Junūn: Mental illness in the Islamic world* (pp. 43–70). Madison, CT: International Universities Press.

Al-Issa, I. (2000b). Religion and psychopathology. In I. Al-Issa (Ed.), *Al-Junūn: Mental illness in the Islamic world* (pp. 3–41). Madison, CT: International Universities Press.

Al-Krenawi, A., & Graham, J. R. (2000). Culturally sensitive social work practice with Arab clients in mental health settings. *Health and Social Work*, *25*, 9–22.

Alexander, B. K., Arasaratnam, L. A., Durham, A., Flores, L., Leeds-Hurwitz, W., Mendoza, S. L., & Halualani, R. (2014). Identifying key intercultural urgencies, issues, and challenges in today's world: Connecting our scholarship to dynamic contexts and historic moments. *Journal of International and Intercultural Communication*, 7(1), 38–67.

Ali, O. M., Milstein, G., & Marzuk, P. M. (2005). The imam's role in meeting the counseling needs of Muslim communities in the United States. *Psychiatric Services*, *56*, 2–5.

Aloud, N., & Rathur, A. (2009). Factors affecting attitudes towards seeking and using formal mental health and psychological services among Arab Muslim populations. *Journal of Muslim Mental Health*, *4*, 79–103.

American Psychiatric Association. (n.d.). Words matter: Reporting on mental health conditions. Retrieved from https://www.psychiatry.org/newsroom/reporting-on-mental-health-conditions

Angermeyer, M. C., & Matschinger, H. (1995). Violent attacks on public figures by persons suffering from psychiatric disorders. Their effect on the social distance towards the mentally ill. *European Archives of Psychiatry and Clinical Neuroscience*, *245*(3), 159–164.

Anglin, D., Link, B., & Phelan, J. (2006). Racial differences in stigmatizing attitudes toward people with mental illness. *Psychiatric Services*, *57*, 857–862.

Bar-On, D. (1995). *Fear and hope: Three generations of the Holocaust.* Cambridge, MA: Harvard University Press.

Blumberg, A. (2015). 7 questions with Muslim mental health professional Kameelah Rashad. Huffington Post Religion, April 9, 2015. Retrieved from https://www.huffpost.com/entry/muslim-mental-health_n_7018428

Brave Heart, M. (1999). Gender differences in the historical trauma response among the Lakota. *Journal of Health and Social Policy, 10*, 1–21.

Brave Heart, M., & DeBruyn, L. (1998). The American Indian holocaust: Healing historical unresolved grief. *American Indian and Alaska Native Mental Health Research, 8*, 56–76.

Breakey, W. R. (2001). Psychiatry, spirituality and religion. *International Review of Psychiatry, 13*(2), 61–66.

Byrne, A., Mustafa, S., & Miah, I. Q. (2017). Working together to break the 'circles of fear' between Muslim communities and mental health services. *Psychoanalytic Psychotherapy, 31*(4), 393–400.

Caplan, S. (2019). Intersection of cultural and religious beliefs about mental health: Latinos in the faith-based-setting. *Hispanic Health Care International, 17*(1), 4–10.

Caruth, C. (1995). Trauma and experience: Introduction. In C. Caruth (Ed.), *Trauma: Explorations in memory.* Baltimore, MD: Johns Hopkins University Press.

Charland, L. C. (2013). Why psychiatry should fear medicalization. In K. W. M. Fulford et al. (Eds.), *The Oxford handbook of philosophy and psychiatry* (pp. 159–174). Oxford, England: Oxford University Press.

Chauvratra, A. (2017, October 2). Managing anxiety after a mass shooting. *Psychology Today.* Retrieved from https://www.psychologytoday.com/us/blog/women-s-mental-health-matters/201710/managing-anxiety-after-mass-shooting

Ciftci, A., Jones, N., & Corrigan, P. W. (2012). Mental health stigma in the Muslim community. *Journal of Muslim Mental Health, 7*(1), 17–32.

Coker, E. M. (2005). Selfhood and social distance: Toward a cultural understanding of psychiatric stigma in Egypt. *Social Science & Medicine, 61*, 920–930.

Cross, W. E. (1998). Black psychological functioning and the legacy of slavery. In Y. Danieli (Ed.), *International handbook of multigenerational legacies of trauma* (pp. 387–400). New York, NY: Plenum Press.

Dale, M., Lauer, C., & Breed, A. G. (2018). "I'm barely breathing": Synagogue survivor recounts terror. Associated Press, October 29, 2018. Retrieved from https://www.apnews.com/017eca5511ec4834b4406ac8c6b5bb13

Davidson, S. (1980). The clinical effects of massive psychic trauma in families of Holocaust survivors. *Journal of Marital and Family Therapy* (January 1980), 11–21.

Disha, I., Cavendish, J. C., & King, R. D. (2011). Historical events and spaces of hate: Hate crimes against Arabs and Muslims in post-9/11 America. *Social Problems, 58*(1), 21–46.

Doucet, M., & Rovers, M. (2010). Generational trauma, attachment, and spiritual/religious interventions. *Journal of Loss and Trauma, 15*(2), 93–105.

Edwards, B.T. (2014). Islam. In B. Burgett & G. Hendler (Eds.), *Keywords for American cultural studies.* New York, NY: New York University Press.

Eyerman, R. (2001). *Cultural trauma: Slavery and the formation of African American identity.* Cambridge, England: Cambridge University Press.

Faaria Aleema Islam, K. (2017). To be Muslim and bipolar–"One time, I told a sister that I was depressed and she told me that depression was from the devil." Retrieved from http://mvslim.com/to-be-muslim-and-bipolar/

Fergus, T. A., Rabenhorst, M. M., Orcutt, H. K., & Valentiner, D. P. (2011). Reactions to trauma research among women recently exposed to a campus shooting. *Journal of Traumatic Stress, 24*, 596–600.

Fifield, A. (2019, March 19). Christchurch, once ravaged by quakes, is re-traumatized by mosque shooting. *Washington Post*. Retrieved from https://www.washingtonpost.com/world/asia_pacific/christchurch-once-ravaged-by-quakes-re-traumatized-by-mosque-shooting/2019/03/19/dad9dafe-49b5-11e9-8cfc-2c5d0999c21e_story.html?noredirect=on&utm_term=.28f9325c0b56

Foucault, M. (1965). *Madness and civilization: A history of insanity in the age of reason*. London, England: Pantheon.

Fromm, M. G. (2012). *Lost in transmission: Studies of trauma across generations*. Abington, Oxon, England: Routledge.

Gary, F. A. (2005). Stigma: Barrier to mental health care among ethnic minorities. *Issues in Mental Health Nursing, 26*, 979–999.

Gat, A. (2017). The other N-word. *Foreign Policy*, April 21, 2017. Retrieved from https://foreignpolicy.com/2017/04/21/the-other-n-word-nationalism-trump-immigration/

Gkiouleka, A., Huijts, T., Beckfield, J., & Bambra, C. (2018). Understanding the micro and macro politics of health: Inequalities, intersectionality & institutions—A research agenda. *Social Science & Medicine, 200*, 92–98.

Gottschalk, S. (2003). Reli(e)ving the past: Emotion work in the Holocaust's second generation. *Symbolic Interaction, 26*, 355–377.

Granello, D. H., & Gibbs, T. A. (2016). The power of language and labels: "The mentally ill" versus "people with mental illnesses." *Journal of Counseling & Development, 94*(1), 31–40.

Greenstein, L. (2016). Community support builds better lives. National Alliance on Mental Illness. Retrieved from https://www.nami.org/Blogs/NAMI-Blog/December-2016/Community-Support-Builds-Better-Lives

Hamdan, A. (2009). Mental health needs of Arab women. *Health Care for Women International, 30*, 595–613.

Hamsyah, F., & Subandi, D. (2017). Dzikir and happiness: A mental health study on an Indonesian Muslim Sufi group. *Journal of Spirituality in Mental Health, 19*(1), 80–94.

Harvard Health Publishing. (2011). Mental illness and violence. *Harvard Mental Health Letter*, January 2011. Retrieved from https://www.health.harvard.edu/newsletter_article/mental-illness-and-violence

Hasanović, M., Pajević, I., & Sinanonvić, O. (2017). Spiritual and religious Islamic perspectives of healing of posttraumatic stress disorder. *Insights on Depression and Anxiety, 1*, 23–29.

Hassouneh, D., & Kubwicki, A. (2009). Family privacy as protection: A qualitative pilot study of mental illness in Arab-American Muslim women. *Research in the Social Scientific Study of Religion, 20*, 195–215.

Hirschberger, G. (2018). Collective trauma and the social construction of meaning. *Frontiers in Psychology, 9*, article 1441, doi: 10.3389/fpsyg.2018.01441

Hopkins, B., & Battin, M. P. (2004). Religion. In J. Radden (Ed.), *The philosophy of psychiatry: A companion* (pp. 312–327). Oxford, England: Oxford University Press.

Hughes, M., Brymer, M., Chiu, W. T., Fairbank, J. A., Jones, R. T., Pynoos, R. S.,... Kessler, R. C. (2011). Posttraumatic stress among students after the shootings at Virginia Tech. *Psychological Trauma: Theory, Research, Practice, and Policy, 3*, 403–411.

Iheanacho, T., Stefanovics, E., & Ezeanolue, E. E. (2018). Clergy's beliefs about mental illness and their perception of its treatability: Experience from a church-based prevention of mother-to-child HIV transmission (PMTCT) trial in Nigeria. *Journal of Religion and Health, 57*(4), 1483–1496.

Jervis, L., & AI-SUPERPFP Team. (2009). Disillusionment, faith, and cultural traumatization on a northern plains reservation. *Traumatology, 15*, 11–22.

Jozaghi, E., Asadullah, M., & Dayha, A. (2016). The role of Muslim faith-based programs in transforming the lives of people suffering with mental health and addiction problems. *Journal of Substance Use, 21*(6), 587–593.

Kaleka, P. (2019). Pardeep Kaleka: Our habituation to mass murder and violence is a bitter soup of inaction. *Milwaukee Independent*, March 29, 2019. Retrieved from http://www.milwaukeeindependent.com/featured/pardeep-kaleka-our-habituation-to-mass-murder-and-violence-is-a-bitter-soup-of-inaction/

Kaleka, P. S., Michaelis, A., & Fisher, R. G. (2018). The gift of our wounds: A Sikh and a former white supremacist find forgiveness after hate. *Serve U Unite.* Retrieved from https://www.giftofourwounds.com/serve2unite/

Kellerman, N. (2001). Transmission of Holocaust trauma: An integrative view. *Psychiatry, 64*, 256–267.

Khan, A. (2019). After Christchurch shooting, Jewish communities share in trauma and healing. *Religion News*, March 18, 2019. Retrieved from https://religionnews.com/2019/03/18/after-christchurch-shooting-jewish-communities-share-in-trauma-and-healing/

Khan, M., & Ecklund, K. (2012). Attitudes toward Muslim Americans Post-9/11. *Journal of Muslim Mental Health*, 7(1). Retrieved from https://quod.lib.umich.edu/j/jmmh/10381607.0007.101/--attitudes-toward-muslim-americans-post-911?rgn=-main;view=fulltext/

Kidron, C. A. (2003). Surviving a distant past: A case study of the cultural construction of trauma descendant identity. *Ethos, 31*, 513–544.

Klain, E. (1998). Intergenerational aspects of conflict in Former Yugoslavia. In Y. Danieli (Ed.), *International handbook of multigenerational legacies of trauma* (pp. 279–295). London, England: Plenum Press.

Latalova, K., Kamaradova, D., & Prasko, J. (2014). Violent victimization of adult patients with severe mental illness: A systematic review. *Neuropsychiatric Disease Treatment, 10*, 1925–1939.

Lazar, A.,Litvak-Hirsch, T., & Chaitin, J. (2008). Between culture and family: Jewish-Israeli young adults relation to the holocaust as a cultural trauma. *Traumatology, 14*, 110–119.

Lengel, L. (in press). Writing the competing first drafts of history: Analysis of UK media coverage of 9/11. In K. Begum (Ed.), *Refracted visions in global media & trauma narratives on 9/11 & terrorism discourses*. London, England: Palgrave.

Lengel, L. (2018). Mediated memory work and resistant remembering of wartime sexual violence, 1992–1995. *Feminist Media Studies, 18*(2), 325–328.

Lengel, L., & Holdsworth, H. (2015). Enacting social change along the cultural identity spectrum: Intercultural identity construction in faith-based community organizations. *Journal of International and Intercultural Communication, 8*(3), 249–267.

Lengel, L., & Smidi, A. (2019). How affect overrides fact: Anti-Muslim politicized rhetoric in the post-truth era. In L. Zhang & C. Clark (Eds.), *Emotion, affect, and rhetorical persuasion in mass communication: Theories and case studies* (pp. 115–130). New York, NY: Routledge.

Lowe, S. R., & Galea, S. (2017). The mental health consequences of mass shootings. *Trauma, Violence & Abuse, 18*(1), 62–82.

Mansour, S. (2019). After the Christchurch massacre, how do we deal with the trauma and outrage? *The Guardian* (UK), March 18, 2019. Retrieved from https://www.theguardian.com/world/commentisfree/2019/mar/19/after-the-christchurch-massacre-how-do-we-deal-with-the-trauma-and-outrage

Mantovani, N., Pizzolati, M., & Edge, D. (2017). Exploring the relationship between stigma and help-seeking for mental illness in African-descended faith communities in the UK. *Health Expectations, 20*(3), 373–384.

Mental Health Foundation. (n.d.). Terminology. Retrieved from https://www.mentalhealth.org.uk/a-to-z/t/terminology

McGinty, E. E., Goldman, H. H., Pescosolido, B. A., & Barry, C. L. (2018). Communicating about mental illness and violence: Balancing stigma and increased support for services. *Journal of Health Politics, Policy and Law, 43*(2), 185–228.

Minsky, A. (2017). Hate crimes against Muslims in Canada increase 253% over four years. Global News, June 13, 2017. Retrieved from https://globalnews.ca/news/3523535/hate-crimes-canada-muslim/

Murphy, D. (2013). The medical model and the philosophy of science. In K. W. M. Fulford, et al. (Eds.), *The Oxford handbook of philosophy and psychiatry* (pp. 966–985). Oxford, England: Oxford University Press.

Muslim Wellness Foundation. (2017). 2017 review: A year of growth & gratitude. Retrieved from https://www.muslimwellness.com/2017

National Alliance on Mental Health. (n.d.). African American mental health. Retrieved from https://www.nami.org/find-support/diverse-communities/african-americans

National Center on Disability and Journalism. (n.d.). Disability language style guide. National Center on Disability and Journalism. Retrieved from http://ncdj.org/style-guide/

Newsom, V. A., & Lengel, L. (in press). Contradicting borderlessness: Tracing the mediated circuitries of ethnonationalist belonging. In K. Silva & M. Franz (Eds.), *Migration, identity, and belonging: Defining borders and boundaries of the homeland*. New York, NY: Routledge.

Overstreet, S., & Braun, B. S. (2000). Exposure to community violence and posttraumatic stress symptoms: Mediating factors. *American Journal of Orthopsychiatry*, *70*(2), 263–271.

Padela, A. I., Killawi, A., Forman, J., DeMonner, S., & Heisler, M. (2012). American Muslim perceptions of healing: Key agents in healing, and their roles. *Qualitative Health Research*, *22*, 846–858.

Phillips, D., & Lauterbach, D. (2017). American Muslim immigrant mental health: The role of racism and mental health stigma. *Journal of Muslim Mental Health*, *11*(1), 39–56.

Pilkington, A., Msetfi, R., & Watson, R. (2012). Factors affecting intention to access psychological services amongst British Muslims of South Asian origin. *Mental Health, Religion and Culture*, *15*, 1–22.

ProPublica. (2017). Documenting hate. ProPublic Projects. Retrieved from https://projects.propublica.org/graphics/hatecrimes/

Qadi, Y. (2018). "Scholars are not psychiatrists!" Dr. Qadhi on faith & depression. Retrieved from http://aboutislam.net/shariah/shariah-and-humanity/shariah-and-life/scholars-not-psychiatrists-dr-qadhi-faith-depression/

Roberts, M. (2005). The production of the psychiatric subject: power, knowledge and Michel Foucault. *Nursing Philosophy*, *6*(1), 33–42.

Rockwood, N. (2013). Muslim ... and Bipolar! Coping with mental illness today. *The Islamic Monthly*, March 13, 2013. Retrieved from https://www.theislamicmonthly.com/muslimand-bipolar-coping-with-mental-illness-today/

Rondelez, E., Bracke, S., Roets, G., & Vandekinderen, C., & Bracke, P. (2018). Revisiting Goffman: Frames of mental health in the interactions of mental healthcare professionals with diasporic Muslims. *Social Theory & Health*, *16*(4), 396–413.

Rose, D., Thornicroft, G., Pinfold, V., & Kassam, A. (2007). 250 labels used to stigmatise people with mental illness. *BMC Health Service Research*, *7*, article number 97. Retrieved from https://bmchealthservres.biomedcentral.com/articles/10.1186/1472-6963-7-97

Rössler, W. (2016). The stigma of mental disorders: A millennia-long history of social exclusion and prejudices. *EMBO Reports*, *17*(9), 1250–1253.

Said, E. (1978). *Orientalism*. New York, NY: Pantheon.

Saleem, M., & Anderson, C.A. (2013). Arabs as terrorists: Effects of stereotypes within violent contexts on attitudes, perceptions, and affect. *Psychology of Violence*, *3*, 84–99.

Saul, J. (2014). *Collective trauma, collective healing: Promoting community resilience in the aftermath of disaster*. New York, NY: Routledge.

Schaefer, D. (2015). *Religious affects: Animality, evolution, and power*. Durham, NC: Duke University Press.

Semati, M. (2011). Communication, culture, and the essentialized Islam. *Communication Studies*, *62*(1), 113–126.

Shaw, I. S. (2012). Stereotypical representations of Muslims and Islam following the 7/7 London terror attacks: Implications for intercultural communication and terrorism prevention. *International Communication Gazette*, *74*(6), 509–524.

Shibre, T., Negash, A., Kullgren, G., Kebede, D., Alem, A., Fekadu, A., … Jacobson, L. (2001). Perception of stigma among family members of individuals with schizophrenia and major affective disorders in rural Ethiopia. *Social Psychiatry and Psychiatric Epidemiology*, *36*(6), 299–303.

Shrira, A., Menashe, R., & Bensimon, M. (2019). Filial anxiety and sense of obligation among offspring of Holocaust survivors. *Aging & Mental Health*, *23*(6), 752–761.

Smidi, A., & Lengel, L. (2017). Freedom for whom? The contested terrain of religious freedom for Muslims in the United States. In E. Miller (Ed.), *The rhetoric of religious freedom in the U.S.* (pp. 85–99). Lanham, MD: Lexington/Rowman & Littlefield.

Smietana, B. (2013). Tackling stigma of mental illness. *The Christian Century*, *130*(11), 14–15.

Smith, A. J., Abeyta, A. A., Hughes, M., & Jones, R. T. (2014). Persistent grief in the aftermath of mass violence: The predictive roles of posttraumatic stress symptoms, self-efficacy, and disrupted worldview. *Psychological Trauma: Theory, Research, Practice, and Policy*, *7*, 179–186.

Southern Poverty Law Center. (2017). Post-election incidents up to 1,372; New collaboration with ProPublica. February 10, 2017. Retrieved from https://www.splcenter.org/hatewatch/2017/02/10/post-election-bias-incidents-1372-new-collaboration-propublica/

Stuart, H. (2003). Violence and mental illness: An overview. *World Psychiatry*, *2*(2), 121–124.

Stuart, J., & Ward, C. (2018). The relationships between religiosity, stress, and mental health for Muslim immigrant youth. *Mental Health, Religion & Culture*, *21*(3), 246–261.

Sultan, K. (2016). Linking Islam with terrorism: A review of the media framing since 9/11. *Global Media Journal: Pakistan Edition*, *9*(2), 1–10.

Tabassum, R., Macaskill, A., & Ahmad, A. (2000). Attitudes towards mental health in an urban Pakistani community in the United Kingdom. *International Journal of Social Psychiatry*, *46*(3), 170–181.

Trein, L. (2017). Islamophobia reconsidered: Approaching emotions, affects, and historical layers of Orientalism in the study of religion. *Method and Theory in the Study of Religion*, 1–16.

Turner, F. (2011). *Social work treatment: Interlocking theoretical approaches*. Oxford, England: Oxford University Press.

Tynes, B. M., Willis, H. A., Stewart, A. M., & Hamilton, M. W. (2019). Race-related traumatic events online and mental health among adolescents of color. *Journal of Adolescent Health* (June 2019). doi: 10.1016/j.jadohealth.2019.03.006

United Nations Office of the High Commissioner for Human Rights. (2002). *Principles for the protection of persons with mental illness and the improvement of mental health care*. Geneva, Switzerland: Office of the United Nations High Commissioner for Human Rights.

Weinstein, E., Wolin, J., & Rose, S. (2014). *Trauma informed community building: A model for strengthening community in trauma affected neighborhoods*. San Francisco, CA: BRIDGE Housing Corporation and Health Equity Institute.

Williams, D. R., & Williams-Morris, R. (2000). Racism and mental health: The African American experience. *Ethnicity and Health*, *5*, 243–268.

World Health Organization. (2008). *Preventing suicide: A resource for media professionals.* Geneva, Switzerland: World Health Organization. Department of Mental Health and Substance Abuse and the International Association for Suicide Prevention.

Youssef, J., & Deane, F.B. (2006). Factors influencing mental-health help-seeking in Arabic speaking communities in Sydney, Australia. *Mental Health, Religion & Culture*, *9*(1), 43–66.

CHAPTER TWELVE

Searching for a Good Death

BY JILLIAN A. TULLIS

Every so often I see a headline or a byline proclaiming, "Death is Having a Moment," and it makes me chuckle. What usually follows is a story about someone who is working in death care, and I'm not talking about a typical feature on a funeral director, although it might be, but someone who is touted as pushing back against the taboos surrounding dying and death. One reason this type of declaration tickles me is because I wonder what the pioneers, like Dr. Ernest Becker, Dame Cicely Saunders, or Dr. Elisabeth Kübler-Ross, would think if they were still alive. Fifty years ago, Kübler-Ross helped death have a moment when her groundbreaking book *On Death and Dying* (1969) was published. While working as a psychiatrist in a Chicago hospital, Kübler-Ross and a small group of graduate students spent time talking with seriously and terminally ill patients (and their loved ones) about their experiences dying and confronting death. The research team's observations led to the now famous stages of dying model. Some of the most important lessons in the book are about communication and for this reason I insist that students in my end of life communication classes read this text. It's foundational to teaching about dying and death, but it also highlights how modern issues surrounding how we care for and communicate with people who are dying are not new. And while this work has been criticized despite its salience and fidelity, we cannot escape its wisdom or influence half a century later. Kübler-Ross called on us to make the time to sit with people who are dying, believing that we had much to gain from listening to their experiences. Perhaps we would fear death less and live life more fully.

Not long after the debut of *On Death and Dying*, Cicely Saunders, a nurse, social worker, and eventually a physician, visited the United States from Britain to discuss a new form of care for terminally-ill people called Hospice (Emanuel & Emanuel, 1998; Saunders, 1996). People who knew their illness could not be cured, and would eventually lead to their death, now had an alternative to dying with intractable pain in isolation in a hospital ward. Hospice care, primarily delivered in a dying person's home, promised to make dying more bearable. Aggressive treatments could cease and a person's physical and spiritual (or existential) pain would become the primary focus of care in hospice. A team of practitioners from medicine to social work to clergy would manage a dying person's last days. Dr. Saunder's visit was the catalyst for the debut of the first hospice in the United States in Connecticut in 1974 (Emanuel & Emanuel, 1998). This method of care was a welcome relief for people who were terminally ill, and while there have certainly been technical medical advances that have fundamentally changed how we die, the role of hospice in that evolution is significant. The introduction of hospice necessitated a change to how physicians would need to communicate with their patients. Rather than practicing paternalism, avoiding or denying the inevitability of death, physicians would need to be forthright with their patients about their prognoses and provide the information necessary to make an informed decision about care. Less than a decade later in 1983, Congress would establish the Hospice Medicare Benefit (Emanuel & Emanuel, 1998). A healthcare organization with a philosophy of care committed to accepting death as a natural part of life was now government sanctioned and supported.

Death had other moments in the courts, with several prominent *Right to Die* cases involving Karen Ann Quinlan in the 1970s, Nancy Cruzan in the 1980s, and Terri Schiavo which began in the 1990s and concluded with her death in 2005 (Colby, 2002; Emanuel & Emanuel, 1998; Quill, 2005; Sabatino, 2010). All three of these women suffered medical emergencies that left them dependent on life support and unable to communicate their wishes for care. Because family members and hospital staff could not agree on the best course of action, the courts were called on to halt medical interventions and allow these women to die naturally. While Karen Ann Quinlan's case was being litigated in New Jersey in 1975, California was working to make living wills legal (Sabatino, 2010). Since 1976, living wills and documents like it, such as an advance directive, healthcare power of attorney, and eventually Physician's Orders for Life Sustaining Treatment (POLST or sometimes called the Medical Orders for Scope of Treatment) forms have provided loved ones and clinicians with the information they needed to carry out a person's last wishes for medical treatment. Experts considered these tools as essential to facilitate conversations about a good death. Moreover, these documents are believed to benefit individuals who do not have or trust next of kin to carry out their wishes, as well as queer people (or unmarried couples) whose relationships (at the time) were not sanctioned through marriage. Unfortunately, despite widespread public support for these documents, research suggests only about a quarter of the U.S. population has completed them, although the numbers are higher among terminally ill individuals (Emanuel & Emanuel, 1998; Pew Research Center, 2013; Sabatino, 2010).

And then in 1994, death had a moment when the state of Oregon became the first in the United States to allow medical aid in dying, another mechanism for someone to accomplish their version of a good death (Death with Dignity, n.d.). Six states and the District of Columbia now have Death with Dignity or Aid in Dying laws, which allow physicians to write prescriptions for a lethal dose of medication for terminally ill people without fear of reprisal, thus affording dying people the chance to end their lives when they choose (Death with Dignity, n.d.). Death certificates in these cases indicate illness and not suicide as the cause of death (Buck, 2016), an important distinction for life insurance as well as avoiding the stigma of suicide. Efforts to pass such laws have pitted aid in dying advocates against religious organizations, especially the Catholic Church, and Disability Rights groups who see these laws as devaluing human life and a slippery slope towards hastening the lives of people with disabilities (Neumann, 2016). While it is not clear that these groups are in dialogue with each other, the debate is part of the larger public discourse about whether aid in dying is necessary for a good death in light of the availability of hospice and palliative care (care focused on pain and symptom management for chronically and terminally ill).

Death is having yet another moment and this time there is a hashtag, #DeathPositive. Caitlin Doughty, star of the popular YouTube channel, *Ask a Mortician* (Doughty, 2011), launched the concept of Death Positivity via Twitter in 2013 (The Order of the Good Death, 2018). Since then, organizations such as The Order of the Good Death, Dying Matters, and events such as Death Salon, EndWell, Dying Matters Awareness Week, Death Café, Death Over Dinner, National Health Care Decisions Day, and The Conversation Project have benefited from social media with the goal of making death less taboo. There are more outlets than ever, face-to-face and virtual, to get information about dying, death, after death care, to mourn, and to learn about grief than ever before. Social media activity has surely made the topic more accessible to a wide range of people with 336 million Twitter users (Statista.com, 2018b) and 2.19 billion Facebook users worldwide (Statista.com, 2018a). It is difficult to determine the impact of this social media content on attitudes and willingness to communicate about dying and death. But a glimpse at Caitlin Doughty's social media accounts suggest the message about death positivity is getting out. Doughty has over sixty-four thousand Twitter followers and nearly eighty-nine thousand on Instagram, the Order of the Good Death, a nonprofit organization founded by Doughty, has a Facebook page followed by 130,000.

In light of the present moment where access to information is widespread and there are more voices advocating for good end of life care, I consider the implications of these turns in this chapter with the goal of broadening the conversation and ensuring a good death is inclusive. To accomplish this, I explore what it means to die well for people on the margins in the United States, and whether or not these features are present in existing end of life care, especially hospice. I also consider the implications of efforts to export Western conceptions of a good death abroad. Alongside literature about a good death, this chapter includes examples from my experience as a researcher and hospice volunteer, ponders questions about who gets to experience a good death, and discusses the problem with definitions of a good death. First, I describe my positionality to better understand the vantage point through which I see and engage the concept of a good death.

Background and Positionality

My interests in thanatology, or the study of dying and death, started when I was earning my Master of Arts in Communication Studies. The conversations I was having with my mother about the then new TV show *Six Feet Under* (Ball, 2001) was the catalyst for my thesis about people's first experiences with death. I continued this work during my doctoral program where I conducted observations for two years in an oncology clinic for older adults, and did an ethnographic study of a hospice team for my dissertation. I have also served as a hospice volunteer on and off since 2002. I have interviewed terminally ill head and neck cancer patients as well (Roscoe, Tullis, Reich, & McCaffrey, 2013). I have hosted Death Café and attended Death Doula training. In September 2018, I had the honor of speaking at Death Salon hosted by the Order of the Good Death. The unit on dying and death in my health communication class is frequently my favorite, and I eventually developed a course about end of life communication. Several of my friends contact me for advice when a family member is seriously ill or when they are worried about a grieving loved one. They also tag me on social media about articles and suggest films and TV shows that include death related topics and themes. These recommendations from friends and family usually arrive with a joke about how when they think of death they think of me. I tell them I don't take it personal, and I don't. I love it. I love talking about, teaching about, and thinking about dying and death. All of this passion coalesces around understanding the role communication plays in quality of life, dying, and facilitating a good death. The latter of which is a concept I have faithfully embraced since it first entered my vocabulary over 15 years ago. Yet after a conversation at a death positive event in 2014 about the absence of people of color in these spaces, I began thinking about a good death with new skepticism. Whether workshops or public talks, I am often the only woman of color in a sea of white faces at death events. Twice, I have been mistaken for the other black woman on the program. While I'm used to being the only person of color in the room, the more I contemplated the absence of people who look like me, the more I questioned whether the issues salient in the death positive community, such as dying well, green burial practices, and managing grief, the more I questioned the relevance of these issues to communities on the margins. And I began reflecting on a few experiences with hospice patients, families, and clinical staff.

Hospice Care and a Good Death

Hospice is a type of care for people who are dying, and their loved ones. In the United States, this usually means a person must have a terminal diagnosis with a prognosis of 6-months or less to live. The focus of care is on pain and symptom management and not aggressive treatment or cure. The philosophy foundational to hospice is an acceptance of death as a natural part of life. The dying person and their loved ones are the unit of care, and this care is delivered by an interdisciplinary team. The members of the team are charged with caring for one of the five-quality of life dimensions, which address a patient's physical, emotional, social, and spiritual needs at the end of life (Byock & Merriman, 1998). In its most basic form, but especially in hospice, a good death is one free of physical and existential or spiritual pain. The Institute of Medicine's (Field & Cassel, 1997) definition is more detailed, "*a decent or good death* is one that is: free from avoidable distress and suffering for patients, families, and caregivers; in general accord with patients' and families' wishes; and reasonably consistent with clinical, cultural, and ethical standards" (p. 24). Such a definition both enables and constrains. On one hand, the ambiguity of the concept affords dying patients, their loved ones, and their carers a great deal of flexibility (Kehl, 2006; Tullis, 2009). On the other, without a more concrete definition, the possibilities for care are limitless. In fact, a review of the scholarship about a good death by Kehl (2006), reveals a dozen attributes of a good death, which include such issues as being in control, being comfortable, a sense of closure, valuing the dying person, and trust in care providers, all of which can vary from person to person. A definition such as the one above then can only serve as a catalyst for a dialogue among the dying person and their clinical team members responsible for care. This is especially true in light of the attributes of a good death that are unrelated to medical care.

After a year of observations with a hospice team, I actually found a lack of communication about what might constitute a good death for patients (Tullis, 2009). This dearth of conversations between team members and patients about dying well also extended to team meetings, (which occur outside the purview of patients) and focused more on Medicare rectification and reporting a list of the patient's symptoms. Instead of meeting patients where they are, a common refrain in many hospice organizations, hospice staff enacted an established and institutionalized mode of hospice care (Whitney, 2015). What can happen as a result, is that patients and families who push back on this hospice narrative are sometimes labeled difficult rather than exercising their autonomy (Tullis, Roscoe, & Dillon, 2017). Ultimately and regretfully, hospices may begin to resemble the very healthcare organizations they sought to resist (Tullis et al., 2017; Whitney, 2015).

It is not just that healthcare and its discourses, described by Whitney (2015), has become standardized, but those tasked with delivering the care and those who receive it are homogeneous. An estimated 1.43 million Medicare recipients received hospice services in 2016 (National Hospice and Palliative Care Organization, 2017). More than 86.5% of these patients were white, just 8.3% were African American, and all other racial groups combined made up the remaining 5%, and 58.6% of these recipients were woman. While I was unable to locate data about hospice staff demographics, the vast majority of clinical staff I have encountered across five Medicare approved non-profit hospices in three states were also white women. Hospice, run primarily by nurses, proclaims an egalitarian approach on teams, but more often than not, I observed teams with clear hierarchies (Tullis, 2009). The team approach promises to provide holistic care, yet the power imbalances and limited participation from lower-ranking, less formally educated staff (who were also frequently women of color), such as nursing assistants, can undermine this objective. So, in addition to focusing on the business of hospice (e.g., whether or not a patient is Medicare eligible), team members in their interactions with each other, as well as with their patients, are shaped by those who have the most autonomy and authority. Interactions in the front and backstage often center around maintaining politeness that stifles conversation and productive conflict (2009). It is also this implicit commitment to politeness that keeps dying and death taboo topics and limit who can experience a good death.

To further illustrate my point about proscriptions related to death consider this experience. During a meeting of an end of life coalition of which I was a member, I proposed hosting a Death Café, an ideology-free public gathering (with cake!), where people can talk openly about dying and death, which I thought fit well with the coalition's mission. After the flyer with details about the event made its way around the conference room, the head of clinical care for a hospice said, "I don't know … I just don't like the word 'death.'" I was stunned. If the leader of all the clinical medical staff at a hospice was uncomfortable with the word *death* and worried that such language was too explicit, the efforts to help patients and their loved ones experience a good death felt compromised.

The inabilty or unwillingess to talk about dying and death happens in the front stage as well. Consider, for example, one of my most recent hospice patients who I volunteered with for five months. A gay man in his 70s with no partner, no children, no family nearby, and living on a very limited budget, John was surprised to learn just days before his discharge (because his health improved) that he was once considered terminally ill. Or the husband and wife I visited during my dissertation research who believed they were receiving hospice care because they "needed more support," not because the husband was dying of lung cancer. During these heighten emotional times, it is possible that patients and their loved ones are not prepared to confront the realities of mortality, and therefore the messages about the goals of hopsice get distorted. Yet, if a patient and their loved ones don't know what hospice is for, it is difficult to see how they could make a meaningful contribution to their plan of care and expereince a good death.

Resources and Socioeconomic Status

Knowledge about what hospice is and information about a person's health status are types of resources that are certainly a piece of the hopsice puzzle, but there are other ways in which socio-economic status plays out in hospice settings, which I was address next. I will discuss some of the structural issues in hospice that hinder care for those on the margins financially. But first, I will consider hospice for those in our community with the least amount of resources, the homeless.

The topic of hospice for homeless has appeared in the media recently, both in the United States and Canada (Hubert, 2018; Stroh, 2018). Most hospice care is currently provided in a patient's home, although some individuals receive care in nursing homes, assisted living facilities, hospitals, and hospice houses. Hospices can and will deliver care to people who are transient, but this is less than ideal for ensuring a continuity of care. One solution is to have hospices specifically designed to meet the special needs for homeless. There are currently just seven such programs in the United States, and Dr. Marlene von Friedrichs-Fitzwater (my former MA advisor) was preparing to move forward with the plans to open an eighth when the neighborhood association where the facility would exist filed an appeal to stop the project, citing quality of life concerns of the residence (Hubert, 2018). Sacramento City Council eventually approved the project unanimously after a public hearing, but the opposition suggests that the universality of a good death is not yet realized and accessible only to those economically advantaged.

Hospice for homeless addresses one barrier to care, but there are other ways in which socio-economic status is a hurdle. Once a person is admitted to hospice they will be assigned to an interdisciplinary team and these staff conduct visits Monday through Friday during typical business hours. Outside of these days and times, patients and families have access to hospice staff on an on-call basis. One family I volunteered for was experiencing the death of its matriarch. The eldest daughter and caregiver to her mother, was in her late teens, and unable to be present for hospice visits because she worked during the day. These visits are important opportunities for information exchange between the caregiver and the hospice team about the patient's status and needs for care. Hospice patients who are not mobile, cannot feed, bathe, or use the toilet themselves are unable to use hospice for these needs, they must also have additional support from caregivers, either family or friends or private-hire aides.

My expereince with John, who I mentioned earlier, contributed to my reexamination of hospice, its mission, and reignited a question about who can most benefit from this model of care. Not long after I began vising him, he was transferred to a skilled nursing facility, what most people recognize as a nursing home. This change was made despite the fact that he had a private hire home health aide. The hospice felt that he needed more around the clock care than what they were able to give him and the transfer was made. And while he was not happy about the decision, he was unable to put up much resistance. He couldn't afford it.

I continued to visit him in the facility, but he no longer lived in a space he recognized, he didn't have any of his belongings, he was struggling to get along with his roommates, and reported to me that he was having issues with his medication. Sometimes he couldn't get it when he needed it, and other times he wasn't able to get the types of medication he required. I reported these challenges each week in my volunteer notes, but there was no substantive change. He was now having to navigate the bueracracy of the nusing home and the hospice. After about three months of weekly visits, and teaching myself to make balloon animals (John was a professional clown) to amuse my new friend, I received word that John was being discharged. Most patients are thrilled to "graduate" from hospice because it means their health has improved. John, however, was devesatated when I broke the news to him that I would not be able to visit any longer. As he said that afternoon, "I've already lost my apartment. I can't go to church. I don't have my things. And now this is another thing I'm losing." We were both in tears. I was sad for John. I knew he looked forward to our visits. But I was also angry, if I'm being honest. The reason for his admission should not have been news, nor should the changes that would happen upon his graduation. He had become dependent upon the organization and he felt let down because they were not forthright with information he needed to prepare for yet another change. While I do now know John's status today, his financial status was a key factor in his hospice experience.

Dying well, and the promise of helping people die at home, if that is their wish, is then predicated on financial resources or job flexibility. The burden on lay or family caregivers is significant. Untrained, and perhaps confronting serious illness or mortality (their loved one's and their own) for the first time, they are frequently unprepared emotionally or physical for the challenges of this level of care. Economically disadvantaged communities may not be able to easily assume these responsibilities, even with additional support and guidance from hospice organizations. My colleagues and I (Tullis et al., 2017) have argued that communities who are economically disadvantaged may resist the hospice approach not because they are being defiant, but because they do not have the resources to make hospice work within hospice structures.

LGBT Needs

Hospice structures are worth considering in detail as they relate to the lesbian, gay, bisexual, and transgender (LGBT) community. The unit of care in hospice is the patient and their family, as defined by the patient. This nonnormative approach to "family" is helpful for unmarried couples or those who have difficult or broken relationships with blood relatives. Yet, organizations are only as good as the individuals within them. As observed in the documentary *Gen Silent* (Maddux, 2011), older LGBT people who have been out for decades are going back in the closet when faced with increasing healthcare needs for fear of discrimination. I once met with an administrator at an assisted living facility who denied they had any such issues, but also did not seem to know if they had any LGBT residences in their charge. Nursing students I have done workshops with have asked for advice about how to get their colleagues to use trans* patients' preferred names without compromising working relations or patient care. Research and reporting mirror these anecdotes, some trans* people, for example, will delay care and once hospitalized endure confusion and further indignities (Cicero & Black, 2016; Ellin, 2016; Welch, 2019). If healthcare practitioners are not prepared to honor the most basic desire to call patients by their preferred names or pronouns then other anxieties related to having end of life wishes respected is reasonable.

Thus far, this chapter has focused on some of the specific behaviors and practices that might stand in the way of a patient and their family experiencing a good death. I've also highlighted some of the structural issues (e.g., timing of the delivery of care). The role of culture, however, is also an important factor with implications in United States and abroad. For people of color and people with disabilities, many facets of a good death as practiced in hospice may clash with the values, attitudes, and beliefs of patients in these communities. While these two groups have specific and unique needs, I discuss their commonalities in an effort to further problematize a good death.

Medical Care and Trust

Ceasing medical treatment considered aggressive or care that is provided with the goal of life extending is prohibited in hospice. Medical care such as chemotherapy or mechanical breathing is not allowed. Some hospices have the resources to cover palliative chemotherapy, which can help with managing pain, but otherwise, such treatment makes an individual ineligible for hospice. One reason for this approach is that the hospice philosophy maintains that death is a natural part of life and medicine should not interfere with this process. The hospice philosophy operates under the assumption that less medical care, especially when treatment is futile, is better, and a good death happens at home, not in a hospital (Kehl, 2006). Quality of life over quantity of life is the focus in hospice, not a long, protracted death in an intensive care unit (ICU) hooked up to machines. For some patients once they have their symptoms managed and their pain controlled, their lives are extended (Connor, Pyenson, Fitch, Spence, & Iwasaki, 2007). Yet, some families remain unconvinced by arguments in favor of shifting treatment goals from aggressive care to comfort care, even with the promise of a better prognosis.

Many people of color and people with disabilities do not necessarily view aggressive medical care or a hospital death as troubling or a sign of a bad quality of life or bad death (Savin, 2018). According to Savin (2018), some people with disabilities have multiple experiences with the ICU and do not conceive of aggressive care as over-treatment, nor is it a sign of poor care. For some people with disabilities, their experience in ICU settings over the course of their lives shapes what counts as quality of life and therefore may differ significantly from people without disabilities (Mitchell, Weigel, Stewart, Mako, & Loughnane, 2017).

For both people with disabilities and people of color, especially African Americans, the issue of trust is significant. People with disabilities have reported experiences with practitioners who don't understand their disabilities and view their lives as less fulfilling because of their limitations (Mitchell, Weigel, Stewart, Mako, & Loughnane, 2017). African Americans similarly experience mistrust informed by a long history of inequities in access, treatment, overt discrimination, and experimentation (Washington, 2006). This lack of confidence in healthcare may actually prompt some to request or continue more aggressive care as a sign that every effort is being made to protect life and that their lives (or their loved ones' lives) are valued. As a result, the suggestion that certain medical interventions should stop to focus on palliative care outside of a hospital setting, is troubling, even frightening.

Rather than find ways to address these issues, perhaps by reconceptualizing a good death, many hospices try to find new ways to frame the care they provide (Savin, 2018). Outreach efforts include educating publics about what hospice care is in the hopes of dispelling myths. Some hospices have tried to craft messages that are more culturally relevant. These efforts are notable and will ensure some who have never considered hospice before will in the future. Reframing or repackaging hospice in these ways will not overcome cultural values, beliefs, and attitudes, and practices foundational to how poor people, communities of color, people with disabilities, or LGBT individuals will define a good death. It would serve hospices organizations well to view these issues from the perspective of their patients and loved ones, then advocate for structures that will meet a broader range of needs and more diverse concepts of dying well, if the goal is to eventually provide care to all seriously ill and dying individuals. Perhaps expanding the scope of hospice is too great a challenge as this type of care is becoming more established (Whitney, 2015). The role of hospice, however, in shaping the definition of a good death is significant and has implications for end of life care both here and abroad.

It is estimated that 20 million people worldwide are in need of palliative care (care focused on pain and symptom management for chronically and terminally ill), which includes hospice care (Connor & Sepulveda Bermedo, 2014). The promise of a good death for so many diverse people will not be found in a one-size-fits all approach, particularly if we consider that the United Kingdom, United States, and Australia have more fully realized hospice and palliative care programs than the rest of the world (Connor & Sepulveda Bermedo, 2014). In other words, we cannot expect to export our vision for a good death easily if we have not attended to the ways in which hospices in these developed countries do not represent diversity and variations in a good death. Advocates for the spread of hospice around the globe should expect to encounter the same issues abroad as here, and then some. For example, in some parts of the Ukraine they have hospice facilities with explicit signage, but telling patients they are terminally ill is not part of standard medical practice. A friend of mine who is Kenyan told me that not taking a family member to the hospital when they are dying would be thought odd. When I traveled to Peru and inquired about hospice, my local host was unfamiliar with the concept. A former student from Ecuador shared stories with me about one of the hospices in her country that is run by the Catholic Church. While hospice was available in the city, she noted that there was still an unmet need in rural and indigenous communities. The presence or absence of hospice is just one hurdle. Some of these countries practice paternalism in medicine, have little or no education for children with disabilities because of stigma, and are not LGBT friendly. So, hospice initiatives abroad will need to overcome more than language or translation challenges, but with attitudes, values, and beliefs about dying, what counts a family, and who deserves care. Relieving suffering (spiritual or existential) is the goal of palliative and hospice care and how to accomplish this when confronted with difference should be regarded an opportunity rather than a challenge or a mode of resistance (Tullis et al., 2017). Hospice, one that is grounded in the promise to come alongside a patient and their family, meet them where they are in the dying process, and create a plan of care to meet their needs is an opportunity (Diversity and difference in communication, 2018). It is not a problem of convincing a patient or family that dying well is only accomplished one way. The chance to provide a good death lies in curiosity and flexibility and it requires asking questions. Here are some:

- How can a good death be accomplished for people who cannot access early diagnostic tools or pain medication?
- How we can minimize emotional and physical pain in communities where dying may be predestined by God or Allah (Tullis, 2010)?
- How do we help people who want "everything done" die well (Roscoe and Tullis, 2015)?
- What structures within hospice need to change to help poor and working class people receive hospice care?
- How can hospices build trust between them and LGBT communities, and communities of color?
- Is a good death possible for immigrants or undocumented? What are some of the challenges or barriers?
- Does a good death look different for individuals in places of global turmoil or war?
- Is denial of death a hinderance to dying well? (Kübler-Ross, 1969)

- How can we start conversations about a good death if such talk can bring bad fortune?
- Can people die well in a hospital setting?
- Is a good death ableist?
- Is a good death a middle class value?

None of these questions have easy answers, but they must at least be considered and addressed if the goal is a good death for all. We may very well conclude after exploring these questions that a good death as it is defined today is only valued by some, or that a good death is only possible under some very specific circumstances. In addition to these questions, I think hospice and good death advocates like myself should find ways for the communities we seek to reach to inform, shape, and even change our thinking about a good death. I am hopeful the boundaries of a good death and how it is carried out in hospice can expand with thoughtful consideration of difference.

Review and Closing Thoughts

Emanuel and Emanuel (1998) assert that we know a great deal about how hospice intervenes when a patient has physical symptoms, but we know less about how staff meet psychological, social, spiritual needs. These are the areas where issues of diversity and difference are most likely to arise, although some have argued that managing physical symptoms, even withdrawing life support and ceasing aggressive treatment may not be a universally held value (Crawley, 2002; Pew Research Center, 2013). If for example, a pain free death is not valued by a community because to suffer is human or expected then the means of accomplishing a good death requires more nuance and a wider range of practices. I have observed many interactions in hospice, from admissions to the verbal and nonverbal communication in the days just before a person's death, and never saw a team member ask a patient what a good death might be for them. This is a missed opportunity for both the dying person and their caregivers. Perhaps more importantly, the issues described here demonstrate that we need a markedly different approach to communicating about what constitutes a good death. While death is inevitable, how we die is not. Advances in medicine have extended life expectancies and we now live longer than ever before (Kübler-Ross, 1969; Puchalksi, 2006). Diseases such as cancer are no longer an automatic death sentence, at least not in the United States, but we have yet to reckon with Alzheimer's. Communities of color, the disabled community, and LGBT individuals still have reasons to feel skeptical towards some healthcare professionals and the organizations that employ them. We also cannot expect the rest of the world to embrace Western notions of a good death without question. In the quest for a good death we have to include these voices and ask what dying well means to them, assuming we are truly committed to this goal. And then, be prepared to come along side those in need and help them navigate the end of their lives. Death is on the precipice of another moment. The question remains if we are ready for this moment to be truly death positive and inclusive.

References

Ball, A. (Producer). (2001). *Six feet under* [Television Series]. Hollywood, CA: Home Box Office.

Buck, C. (2016, June 6). Eight things you should know as California's new aid-in-dying law takes effect. *Sacramento Bee*. Retrieved from https://www.sacbee.com/news/local/health-and-medicine/article82660497.html

Byock, I. R., & Merriman, M. P. (1998). Measuring quality of life for patients with terminal illness: The Missoula–VITAS® quality of life index. *Palliative Medicine*, *12*, 231–244.

Cicero, E. C., & Black, B. P. (2016). "I was a spectacle … A freak show at the circus": A transgender person's ED experience and implications for nursing practice. *Journal of Emergency Nursing*, *42*(1), 25–30. doi: 10.1016/j.jen.2015.08.012

Colby, W. H. (2002). *Long goodbye: The deaths of Nancy Cruzan*. Carlsbad, CA: Hay House.

Connor, S. R., Pyenson, B., Fitch, K., Spence, C., & Iwasaki, K. (2007). Comparing hospice and nonhospice patient survival among patients who die within a three-year window. *Journal of Pain and Symptom Management*, *33*(3), 238–246.

Connor, S. R., & Sepulveda Bermedo, M. C. (Eds.) (2014). *Global atlas of palliative care at the end of life*. World Palliative Care Alliance. Retrieved from https://www.who.int/nmh/Global_Atlas_of_Palliative_Care.pdf

Crawley, L. M. (2002). Palliative care in African American communities. *Journal of Palliative Medicine*, *5*(5), 775–779.

Death with Dignity. (n.d.). Death with dignity acts. Retrieved from https://www.deathwithdignity.org/learn/death-with-dignity-acts/

Diversity and difference in communication. (2018). *The Open University*. Retrieved from http://www.oercommons.org/courses/diversity-and-difference-in-communication/view

Doughty, C. (Producer). (2011). Ask a mortician, episdoe one. *Ask a Mortician*. Retrieved from https://www.youtube.com/watch?v=JTCg6PGaOkM

Ellin, A. (2016, January 16). Transgender patients face challenges at the hospital. *New York Times*. Retrieved from https://well.blogs.nytimes.com/2016/02/16/for-transgender-patients-challenges-at-the-hospital/

Emanuel, E. J., & Emanuel, L. L. (1998). The promise of a good death. *The Lancet*, *351*, SII21–SII29. doi: https://doi.org/10.1016/S0140-6736(98)90329-4

Field, M. J., & Cassel, C. K. (1997). Introduction. In M. J. Field & C. K. Cassel (Eds.), *Approaching death: Improving care at the end of life* (pp. 14–32). Washington, DC: Institute of Medicine.

Hubert, C. (2018, May 16). 'It's the right thing to do.' City approves homeless hospice, despite objections. *Sacramento Bee*. Retrieved from https://www.sacbee.com/news/local/homeless/article211262204.html - storylink=cpy

Kehl, K. A. (2006). Moving toward peace: An analysis of the concept of a good death. *American Journal of Hospice and Palliative Medicine*, *23*(4), 277–286.

Kübler-Ross, E. (1969). *On death and dying*. New York: Macmillan.

Maddux, S. (Writer). (2011). *Gen silent*. In S. Maddux & Applebaum (Producer): Iterrobang Productions.

Mitchell, S. E., Weigel, G. M., Stewart, S. K. A., Mako, M., & Loughnane, J. F. (2017). Expereinces and perspectives on advance care planning among individuals living with serious physcial disablities. *Journal of Palliative Medicine*, *20*(2), 127–133. doi: 10.1089/jpm.2016.0168

National Hospice and Palliative Care Organization. (2017). *NHPCO facts and figures: Hospice care in America*. Retrieved from https://www.nhpco.org/sites/default/files/public/Statistics_Research/2017_Facts_Figures.pdf

Neumann, A. (2016). *The good death: An exploration of dying in America*. Boston, MA: Beacon Press.

Pew Research Center. (2013). *Views on end-of-life medical treatments*. Retrieved from http://www.pewforum.org/2013/11/21/views-on-end-of-life-medical-treatments/

Puchalski, C. M. (2006). *A time for listening and caring: Spirituality and the care of the chronically ill and dying*. USA: Oxford University Press.

Quill, T. (2005). Terri Schiavo—A tragedy compounded. *New England Journal of Medicine*, *352*, 1630–1633. doi: 10.1056/NEJMp058062

Roscoe, L. A., & Tullis, J. A. (2015). The meaning of everything: communication at the end of life. *Journal of Medicine and the Person*, *13*(2), 75–81.

Roscoe, L. A., Tullis, J. A., Reich, R. R., & McCaffrey, J. C. (2013). Beyond good intentions and patient perceptions: Competing definitions of effective communication in head and neck cancer care at the end of life. *Health Communication*, *28*(2), 183–192. doi: https://doi.org/10.1080/10410236.2012.666957

Sabatino, C. P. (2010). The evolution of health care advance planning law and policy. *The Milbank Quarterly*, *88*(2), 211–239. doi: http://doi.org/10.1111/j.1468-0009.2010.00596.x

Saunders, C. (1996). Hospice. *Mortality*, *1*(3).

Savin, K. (2018). A death by any other name: When are health dispartieis call for assimilation to a medicalized norm? (Qualifying Paper), University of California, Berkeley.

Statista.com. (2018a). Number of Facebook users worldwide 2008–2018. Retrieved from https://www.statista.com/statistics/264810/number-of-monthly-active-facebook-users-worldwide/

Statista.com. (2018b). Number of monthly active Twitter users from 2010 to 2018. Retrieved from https://www.statista.com/statistics/282087/number-of-monthly-active-twitter-users/

Stroh, P. (2018, July 2). Life on streets 'a killer': New hospice offers end-of-life care to the homeless. *CBC News*. Retrieved from https://www.cbc.ca/news/health/journey-home-hospice-toronto-homeless-end-of-life-care-1.4715540

The Order of the Good Death. (2018). Death positive movement. Retrieved from http://www.orderofthegooddeath.com/resources/death-positive-movement

Tullis, J. A. (2009). *Communicating spirituality, dying and a "good death" at the end-of-life: The role of hospice interdisciplinary team members* (Doctoral Dissertation). University of South Florida, Tampa.

Tullis, J. A. (2010). Bring about benefit, forestall harm: What communication studies says about spirituality and cancer care. *Asian Pacific Journal of Cancer Prevention*, *11*(MECC Suppl), 67–73.

Tullis, J. A., Roscoe, L. A., & Dillon, P. J. (2017). Resisting the hospice narrative in pursuit of quality of life. *Qualitative Research in Medicine & Healthcare*, *1*(2), 63–72. doi: https://doi.org/10.4081/qrmh.2017.6152

Washington, H. (2006). *Medical apartheid.* New York: First Anchor Books. Publishing, Inc.

Welch, A. (2019, January 16). Most cancer doctors don't know enough about LGBTQ patient care study finds. *CBS News*. Retrieved from https://www.cbsnews.com/news/cancer-doctors-oncologists-lgbtq-transgender-patient-care-survey/

Whitney, A. (2015). Discourse "on or about" dying: Palliative care. In J. F. Nussbaum, H. Giles, & A. K. Worthington (Eds.), *Communication at the end of life*. New York: Peter Lang Publishing, Inc.

PART 5

Engaging Classrooms: Meaningful Complexity of Teaching and Learning

CHAPTER THIRTEEN

Critical Intercultural Health Communication Pedagogy: An Autoethnographic Approach

BY SATOSHI TOYOSAKI, PATRICK SEICK, SHELBY SWAFFORD, DARREN J. VALENTA, AND LINDY WAGNER

The siren goes off. My mother once told me that she hated the siren because it reminded her of the Tokyo air raid. The loud siren cuts the air on a sunny summer day. For a brief moment, it feels like time has just stopped as my friends and I drop everything we are doing outside and we switch our gear from a fun mode to an evacuation mode. It is the time for us to run from what we don't see that surrounds us. Quickly do we say good-byes, run home, and close windows if they are not already. My family lives in this old apartment without air-conditioning near industrial areas, something a middle-to-low socioeconomic class family with three children can afford. Inside the old apartment, I wonder if this old window is going to protect me as I look outside through it, feeling sweat droplets run down my spine under my t-shirt. I am trying to hide from 光化学スモッグ, which my mother has taught me over and over is a very bad thing.

***

I was born and grew up on the outskirts of Tokyo Prefecture in the 1970s. Much of my childhood was in the last part of Japan's post-World War II (WWII) reconstruction era from 1945 to somewhere around 1980 (Graburn, Ertl, & Tierney, 2008). During those thirty some years, many things happened in Japan. Japan reconstructed itself from the defeated and flattened nation to a highly industrial and technological nation with high productivity. In the 1970s, Japan experienced high levels of various air pollutants (Wakamatsu, Morikawa, & Ito, 2013), prompted by Japan's urbanization and industrial developments, which led Japan to tremendous and acute economic growth in the 1980s which we now call the "bubble" (Graburn & Ertl, 2008).

Those sirens alarmed residents of the high level of 光化学スモッグ or photochemical smog in the air. Photochemical smog symbolized Japan's "growth," while being hazardous to those living there. Photochemical oxidants, for example, are "secondary air pollutants" (Wakamatsu et al., 2013, p. 182); a high level of O3 (also known as ozone) is observed on the ground, which is reported to "irritate mucous membranes and affect respiratory organs … . In Japan, the first report of health damage attributable to [photochemical oxidants] in the Tokyo metropolitan area appeared in 1970" (p. 182). My childhood doctor often informed my mother that I had hypertrophy of tonsils.

While the causality of my childhood tonsil hypertrophy to photochemical smog could not be proven, I think it is productive for intercultural health communication scholars to pay close attention to cultural contextuality of human health and how we experience health. Such cultural contextuality includes but is not limited to inter/transnational politics (e.g., WWII), cultural politics (e.g., power), global economy (e.g., Japan's bubble), histories (e.g., Japan's industrialization and my birth into a particular time and place), environmental issues (e.g., various pollutions), institutionalizations (e.g., the biomedical model), organizational systems (e.g., work, school, hospital, and family contexts), geopolitical locations (e.g., Tokyo), temporal locations (e.g., the 1970s), ones' idiosyncratic and intersectional experiences (e.g., how I experienced the siren), ones' perceptual experiences (i.e., a "bad" thing), and so on. Some contextual factors are salient while others are subdued and/or ignored in our idiosyncratic health experiences.

Contextual factors—the ones we are aware of in the way we are now and the ones we are not aware of yet in the way we are not—are all significant, temporal, and contingent aspects of what constitute our lived and situated experiences of our own and other's health. Our awarenesses continue to shift in flux, which renders a renewed sense of cultural contextuality. Such critical attention to cultural contextuality renders our analysis of human health nuanced and complex. Understanding health is messy. In the following, I, along with my coauthors, struggle to understand a pedagogical juncture between critical intercultural communication and health communication, while meaningfully engaging human health as an inherently messy experience—contextual, nuanced, and complex.

An Autoethnographic Approach to Critical International Health Communication Pedagogy

Critical intercultural communication recently emerged as a sub-discipline of intercultural communication studies (see Nakayama & Halualani, 2010). Historically speaking, intercultural communication studies has a tendency to treat culture as nations and cultural groups and conceptualizes them as independent nominal variables that help researchers to predict human communicative choices. Critical intercultural communication studies departs from this conceptualization of culture, adhering to critical theory. "Critical theory suggests that rigorous and insightful research is only made possible by its being grounded in the realities of the social world, including the power relationships, the distortions and the pathologies that affect how we live" (McArthur, 2013, p. 10). Critical intercultural communication research interrogates power and social injustice and produces complex and context-oriented analyses of cultures, such as race, gender, ability, sexuality, class, and other various intersectional identities within inter/transnational and inter/transcultural contexts. It helps envision social justice.

There are many health communication scholars, who have made a turn to investigate the essential juncture between intercultural communication and health communication. For example, Dillon and Basu (2014) study minority men who have sex with men, and Dutta and Jamil (2013) Bangladeshi immigrants. The most influential work that situates the (inter)cultural turn in health communication research is Dutta's (2008) culture-centered approach. This approach is conceived with a critical research agenda, which is intended to challenge the biomedical and Eurocentric underpinnings of health communication studies. Dutta writes;

> This approach questions the very values which underlie the universal logic of the biomedical model and of the cognitive-behavioral model, bringing out the hidden agendas embedded in the top-down frameworks underlying health communication and providing a critical entry point for interrogating them. (p. 3)

This approach invites those situated within global and domestic cultural marginalities into our health communication research.

Dutta's (2008) culture-centered approach engages three aspects of our health-being: structure, culture, and agency. Structure, to him, means "those aspects of social organization that constrain and enable the capacity of cultural participants to seek out health choices and engage in health-related behaviors" (p. 6). The approach focuses on the cultural—various local contexts where meanings of health are constituted, negotiated, contested, and competed. "Agency refers to the capacity of cultural members to enact their choices and to participate actively in negotiating the structures within which they find themselves" (p. 7). Human health, as experienced in our everyday communication and interactions in particular contexts, is complex as it is comprised simultaneously of these factors at the macro, meso, and micro levels.

It is evident that critical intercultural communication studies and culture-centered health communication studies share axiological commitments to complex analysis of power, social injustice, and communicative contexts. Both believe in research activities' potentiality in transforming the ways through which we participate in world-making and, consequently, the world in which we live. There are various ways to engage the critical intersection, conceiving critical intercultural health communication research and pedagogy.

We endorse autoethnography as a productive way to engage the epistemological significance of "context" for critical intercultural health communication research and pedagogy. Ellis (2004) describes autoethnography as "an autobiographical genre of writing and research" that focuses on "the personal and its relationship of culture" (p. 37). She continues;

> Back and forth, autoethnographers gaze: First they look through an ethnographic wide angle lens, focusing outward on social and cultural aspects of their personal experience; then, they look inward, exposing a vulnerable self that is moved by and may move through, refract, and resist cultural interpretations. As they zoom backward and forward, inward and outward, distinction between the personal and cultural become blurred, sometimes beyond distinct recognition. (pp. 37–38)

Ellis and Bochner (2014) write that autoethnographic stories "blur the boundaries between humanities and social science, expressing concrete lived experience in novel and literary forms, depicting local stories and including authors' critical reflections on their lives and writing process" (pp. 9–10).

Many intercultural communication scholars have realized the importance of autoethnography investigating the cultural. For example, see Boylorn and Orbe's (2014) collection entitled *Critical Autoethnography: Intersecting Cultural Identities in Everyday Life*. Dutta (2008) reveals characteristics of the culture-centered approach of health communication: power, marginalization, context, stories, and resistance (pp. 12–14). Autoethnography can function as an epistemological vehicle for culture-centered health communication studies. Such labor has already begun. For example, among many, Ellis and Bochner (1992) use autoethnography to explore their abortion experience. Mingé and Sterner's (2014) relational autoethnography, entitled "The Transitory Radical: Making Place with Cancer," stories their love and trust while moving through a diagnosis and treatments of cancer and gets at the complexity of illness in contexts. They write, "Illness incoherently reorders the sensible into nonsensical place making and marking in transition" (pp. 45–46). Autoethnography has capacity to pay due attention to the significance of communicative contexts for critical intercultural health communication studies. It also responds to Parrott and Kreuter's (2003) push toward multi-, inter-, and trans-disciplinary approaches to health communication.

Pedagogical potentiality of autoethnography is grand (Toyosaki, 2013). Both autoethnographic pedagogy and critical pedagogy (Freire, 2000) focus on the transformative potentiality of selfhood as it is the human mechanism that both internalizes and externalizes macro-, meso-, and micro-socialization and globalization. In *Pedagogy of the Oppressed*, Freire explains that "the term *conscientização* refers to learning to perceive social, political, and economic contradictions, and to take action against the oppressive elements of reality" (p. 35). For him, a praxis of *conscientização* is a self-affirming process through which we participate in histories and world-making. Doing autoethnography functions as a site where we understand situated selves-in-the-world in their particularity and complexity through analyzing our lived experiences. Autoethnography serves as a vehicle through which we transform our situated selves in the world.

Employed as a teaching method, autoethnography invites several pedagogical turns. They are (1) narrative/autobiographic (see Bochner & Ellis, 1995; Langellier, 1989), (2) performative/corporeal (see Kiesinger, 2002; Lockford, 2002; McLaren, 1999; Pineau, 2002), (3) self-reflexive/therapeutic (see Davies, 1999; Goodall, 2000), (4) empathic/aesthetic (see Pelias, 1999), and critical/transformative (see Banks & Banks, 2000; Ellis, 2004). Toyosaki and Penseneau-Conway (2013) understand autoethnography as a praxis of social justice: Autoethnography connects people through its relational and communal implications. Autoethnographies, produced by various people of various identities in various contexts in the world, have potentiality in coming together to create a global literary/interpretive network and to understand the world we live in together—both the beautiful and dirty sides and many things in between—from a bottom-up approach, privileging our lived concrete experiences. Autoethnographic pedagogy treats our intersectional identities and our concrete lived experiences as teaching/learning materials to study the intersectional complexity of health and culture.

Critical Intercultural Health Autoethnographies

One semester brought an opportunity for several graduate students/co-authors and me to interrogate cultural health politics in various domestic US-American and global contexts. During the semester, we together studied various topics, such as health narratives, identity politics in health, cultural and health marginalization/stigmatization, health disparity, community-centered health promotion, nuclear/

radiation politics, and health pedagogy. Using autoethnography, we engaged our own selfhood and lived experiences in order to understand the complex intersection between health and cultures. In the following, we share our autoethnographic pieces and unpack the significance of autoethnographic pedagogy for critical intercultural health communication studies/teaching.

Valid Misidentification: (Possible) Intersectional Meanings in the Layering of Hands (By Satoshi Toyosaki)

I am a checker.
I check my power strips, many times.
Repeat.
I check my doors and windows, many times.
Repeat.
I check my driver's license in my wallet, many times.
Repeat.
I am a counter.

1. One, two, three, four, five.
2. "Right Front burner, off!"
3. One, two, three, four, five.
4. "Right back burner, off!"
5. One, two, three, four, five.
6. "Left back burner, off!"
7. One, two three, four, five.
8. "Left front burner, off!"

I am a washer.
I wash my hands, many times.
Repeat.
I sanitize my hands, many times.
Repeat.

***

It is a chilly cloudy day. Here in the North, people have an expression, "It's too cold to snow." As a new transplant, I am still trying to figure out the saying; meteorology is not my thing. "It is not that cold. So, it may snow," I wonder as I drive. I am a bit worried about driving in the snow. It feels like the low hanging clouds are mounting over my anxious shoulders; my self-diagnosed obsessive compulsive disorder (OCD) is flaring. Tired from working late last night, I wanted to sleep ten more minutes this morning. I retrospectively think, "I should not have done that," as I drive up to a fast-food drive-through. The ten more minutes threw me off of my morning ritual of checking all the burners, doors, windows, and power strips. Something in my body is nagging me to go back and to check, check, check, check. It almost feels like something is poking from the inside of me and coordinating my muscle fibers, like a puppet, to drive back home to check, check, check, check. My mind tells it to shut up. But standing hairs on my forearms try to convince my mind otherwise. My mind tries to convince my body, "I have to go to work."

I get nervous when I order at a drive-through because I have an accent. My Japanese ears are not trained to discern English that comes out of unfriendly audio-speakers at drive-throughs. I often fail to order. This time: Success! I drive up to the window wondering which type of experience I will have this morning. See, I have my own OCD ritual, which starts after getting the change:

1. I get my change.
2. I put the change in my wallet.
3. I check and count my driver's license and other things in my wallet.
4. I sanitize my hands.
5. I reach out to get the food with my clean hands.
6. (I sanitize my hands again sometimes.)

I have a typology of my drive-through experiences.

Type 1: I drive up to the window, I pay, I get the change, I do my OCD ritual while waiting, the window person goes to prepare/get my food, they come back, and I get my food.

Type 2: I drive up to the window, I wait, the window person comes to the window with my food, they tell me how much, I pay, I get the change, I do my OCD ritual very quickly, and the window person hands over my food. Type 2 does not give me enough time for me to perform my OCD ritual between the change and the food.

I really don't like Type 2. I prefer performing my OCD ritual in private to in public. Type 2 exposes me; I am afraid of being marked and stigmatized (Link & Phelan, 2001). The window person holding my food in the air out of the drive-through window is an indication that I am inconveniencing them. I apologize.

I drive up to the window. The window person is not there this morning. This is a bad sign; it will be Type 2. I open the lid of my Aloe-hand-sanitizer bottle and place it in between my legs so that I can perform my OCD ritual quickly between the change and the food. My OCD ritual performance requires precision this morning. I pay, and the window person places the change on my left hand. I take the change and put my left hand quickly into my car so that I can start my OCD ritual.

	I am putting the change in my wallet, fast.
	I am counting things in my wallet, fast.
	I am miscounting, fast.
	I am counting things in my wallet, again, fast.
The Window Person	I am putting several drops of my Aloe hand sanitizer with my right hand on my left hand, fast.
	I am rubbing my hands together, fast.
	(I hope that the window person is patient with my OCD ritual.)
	I am rubbing my hands together, fast.
	(I wonder if I look like a fry rubbing its legs to the window person.)
	I am rubbing my hands together, fast.
	(I wonder what the window person thinks of my OCD ritual.)

I reach two clean hands out of my car to get the brown bag and a drink. The window person puts my food and drink on the window shelf inside and reaches her two hands out of the drive-through window. "This is neither Type 1 nor Type 2." She grabs my two hands with her two hands. Without knowing how to make sense, my hands rest motionlessly in her hands.

She smiles.		
She smiles with a hint of sorrow.		
She looks into my eyes.	Her/My Layered Hands	Me
She takes a pause.		
She says, "It won't rub off of me."		

My mind spins fast, "What won't rub off of her?" My English-as-a-Second-Language mind thinks, "What does the third-person singular pronoun stand for?" As she lets go of my hands, my hands suddenly feel the gravity. I see my hands. As her hands slowly retrieve into the window, my eyes follow them. Her hands suddenly become racialized to my eyes. The window person's hands were once raceless to my eyes. She "becomes" an African American middle-aged woman phenotypically to my eyes. She hands me over my food and drink. I look at her hands and her face.

The only thing that my mind can squeeze out at this moment is that this is her cultural critique of interracial conflicts, maybe between African Americans and Asian Americans. My OCD, unidentifiable and invisible to her, may have become visible possibly as a racist act. My mind goes again, "She has a valid critique. I agree with her if my assumption is somewhat close. What should I say? Should I say anything at all?" The drive-through window closes.

***

I now drive to my work. My mind does not stop: My OCD is a powerful framework with which I make sense out of my experienes. I have two types for my drive-through experiences: Type 1 and Type 2. I have not thought of my OCD intersectionally with race in context. Intersectional implications on class, gender, sexual orientation, (dis)ability, and more? My OCD is not culturally isolated in contexts. I park my car and hurry into the building. As I climb up the stairs in front of the building, I wonder if I will see her, again. I am forever appreciative of her critical social labor and lesson on intersectionality.

Chasing Perfection in Pitching: An Autoethnographic Account of Anger and Anxiety on the Baseball Diamond (by Darren J. Valenta)

I stared in at my dad from the pitcher's mound, my eyes smoldering from beneath the slightly curved brim of my dusty royal blue baseball cap. I gripped the red-stitched baseball tight in my right hand, which I'd planted rigidly in the middle of my right thigh. I was in the stretch, as they say in baseball parlance, with my feet shoulder-width apart, my black A2000 infielder's glove tucked against my left armpit, and my head turned over my left shoulder so that I could glare in at home plate. That's where my dad sat on an overturned old white bucket we typically used to store dozens of baseballs. His left arm was extended in front of his chest, slightly bent as he presented the toothless maw of his ancient catcher's mitt.

I never threw a perfect pitch, although my driving mission was to do so. I always missed my target slightly, or forgot to follow through correctly, or bungled the leg kick. My dad didn't always mind or even notice those small imperfections, but I did. They were all I noticed. The accumulation of these seemingly minor mistakes made my blood boil, pushing me closer to the kind of fury that made me wholly incapable of throwing any pitch, let alone a perfect one. Perfection, for me, represented a serene happiness, a comfort in knowing that I'd reached the pinnacle of pitching. Perfection was the standard I set for myself because I hoped that it would come with a relief from the inner turmoil created by its pursuit. In baseball like in life, I've always doggedly chased my potential, trying to mold myself into the image of what I think I should be. The possibility of failing to live up to my "potentiality-for-Being," however, often creates a worry that I'll never get there (Hyde, 1980, p. 147). Baseball was a microcosm in which I could concretely measure progress toward my ideal self. With each pitch, I submitted myself for evaluation from others, exposing the idealized image of myself as a pitcher to the physics and logics of my environment. Those moments of expression, embodied in my repeated deliveries to home plate, created an overwhelming anxiety, a dread that I'd be found wanting (Bhabha, 2008; Lacan, 2014). I wanted to demonstrate to my dad, to my teammates, and to myself that I was perfect because maybe then I'd achieve my ideal self and feel good enough. The continual failure to achieve that perfection felt like a grievous mistake, one which made me incredibly angry.

We were at the local elementary school on a cold spring day practicing, yet again, for the upcoming baseball season when the anxiety and anger detonated, indelibly imprinting this particular session on my brain. There was always an underlying tension to these trips because I wanted to be anywhere else; I loved playing baseball, but, as a kid, I assumed I'd play forever, meaning venturing out into the deceptively chilly Oregon spring wasn't ideal when there were video games to play. My dad drug me out to the field anyway, though, using a combination of guilt and parental do-as-I-say-ism. I'd like to report that I remember the father-son bonding that took place during those practice sessions, or the profound wisdom my dad bestowed upon me between grounders and line-drives, but what I remember most vividly is the rage.

On this day, I must not have been performing particularly well. Truth be told, I don't remember exactly what set me off. It's strange how, all these years later, I don't remember why I was actually mad; the heat of the fire lingers, but the origin has faded with time. I do remember all of my classic angry mannerisms: punching my right thigh repeatedly, slapping my left thigh with my mitt, and yelling incoherently. Crying was the reaction I despised the most, though, because it felt like my body betraying me. Tears indicated sadness or desperation, which is not what I felt. I was furious, incensed. Why did my eyes well up with tears, then, blurring my vision and causing me to wipe them clear with my throwing hand? When my heroes and idols got angry, they didn't cry.

I wasn't in a full rage, but I was certainly headed that way as the crisp wind whipped my grey sweatpants against my legs and I received the ball back from my dad. I was not pitching well, certainly not up to my own unrealistic standards, and my dad could tell that I was in the midst of a temper tantrum. My dad, while much more adept at controlling his anger, still showed flashes of it. When I began exhibiting symptoms, he was usually quick to follow, which only made me more frustrated. The tension between us often stemmed from this symbiotic relationship; it often felt like a stand-off, each of us waiting for the other to begin the cycle over again. One of his typical responses to my irritation at my pitching performance was to try and help by critiquing my form. He probably assumed that fixing whatever issue that inhibited me would alleviate my irritation, but I just saw it as nagging. When this tactic didn't work, my father would often lose his patience and begin criticizing my inability to control my emotions, which he identified as the reason for my poor performance. This approach would usually just exacerbate the situation, leaving us both fuming at each other.

We had reached this point on this particular afternoon, and my dad chose to alter the context in which I was pitching. He rose from his seat behind home plate, gathered our baseballs back into the bucket, placed them near my position on the mound, and took his place in the right-handed batter's box. The previous pitching drill had grown stale so he wanted to change my view of the strike zone and offer me a facsimile of a situation I might actually face in a game. His choice would have made sense on most days, but, on this afternoon, it merely exposed him to the brunt of my anger. To properly throw at a hitter and ensure that the baseball will make contact, a pitcher is instructed to aim at the batter's front hip. Baseball lore maintains that aiming at this specific spot makes it nearly impossible for the batter to dodge out of the way in time. It's also widely accepted that hitting a batter in the hip is the proper way to send a message without endangering their health.

My dad got the message. As the pitch approached, I saw the recognition dawn in his eyes. He quickly realized there was nothing he could do to avoid the pitch, but he still attempted to back out of the way anyway. My father took the blow to the hip and let out a low grunt. It hurts, certainly, but the pain isn't the most jarring part of being hit by a baseball in this manner. The symbolism is what has the greatest impact. This act is meant to demonstrate dominance, showcasing a level of precision and skill designed to intimidate and impress the person on the receiving end of the beaning (Trujillo, 1991). Had I known at the time that my anger was perhaps triggered because of my fear of failure or anxiety, I may have been able to communicate that much to my father and avoid the ensuing blow-up. A teenager is not always equipped with that level of reflexivity, however, and I certainly was no exception.

I don't remember exactly how we transitioned into a hitting drill, but we did. We switched positions, me now in the batter's box and dad on the pitcher's mound. I stood poised to take my pent-up aggression out on the pitches lobbed in from my father, ready to drive ball after ball out into the outfield. Again, I don't remember if it happened right away or if dad threw a few regular pitches to lull me into a false sense of security, but I do remember that he retaliated. Just as he had previously, I attempted to dance out of the way of an incoming baseball aimed directly at my left hip, but proved unsuccessful. Even amidst my irritation at being hit, I accepted the retaliation as the consequence of my previous action. The retribution felt only fair. The batting drill continued, and, just as I had during the pitching drill, I grew enraged with my lack of productivity. I slammed the barrel of my bat into home plate repeatedly with unnecessary ferocity, grunted and moaned with each unsuccessful swing, and fought back angry tears.

My father, having had enough of my outbursts for the day, gruffly suggested we wrap up our practice session. I refused, demanding that he throw more pitches so that I might achieve some level of success, some level of perfection instead of leaving in disgrace. I couldn't stand the thought of not being good enough. Each swing of the bat that didn't result in a solid drive into dead centerfield was an indictment of my character, a commentary on my shortcomings as an athlete and a human being. With these failures came wave after wave of anger, shame, and disappointment, which only made the situation worse.

Finally, my father ended our misery, refusing to throw another pitch despite my protests. Resigning to this decision, I began collecting the baseballs that were scattered around the backstop and field. Again, my recollection of how this happened isn't clear. Perhaps I continued to spew anger and hatred because of my father's decision to end our practice session. Maybe I was more petulant than I remember, causing my dad more frustration than I knew at the time. Whatever the cause, I remember collecting baseballs against the backstop with my back turned to my dad who was gathering balls out near the pitching mound. I knelt down to make retrieving the balls easier and heard the distinct sound of aluminum striking rocks and dirt. I began to turn my head to my left in search of the cause of the sound when I saw my long, slender metal bat skip across the ground and crash into the chain-link fence not six inches from where I knelt. I turned to face my dad aghast, completely overtaken with a renewed rage at the fact that he'd do such a thing. Clearly he'd been battling his own anger throughout the practice session and had finally lost control. The rest of that day is a blur of yelling, silence, and tension as he and I piled the rest of our gear into his truck and drove the short distance back to our house.

***

Recalling this day and all the fury I felt makes me deeply sad. My father and I have a wonderful relationship now, and, really, always have. The tension that surrounded those baseball outings was not typical of the rest of our interactions, perhaps because I felt the anxiety of pursuing perfection so acutely in those times, or perhaps because my anger and disgust turned more inward when it came to schoolwork or my social life. I took my frustration at my imperfection out on my father in those moments, and I regret that. I'm also ashamed of the role that anger has played in my life leading up to and following this episode. In many respects, I feel this toxic cocktail of anxiety and anger now more acutely than I ever did as a teenager, and that trend scares me. Scholars have continued to link conformity to stereotypically masculine gender roles and traits of toxic masculinity to depressive symptoms in men (Genuchi & Valdez, 2015). Additionally, researchers have established that current diagnostic criteria often miss depressive symptoms in men, and that anger and aggression continue to be endorsed as effective coping mechanisms by men who adhere to more traditional conceptions of masculinity (Nadeau, Balsan, & Rochien, 2016). I fear that the anger I often feel when trapped in a situation that makes me doubt my ability or worth as a human being will begin to ruin my relationships and take a significant toll on my mental health. It remains difficult, however, to admit to my anger and anxiety issues because of the stigma still surrounding conversations about mental health (Corrigan, 2004). Stigma, as applied to issues of health and health communication, discredits, devalues, and disgraces the stigmatized (Smith, 2011). To admit to mental health issues like anxiety or depression or to anger issues, then, is to subject myself to a level of delegitimization that may have social and cultural consequences. Furthermore, to admit an inability to control my own emotions is to violate the expectations of the kind of masculinity I've been socialized into, which only increases my aversion to seeking help.

These factors don't mean that I won't seek help, or that doing so is impossible for me. They do, however, mean that the process will be difficult. Writing this narrative offers a beginning means of growth, though. Dutta (2011) argued that "narratives are sites of contestation where cultural meanings are played out through dialogues among cultural participants" (p. 91). Diving back into this narrative and dissecting the various interests and influences at play enables me to identify and perhaps offer resistance to dominant ideologies like hegemonic masculinity and biomedical models of disability that inform and exacerbate my struggles with anger and anxiety. Ultimately, I undertake these kinds of efforts because I've grown tired of losing moments in my life to an overwhelming rage that blots out everything else. How might my recollection of that day with my father change if my understandings of anxiety and anger had been different at the time? How might my relationship with anxiety and anger differ if the social and cultural interests that shape the dominant conceptions of these phenomena were different? In his culture-centered approach to health communication, Dutta (2011) presented an epistemological perspective that endeavors to question the structural and communicative factors that marginalize populations of people and their health experiences. Applied to my lived experience, this culture-centered approach will enable me to investigate the social and cultural factors that construct my experiences of anxiety and anger and how I might resist those through narrative or otherwise. Those moments with my father are gone to my memory, and, while I've been able to recontextualize some of them as positive or instructive given my temporal distance from them, a significant portion of my memories with him are singed with bitter rage. I don't get to see him as often as I used to, making the moments I do spend with him even more precious. Reframing my relationship with anger and anxiety might help me prevent other moments from being stolen from me as some of my time on the baseball field with him has been.

The Legacy of "I'm Okay:" Navigating the Performance of Health and Gender between Mother and Daughter (by Lindy Wagner)

A sharp pain emanates from the base of my spine, down my leg, and into my toes. Tears spring immediately to my eyes and my trainer asks, "Are you okay?" I don't tell him what is happening. I don't think he'll understand, and I don't want to be judged as an emotional or weak woman. Too late. Tears well up in my eyes and I remember lying in a hospital bed for days without hope of walking, running, or working out again. He repeats, "Are you okay? Did something happen to your back?" I snap out of my memory of the cold, sterile hospital room and back to the gym floor and explain that something did happen, but "I'm okay." That statement, one that I use over, and over again, especially when it comes to my health and being a whole, healthy, woman. A statement so laden with how I am not okay, that I know when I say it, I really mean, "Don't ask me more questions, don't ask me how I really am, don't be interested in my health because I will just lie."

***

Roter and Hall (2011) highlight that the emotions of both physician and patient are involved in the medical care process (p. 58). I wonder what the physician thinks when they encounter me. I try to be pleasant, but because I want them to treat me effectively, I assume my behavior in the interaction matters. I often try to present a pleasant façade. One that says, "I'm okay," even when I may not be feeling that way.

***

August 2013; Dance steps running through my head. I am responsible for choreographing our staff's lip sync dance that we perform on the last day of resident assistant training. It's a big deal and it is my responsibility to teach and practice with our staff that evening. All I was thinking was how much pain I would be in, but I wasn't going to tell anyone that. I've been told my whole life to be strong; don't let people think just because you are a woman that you can't do as much as a man. I want to prove that I am strong, I am capable, and my physical body is a testament to that. Admitting my pain counters my proof that a woman is strong and really can do it all. After hours of practice and smiling through the pain, I retreat back to my bunk for the evening and quietly cry myself to sleep. If ibuprofen doesn't help, I'll head back to urgent care for another pack of steroids.

***

I witness a decline in my mother's health. She didn't age overnight, but she moves slower, she needs a minute standing up, she needs help getting up and down stairs sometimes, and she can't walk long distances without it causing her pain. I struggle watching this because I looked to her growing up as my example of a woman who is strong and can do it all. After all, she was the one telling me my body was strong and that I could do anything a man could do. I attribute my strong character and independence of thought to my mom, but I've often wondered when this affirmation has helped and when it has hindered. Even now, as my mom and I acknowledge her aging, she insists she can still do everything for herself and won't ask for help unless she absolutely must. I wonder if the expectation that women be mother, sister, aunt, professional, strong, attractive, charming, and every other construction society has created also leaves women vulnerable to hiding health problems for fear that their health will somehow expose weakness; a soft underbelly that, once exposed, leaves room for a striking blow. These are my thoughts. I assume if others know, especially if any of the men I work with have an inkling that I am sick or weak, I'll be overlooked the next time an opportunity arises, or I'll be seen as inferior to them. I understand why my mom doesn't expose her belly to others, she knows the feeling.

***

I give up. I can barely walk, pain up and down my left leg. I leave work early and go to urgent care, but only because the pain is unbearable. I arrive at Urgent Care and hope the doctor who was there the first time isn't. He barely asked me questions, heard I had leg pain, asked if I sat a lot in my job, then gave me a pack of steroids. This is my experience with most doctors who are men. In my experience they assume I am exaggerating, or that I am just there for attention. They have no idea that coming to them is a last resort and I would only go to a doctor if I absolutely must.

Relief. When the door opens, a woman walks in. When interacting with women doctors, my perception is they actively listen and ask questions not just about the pain. They establish other factors playing a part in what brought me there that day. Today, while I appreciate her attentiveness, I want the pain to go away and explain that, last time, I received a steroid pack and the pain subsided for a while. "Can I just get another steroid pack?" She smiles and explains to not be too hasty because my health is important, and she wants to be thorough. What a difference from the first doctor, I think to myself, so I let myself settle in for a more extensive inquiry. After about fifteen minutes of in-depth questions, she asks if she can touch my back. I explain the pain is in my leg and after a thorough WebMD search, I know my pain comes from sciatica. She smiles and says that while that may be the case, she wants to try something. She comes alongside me and pushes just above my tailbone alongside my spine. Stinging. Hot, searing pain rushes down my leg and up my spine, my eyes feel watery. I have never experienced pain like this. She sees me flinch and asks if that can be the source of the pain. I nod and say that I had no idea my back was the problem all along. She nods politely and sends me for extensive tests.

***

"What did the doctor say?" I ask this of my mother more and more frequently. I remember, as a child, not understanding why adults were always asking about blood pressure, cholesterol, blood tests, doctor visits, and health. I am not sure when it happened, but it did. I am one of those adults, and as the words leave my lips, I genuinely am interested in what my mother has to say. She has been shuffled from doctor to doctor in the last few months and I am frustrated on her behalf. Since when have I become so intent on what doctors say about one's health? Why is this at the forefront of my mind so often during the day?

My mother, a normally sunshiny and positive person has been suffering from pain in her legs. She describes it as excruciating and debilitating. She went to the primary care physician she and my father had seen for several years, but the doctor never really listened to her. The doctor dismissed her explanations of pain and discomfort, said she needed to lose weight, gave her a prescription for a strong anti-inflammatory and sent her on her way. As we talk, she mentions the doctor felt cold, distant, and not invested in her care. Because of my experience with leg pain and doctors, I encourage her to change the primary care doctor if she isn't satisfied. This is something I never considered until I was in a comparable situation early in my adult life.

Early in my career, I saw a doctor recommended by a colleague. I was met with sarcasm and disdain by this male doctor when I expressed that I was concerned I may have depression. He scoffed and said I could go talk to someone, but I should just find some hobbies, so I had something to do outside of work … and lose some weight. That is always tacked on at the end.

My mind wandered to that moment as my mother continues expressing her frustration. Over the course of the next few months, she went to multiple specialists to receive some level of diagnosis. She saw a variety of men and women doctors, and the doctor finally able to help her was indeed a man. However, this did not exempt her from experiencing callous behavior from at least one other male doctor, who rolled his eyes and assumed her pain was simply because she was getting old.

***

Several studies have shown women health care providers present more patient-centered behavior than the men who are their counterparts (Roter, Lipkin, & Korsgaard, 1991; Roter & Hall, 1998; Roter, Hall, & Aoki, 2002; Roter & Hall, 2004). I consider that there are men who can be empathetic and actively listen and I try to be open to this possibility because as my mother gets older and she encounters more health problems, I know she and I will negotiate care from a distance. Scholars indicate this type of long distance caregiving can be challenging (Bevan, Vreeburg, Verdugo, & Sparks, 2012). Caregiving involves many things, such as help for another, the time spent assisting, and the amounts of tasks performed for the betterment of an individual in need (Ellis, Miller, & Given, 1989). When one is a distance caregiver, the engagement with caregiving is a little different. Although distance presents an additional caregiving burden (Kelsey & Laditka, 2009; Mitnick, Leffler, & Hood, 2010), it is something that can be managed. With my mother, I consider geographical distance, but also the doctors we will interact with for appointments. I consider my caregiving approach to my mother because she takes a very serious approach to caregiving of me.

***

Through a barrage of tests and doctor's appointments I learn my L3 and L4 vertebrae are quite off-center. If my vertebrae are supposed to be building blocks perfectly aligned to create a strong tower, my tower is on the verge of collapse. My neurosurgeon upon entering the exam room for the first time, laughs loudly, "You shouldn't be able to walk because your back is so messed up." He explains he wouldn't have known I was in pain unless I had told him and that I must have a high tolerance of pain because an average person would have come much sooner. Was I so jaded by male doctor's lack of empathy that I fooled doctors into believing that "I'm okay." If that's the case, who am I hurting in the process? He goes on to say there is no reason for therapy, shots, or other remedies. My back needs surgery immediately. Despite his terrible timing with humor, I connected with him. I wonder how many male doctors I will encounter like him. What are the chances I will have a positive experience again?

***

Upon waking from surgery, I discover my routine three-hour surgery was an eight-hour surgery. Difficult, unexpected, but successful. I also have an endless stream of caretaking by those in the hospital, friends, and loved ones. The shining star? My mother. She, who lives 515 miles away, is with me for two weeks; in the waiting room during surgery, driving me home when I am released, bathing me, changing my bandages, cooking for me, keeping me company, and counting out endless pills. She is a rock. I can't imagine the patience, love, and dedication it takes to be such an empathetic and attentive caretaker.

***

"I'm okay." That simple, yet context laden statement I hear so many times. A statement I surely got from my mother and she surely got from hers. That statement immediately screaming the opposite. This is what goes through my head as my mom tells me that she has a diagnosis, but that "I'm okay." She needs her knees replaced and it's just routine surgery. I am all too familiar with "routine" surgery. I worry. She, like me, resisted a diagnosis for so long. I reflect on the tender and purposeful way she cared for me after my back surgery. There were so many days and nights that without the help of my mother, I would have been in pain, starved, or suffering alone. I know she is most certainly not okay and I make plans to be with her for her first knee surgery. While I know she has her husband and my sister to help her recover, I know I must be there. There is something about our relationship that dictates I must be present. My mom taught me to be strong and this is how I must be for her.

***

A mother-daughter relationship is tenuous at times. Always ups and downs. Always things you say that you regret, but also always things you wish you would've said. Caretaking, long-term care, distance care, elder care; all the words describing what is often on my mind when my mom says, "I'm okay." I wonder, "When will I be making decisions?" The ones about type of care, location of care, when should care stop, and my role in it all. I wonder what our mother-daughter relationship will encounter when we both have negative male doctor experiences. How do I negotiate care for my mother that works for both of us? How do I consider my mother's autonomy and consider what may be best?

Pecchioni and Nussbaum (2000) define autonomy as "having control over and being responsible for one's life. Autonomy can be divided into two subtypes—independent autonomy and shared autonomy" (p. 320). Cicirelli (1992, 1993) explains that independent autonomy means an individual may utilize information gained from others but will make the final decision on their own; in shared autonomy, an individual will seek information from others and willingly abide by the decision of another. What I hope to avoid, if possible, is paternalism. Cicirelli (1992, 1993) notes this is when a person holds the belief that they may impose a decision on another for the welfare of that individual. My worst fear; being paternal towards my mother. We grow together in the understanding that not only are we strong women in a system that doesn't favor us, but at some point, we will negotiate decisions regarding her care. I never want to take away her autonomy, but perhaps there will be a day when I become the system she resists? All I can hope is that as time goes on, I can learn how best to develop a successful decision-making process alongside my mother—a decision-making process which allows for the best possible understanding of her care within the patriarchal system of which we are a part.

War in Our Blood: Illness, Peace, and Dis/Connection with the Story of Sadako Sasaki (by Shelby Swafford)

There are stories in my bones. In my blood. Stories I feel, but don't really understand. I have been in pain for years. I have been sick for years. The trouble with living with chronic pain and illness is that the longer you live with it, the harder it becomes to remember a time without it. I don't remember exactly where my story begins. The closest I can come to marking the "start" of this experience is August 2016, when I went to my university's student health center for a persistent swollen lymph node on the right side of my face which accompanied a new level of full-bodied exhaustion and body pains I hadn't ever experienced, although I had been in graduate school for two years already. The doctor told me I had mono, which I knew wasn't the case, because I've had mono before and this was different. I told her as much. I told her about the pain. She didn't believe me.

I got sicker. My joints began to swell and throb. My knees buckled under the weight of my body as I walked. Daily migraines. Night sweats. My mouth and eyes dried out. Roughly eight months later I saw my first rheumatologist. When I described my symptoms, he sent me off for a series of complicated tests without telling me what they were for. I was poked and prodded and scanned, analyzed and pathologized and prescribed—over 60 pills per week. He diagnosed me with fibromyalgia with no further question or interest. When I called his office to schedule follow up appointments, they never returned my call.

A few months later, small red dots begin to appear all over my body, collecting in constellations which swell into bruised blotches. At first I think it's an allergic reaction, and so do the doctors, until I get a blood test to check. And then another. And then one more to be sure. Something is wrong in your blood, they say, and admit me to the hospital.

Hospitals are places of healing, where we go to cure the inevitable ailments of our living with the gifts of Western medical technologies. Hospitals are also places of hurt, houses of disease and decay confronting our bodies' mortal limits. Hospitals are where many of us take our first breath, sterilized sanctuaries of birth in the modern age. And hospitals are where many now wish to take their last breaths, in the best-case-scenario of succumbing to peaceful deaths from natural causes at an ever-increasing "old age," surrounded by a bounty of arranged bouquets and a circle of our loved ones, under careful and compassionate medical supervision. I fucking hate hospitals, I think to myself over and over again, laying uncomfortably in the small cot awaiting the on-call hematologist to tell me what's happening in my blood.

***

Storying my experience of health and illness is complicated and messy. When the story is your body, language often seems to fail. I hesitated to write about my diagnoses and hospitalization as it was happening because I didn't understand it, even though I desperately wanted to understand. On the surface this may seem strange, but nuclear politics brought me to story my experience. When I learned more about Hiroshima and Nagasaki, I was struck by the stories of the *hibakusha*, those survivors whose health was affected by the atomic bombs and subsequent radiation. Sadako Sasaki is one of the most well-known *hibakusha*, whose story has become a part of international peace education. Masamoto Nasu's (2015) biographical account of Sadako's struggle with the A-Bomb disease constructs Sadako's story using extensive research and interviews with her family and classmates. Using Nasu's account as a basis for my research and inspiration, I autoethnographically engaged with Sadako's story while using creative writing to performatively reconstruct her experience with illness. Through these performative engagements, I aim not only to better understand my own illness/health experience, but to highlight moments of dis/connection between our stories, voices, and bodies—dis/connection which is symptomatic of the complex network of global systems which bring our histories together.

***

It's been five months since I first arrived at the hospital, longer than I thought I would have to stay. When I first got here, I was hoping I'd be able to go to

Michiko's house for spring break. Now it is July, and my friends are going off to Junior High while I am still here trying to get well. The swelling in the lymph node on my neck went down for a while, but it has returned, and I am beginning to feel pain in my knees and knuckles. I try to be strong and not show my pain in front of my family. My illness has caused them so much pain already. They gave me their blood for the transfusions until they couldn't any longer, and even though Father wouldn't admit it, I know he sold his watch to pay the blood bank. It is only because of the costs of the transfusions and the chemical pills that they sold the family home and moved into the barracks next to the bus line. They do not know that I know about my disease, what it really is. But I am not a little child anymore. I am almost twelve years old, and I have heard grown-ups talk about A-bomb disease.

***

The IV sticking out of (or into) my left arm somehow itches and burns and stings and stabs all at once, as if the needle were simultaneously sucking out my blood and filling my veins with liquid nitrogen. The bruising seems to be getting worse, the deep purple blotch in my elbow crease spilling out from the edges of the bandage holding the IV in place. Maybe if they didn't insist on doing three separate blood panels (almost four, because they said they didn't get enough in the third round to run the tests), all requiring fresh drawls of blood, or maybe if they could get the needle in on the first or second or third poke instead of the eighth or ninth or tenth, the IV wouldn't hurt so damn bad. But who am I kidding? Everything hurts.

***

The first time they put blood into my arm after I came to the hospital in February, it hurt. I remember writing to Michiko about it when I asked her if I could stay at her house during spring break. The doctor told me then if you don't hurt a little when you're sick you won't get well. I wonder now if this is still what he meant. It seems like since I came to the hospital, I have only gotten sicker. My gums have started to bleed and the red dots on my skin have come back. The nurses' charts say my white blood cells have increased and my platelets have dropped. I know my parents and the doctor do not want to tell me about my blood, but I have been recording my numbers in secret since I arrived. I have heard a rumor that if your white blood cell count exceeds 100,000, you die. Mine are above this and I have not died, but I keep thinking about the pale face of the little girl who died last month, who Kiyo and I visited in the mortuary. She looked so peaceful, as if she were sleeping in her tiny coffin. I know I stunned Kiyo when I said I wonder if I am going to die like that, but it is true. Still, I am encouraging for my family and friends. Just like in the relay races at school, I do not want to give up.

***

New patches of petechiae are popping up over my body, small hemorrhages underneath the skin caused by a lack of platelets in the blood that help form clots and keep your veins from popping like suffocating balloons. They appear symptomatically in medical conditions ranging from serious viral infections to blunt force injuries to malnutrition to blood disorders to leukemia. The hematologist tells me in my case, he foresees two possible causes to the sudden onset of my petechiae: leukemia, and a rare blood disorder called ITP. He would need run more tests to "rule out the worst case scenario."

***

There are many people wishing for my recovery, and the recovery of those like me. Today the hospital received a box from high school girls in Nagoya containing one-thousand rainbow paper cranes to distribute to the A-bomb patients. Most of them went to the internal ward, but a nurse brought me a string of them, too. They are so beautiful that Kiyo and I decided to make some ourselves. They say if you fold one thousand, you will get well. Kiyo says I will get well whether or not I fold them, but it couldn't hurt to try. It is tedious work, but I don't mind. It reminds me of how I used to braid sandals back at home. I think both Kiyo and I are grateful for the distraction. I try not to think about my disease, but the image of the young girl keeps coming back to me. She was only five, not even born yet when the atom bomb dropped on Hiroshima, but she had the A-bomb disease like me. The night after she died Kiyo and I went up to the rooftop to look at the sky. I hoped she was at peace with the stars.

***

Hospitals have always made me anxious, but I am terrified. I feel hopelessly vulnerable in my ignorance of my own body. I am only twenty-four, but I have heard stories of cancer claiming lives much younger than mine. But this fear, too, is short-lived. When my tests come back, the hematologist tells me my white blood cell count is fine, considering the condition my body is in. The good news is I don't have cancer. The bad news, he says, is that what I do have is rare, and they don't know a lot about it. He calls it immune thrombocytopenic purpura, or ITP for short. He can't tell me what has caused it for sure, other than it is immune-related. Your body has just become confused, he explains, and is attacking itself. My body is fighting a war of its own making. I have been thinking recently about the "making" of war, and how war "makes" our bodies. War connects us on a global scale, implicating us all in a complex system of fragile relationships between constructed borders. My country dropped an atomic weapon. A two-year-old girl living about 1.7 kilometers from the hypocenter escaped her burning home in the arms of her mother. She grew up to love music and roses and pears and became the fastest runner in her school. And then, at age twelve, the war erupted again in Sadako Sasaki's body. She died of "A-bomb disease" a little over eight months after her diagnosis. My country dropped an atomic weapon and a young girl died of leukemia. But her story has lived beyond her body (Chordas, 2018). "The Paper Crane Project" has become a part of the International Campaign to Abolish Nuclear Weapons. Her paper cranes have been donated to a peace museum in Austria, the 9/11 Peace Memorial in NYC, the Truman Library, and the USS Arizona Memorial in Pearl Harbor. President Harry Truman's grandson said Sadako's was the first human story he had seen of Hiroshima, and has since spoken out against the use of nuclear weapons. My country dropped an atomic weapon and a young girl died of leukemia, but her story has become, in itself, a message for peace, a warning of the war in our blood. I hope she is at peace with the stars.

Medical Un/Certainty: Culture, Religiosity, and Agent Orange (by Patrick Seick)

When I was a child every Sunday was marked by solemn processions and a man in a funny outfit overseeing a group of quiet people who spent much of the time with their heads bowed. Without a doubt, my favorite part of the day was when everyone would spontaneously break into, "peace be with you"s and shake hands with each other. In that moment, everyone was substantially nicer than they normally were. My mother specifically chose a church 30 minutes away that had pews with unpadded kneelers. It was only ever us in that cavernous space, where my Mom's whispered incantations bounced off the many statues of St. Mary. When we would approach the end of the rosary, we were given a chance to implore God to listen to our prayers. Inevitably, my Mom would end her specific pleas with her eyes closed praying for me to be cured—of what, she never really said. At the time of this writing, her prayers, it would seem, have gone unanswered.

My mother clung to her Catholicism with the kind of conviction that made the priest of our church blush. In many ways, I shouldn't have been surprised: Lipka (2015) says over 80% of Filipinos and that nearly two-thirds of U.S. based Filipinos identify as Roman Catholic. As Aguilar (2015) explains, the deep-seated roots of Roman Catholicism of the Philippines can be traced back to Spanish colonization of the fledgling country. Since then, Catholicism continues to structure Filipinos' understanding of their world. Indeed, Sanchez and Gaw (2007) warn that despite the enormous influence of spirituality over Filipinos' relationship with mental health, it has largely gone ignored. Moreover, Guzman, Dalay, Guzman, Jesus,

Mesa, and Flores (2009) contend that though the relationship between spirituality and health has been established by the medical community, Fililpinos' Roman Catholicism is largely unaccounted for in holistic approaches to healthcare.

I wish my doctor had known all of this because he strode in looking as most of my doctors did: white, bearded, and a face lined with exhaustion. My geneticist had overseen my case since I was ten years old, so it was something remarkable when he called my house and told my parents that he finally had a diagnosis. He asked me to strip down to a linen, thin hospital gown and ignored my reddened knee caps. Before stressful hospital visits my mother would demand that the entire family visit the Church to do the rosary. This all became relevant because several moments into his explanation of my genetic condition, he asked if it hurt my knees when I had to kneel. The truth was that it did and it had begun hurting more the older that I got. Recently, by the end of our prayer my eyes were lined with tears and I only mouthed the words of prayers to keep my shaky breath from being heard. I told him that it did and he looked unsurprised; he went on a lot longer about my extremely rare skeletal disorder that would keep me from being taller than five feet and would make certain tasks (like kneeling) extremely difficult. He explained that I had early onset osteoarthritis. He noted my extraordinary odds to even survive with the condition and that, on balance, I was lucky. I thought it strange that lucky and osteoarthritis could go together in the same sentence.

The entire time he talked at us my mother's face was stone still. At the end she asked the question that I know burned at her: how did this happen? The kind doctor tried to explain the nature of a genetic mutation and she interrupted: but how? He just repeated his "I don't know" and let silence hang in the air. He looked like an honest man searching for the right thing to say. He knew my mother was devoutly religious and so I wonder if he thought his expertise was an exercise in futility. My mother got up from the room and left my father with the doctor. When I saw her again her eyes were puffy and all four feet eleven of her was wired with tension.

The ride home was silent save for the radio playing. When we got to my house that was too small for five people, she scolded my brothers to leave the living room to her and me alone. As she watched my brothers walk away she beckoned me to the screen door. We could see my dad and neighbor still making conversation that they would inevitably repeat again days from now.

"Did you know that she smokes a pack a day and drinks all day long? She doesn't have a job. Her boyfriend doesn't live with her and she's pregnant again."

I did know these things. I knew that our neighbor treated her porch stoop like a soldier treats his post. I knew that she watched more TV than any person should and I knew that she traded in neighborhood gossip as if that was actually worth something. And I knew that she liked cigarettes and alcohol and men. I knew that my mom had never smoked, only had the rare glass of wine, and had been married to my dad for years. I knew that my neighbor had never graduated high school and had lived in the same town since she was born. I knew that she had three boys, same as my mom and I knew none of them were disabled or unhealthy like me. Most of all I knew we were neighbors and that my mom hated that she compared herself to a woman who never bothered to pick up a rosary.

In that moment my mom promised that she did everything right during her pregnancy with me, right down to the headphones with Mozart blaring out of them. Her result: a son with misshapen bones and diagnoses that could not be translated to her native tongue. I know and knew that I am and was her greatest pride and shame, that whatever accomplishments I might achieve are outstripped by the inexplicable sin that my body signifies. As I write now I realize that those doctor's visits felt more like a courtroom that was offering judgement on her morality. I don't know that for sure, but I do know that a lot of weight was carried in her silences that day.

While we're staring outside we saw our neighbor's three boys explode out of their front door in a playful hysteria. After a stretch of just watching them run non-stop my mom apologized for her outburst at the hospital. She implored me to wash up because she was just going to throw a frozen pizza in the oven and it would be ready shortly. After dinner, my mother went to her bedroom. I followed her and already her rosary was in her hand: I kneeled down to join her. After awhile, she grabbed a pillow and placed it in front of my knees.

***

When my mother left the hospital room my father apologized profusely for my mother. With the wave of authority I imagine cannot be learned in medical school the doctor gently explains that these conversations are difficult. My father who is more sensible than smart tries to understand how genetic mutations function. The white walls and fluorescent lights make for an intimidating classroom. Eventually, he arrives at the same question my mother did: How did this happen? The doctor pushes forward that the nature of genetic mutations is their randomness, their mere happenstance that can result in any range of result.

As if to one up the doctor's randomness, my father asks, "Could this be the result of Agent Orange?"

My doctor's face does impressive acrobatics and settles on the simple, "I'm not sure how this is relevant. Very little testing has been done on the kind of genetic mutation your son has, certainly not in relation to Agent Orange."

"So you don't know? It could be the result of Agent Orange."

"I suppose it's theoretically possible."

My father served in the Vietnam War for almost its entire duration and so he had an acute awareness of the question he was asking. More than anything from the war—the guns and the killing and the senselessness—he seemed most angry about Agent Orange. Hynes (2016) explains that Agent Orange was a weaponized herbicide used to "destroy enemy forest cover and crops, and to clear vegetation around U.S. bases for visibility" (p. 115). Hynes points out that by the end of the war the United States had sprayed well over 7 pounds of herbicides, the majority of which was Agent Orange, for every woman, man, and child in Vietnam. Because very little testing was done to determine the effect of the weapon on human bodies, it was sprayed often and indiscriminately, including on U.S. soldiers. I knew from outbursts of frustration and anger that my father felt strongly; after all, during the war, the military explicitly declared Agent Orange harmless.

At best, the military was clueless, at worst, they outright lied. The Committee to Review the Health Effects in Vietnam Veterans of Exposure to Herbicides (2014) ruled that exposure to Agent Orange has been tied to several types of cancers, immune system disorders, neurologic impairment, cardiovascular and metabolic complications, respiratory disorders, fertility and gestational issues, and birth effects and defects in the children of those exposed. This is all to say that my father's pointed question to my geneticist was perfectly relevant. Reagan's (2016) work, poignantly titled "My daughter was genetically drafted with me," details the decades of social and legal activism that has sprung up to include children of soldiers to be included in those impacted by the Vietnam War through Agent Orange. In other words, my father is not alone in believing the "deformities" experienced by his son are the direct result of his involvement in a war decades ago.

My dad continued to badger the doctor with questions and detailed for him what he had never told me. During his years long engagement in Vietnam my dad completed several jobs. He was an infantry man, he cleared out foliage, and, often, he served as culinary staff. Despite the enormous time I have spent with my father, he has rarely ever discussed what happened to him in Vietnam. A normally talkative man with the sense of humor of a 13-year-old boy, when it comes to the topic of war his jaw becomes heavy with the weight of unspoken horrors. He talked about how he would often cook in open spaces when planes would fly overhead spraying herbicides. The scene is almost other-worldly to imagine: thick forestry beaten back temporarily so that a military can make base, a blistering sun that can only be damped by vicious rains, insects buzzing about stinging the reluctant visitors. He talked about having to drink water at times wherever one could find it. What was most sad about all of this is the seeming innocuousness of Agent Orange: he slept on the soil, drank the water, breathed the air that was all (and in some cases, still is) laced with devastating compounds. He didn't know then and here he was trying to understand the full extent of his ignorance. Surely, all of these experiences meant that he reached a critical mass of exposure to Agent Orange, a nefarious compound that resulted in his son being sick. That was what he kept saying, "He didn't just get sick on his own."

The doctor was patient, seeming to treat my father's arguments and experiences like a rational game of whack-a-mole. From the very beginning, he seemed intent on proving to my dad that while his experiences in the war were unfortunate, they were in no way related to the genetic mutation that characterizes my genetic condition. After about 15 minutes, his normally neutral face is colored with overt impatience and frustration. He asks me to stand up, pointing out the range of "deformities" that plague my body. He pointed to all of these as if I was one of those hanging skeleton models that joined forces with muscles and could now walk. He explained that his understanding of the literature described non-skeletal impacts of Agent Orange. My father was soon showing the same annoyance that he was not being heard or considered. I was mostly quiet, popping in every now and then to ask my own questions but fully aware what my doctor's almost rhythmic checking of his watch suggested. Eventually, the conversation ended abruptly, and the doctor stood up. He made some vague declaration that he would continue surveying the research and would be ordering a range of tests to get to know more about my diagnosis.

My parents have always done the best they can to make sense of my body. For the past 26 years they have doggedly collected every piece of documentation my doctors provide, and they have become fluent in medical-lese. Yet still, my mother prays and my father continues to voraciously research the most contemporary findings about Agent Orange. I continue to see the same doctor and he has become markedly more kind and understanding. Still, his eyes betray a glaze when his expertise is questioned or when the limits of his answers are exposed. I can't blame him exactly; this treatment is probably incredibly rare for him.

Even long after that experience my doctor gives learned answers and my parents stare long and hard at him. The whole performance is obligatory and awkward and will happen again and again. I'm still trying to figure out what to do with all of this. For the time being I will put down a pillow and pray; not because I believe it will bring answers, but because it is better than resisting the obvious: We are still figuring out what else to do.

Autoethnographically Engaging the Intersection of Health and Culture

Satoshi: How does autoethnography engage us while learning the intersection between health and culture?

Lindy: By learning health and culture simultaneously, I better understood my experiences with health in alignment with my mother's. It was therapeutic to realize our experiences weren't singular, but it also created a critical moment.

Patrick: As I sit and write my autoethnography, it is fascinating to me how unwilling my doctor was to simply say, "I don't know."

Satoshi: I am reminded how complex our communicative interactions are. Such a short time of the interaction between two people was complex, packed with health politics and cultural politics. Unpacking was pedagogical, which helped me to be more reflexive of my own OCD behaviors.

Darren: That day on the baseball diamond is not indicative of my entire relationship with my dad, but it is informative as a manifestation of the cultural influences that drive his and my behavior. Analyzing those moments and those influences improves my understanding of myself, my father, and our relationship.

Shelby: Living with chronic pain and illness teaches me about the limits of biomedical discourse. My experience with medicine has often been alienating and dehumanizing; I frequently leave my doctors' appointments feeling defeated, isolated, and left to sift through highly specialized technical language to piece together a sense of understanding about my own body.

Lindy: I recognize the ways our legacy and performance of being "okay" is part of a much larger and more complicated health picture. I saw with fresh eyes the structures of health and health care and the ways we were both complicit and resistant to this system.

Darren: By delving back into my own experience and identifying emerging themes, I gained a better understanding of the recurrent interactions between anger and anxiety and how toxic masculinity valorizes violent and aggressive coping mechanisms. Additionally, autoethnography, in this case, allowed me to reflect on a set of experiences with my father and recontextualize them as moments where I learned something valuable.

Lindy: While I know autoethnography serves as an opportunity to reflect on self within the layered complexities of the world, I had not been very self-reflexive regarding my health. This autoethnographic writing created an essential and thoughtful mother-daughter moment from which I have an opportunity to consider my continued performance of gender in the biomedical world.

Patrick: This autoethnographic piece has demonstrated the potentiality for autoethnographic writing to explore intersections of health and culture. This kind of research is well suited to imagine what happens beyond blood samples and MRI scans.

Satoshi: Our autoethnographies layer to capture the complex and intersectional landscaping of health and culture in, through, and beyond us. We labor toward a network of narratives which helps us understand the world which we live in, through which we are constructed, and which we construct. To me, autoethnographic pedagogy allows us—our intersectional identities and lived experiences—to become pedagogical instruments for each other.

Shelby: Storying my experience in this way reveals the complex co-constitution of health and culture while offering a self-reflexive and therapeutic method to (re) construct that experience.

Patrick: As I continue to think this through, I am struck by how this project has driven me to unearth a static autobiographic past and reflect upon the taken-for-granted performances that medical professionals embody and the ones ignored by their patients.

Darren: Autoethnographic writing offers the opportunity to slow down and meditate on the subtle influences that shape and guide our everyday lives (Adams, 2011).

Shelby: Autoethnography affords a pedagogical space for experimenting with that sense-making. In a pivot back and forth between self and culture (Ellis, 2004), autoethnography provides critical and creative potentials for storying our intercultural health experiences by situating cultural knowledge production within the messy realm of our intersectional, corporeal bodies.

References

Adams, T. E. (2011). *Narrating the closet: An autoethnography of same-sex attraction*. Walnut Creek, CA: Left Coast Press.

Aguilar, F. V. (2015). Church-state relations in the 1899 Malolos constitution: Filipinization and visions of national community. *Southeast Asian Studies*, *4*(2), 279–311.

Banks, S. P., & Banks, A. (2000). Reading "the Critical Life": Autoethnography as pedagogy. *Communication Education*, *49*, 233–238.

Bevan, J. L., Vreeburg, S. K., Verdugo, S., & Sparks, L. (2012). Interpersonal conflict and health perceptions in long-distance caregiving relationships. *Journal of Health Communication*, *17*, 747–761.

Bhabha, H. K. (2008). *The location of culture*. New York, NY: Routledge.

Bochner, A. P., & Ellis, C. (1995). Telling and living: Narrative co-construction and the practice of interpersonal relationships. In W. Leeds-Hurwitz (Ed.), *Social approaches to communication* (pp. 201–213). New York, NY: Guilford Press.

Boylorn, R. M., & Orbe, M. P. (Eds.). (2014). *Critical autoethnography: Intersecting cultural identities in everyday life*. Walnut Creek, CA: Left Coast Press.

Chordas, P. (2018, August 1). 60 years after Sadako Sasaki's death, the story behind Hiroshima's paper cranes is still unfolding. *The Japan Times*. Retrieved from https://www.japantimes.co.jp/community/2018/08/01/issues/60-years-sadakos-death-story-behind-hiroshimas-paper-cranes-still-unfolding/

Cicirelli, V. G. (1992). *Family caregiving: Autonomous and paternalistic decision making*. Newbury Park, CA: Sage.

Cicirelli, V. G. (1993). Intergenerational communication in the mother–daughter dyad regarding caregiving decisions. In N. Coupland & J. F. Nussbaum (Eds.), *Discourse and lifespan identity* (pp. 215–236). Newbury Park, CA: Sage.

Committee to Review the Health Effects in Vietnam Veterans of Exposure to Herbicides. (2014). *Veterans and Agent Orange: Institute update 2012 of medicine of the national academies.* Washington, DC: The National Academies Press.

Corrigan, P. (2004). How stigma interferes with mental health care. *American Psychologist, 59*(7), 614–625.

Davies, C. A. (1999). *Reflexive ethnography: A guide to researching selves and others.* London, UK: Routledge.

Dillon, P. J., & Basu, A. (2014). HIV/AIDS and minority men who have sex with men: A meta-ethnographic synthesis of qualitative research. *Heath Communication, 29*(2), 182–192.

Dutta, M. J. (2008). *Communicating health: A culture-centered approach.* Cambridge, UK: Polity.

Dutta, M. J. (2011). *Communicating health: A culture-centered approach* (2nd ed.). Malden, MA: Polity Press.

Dutta, M. J., & Jamil, R. (2013). Health at the margins of migration: Culture-centered co-constructions among Bangladishi immigrants. *Health Communication, 28*(2), 170–182.

Ellis, B. H, Miller, K. I., & Given, C. W. (1989). Caregivers in home health care situations: Measurement and relations among critical concepts. *Health Communication, 1*, 207–226.

Ellis, C. (2004). *The ethnographic I: A methodological novel about autoethnography.* Walnut Creek, CA: AltaMira.

Ellis, C., & Bochner, A. P. (1992). Telling and performing personal stories: The constrains of choice in abortion. In C. Ellis & M. Flaherty (Eds.), *Investigating subjectivity: Research on lived experience* (pp. 79–101). Newbury Park, CA: Sage.

Ellis, C., & Bochner, A. P. (2014). Merging culture and personal experience in critical autoethnography. In R. M. Boylorn & M. P. Orbe (Eds.), *Critical autoethnography: Intersecting cultural identities in everyday life* (pp. 9–10). Walnut Creek, CA: Left Coast Press.

Freire, P. (2000). *Pedagogy of the oppressed* (30th anniversary ed.: M. B. Ramos, Trans.). New York, NY: Continuum.

Genuchi, M. C. & Valdez, J. N. (2015). The role of anger as a component of a masculine variation of depression. *Psychology of Men & Masculinity, 16*(2), 149–159.

Goodall, Jr. H. L. (2000). *Writing the new ethnography.* Walnut Creek, CA: AltaMira.

Graburn, N., & Ertl, J. (2008). Introduction: Internal boundaries and models of multiculturalism in contemporary Japan. In N. H. H. Graburn, J. Ertl, & R. K. Tierney (Eds.), *Multiculturalism in the new Japan: Crossing the boundaries within* (pp. 1–31). New York, NY: Berghahn Books.

Graburn, N. H. H., Ertl, J., & Tierney, R. K. (Eds.). (2008). *Multiculturalism in the new Japan: Crossing the boundaries within.* New York, NY: Berghahn Books.

Guzman, A. B., Dalay, N. J. Z., Guzman, A. J. M., Jesus, L. L. E., Mesa, J. B. C., & Flores, J. D. (2009). Spirituality in nursing: Filipino elderly's concept of, distance from, and involvement with God. *Educational Gerontology, 35*(1), 929–944.

Hyde, M. J. (1980). The experience of anxiety: A phenomenological investigation. *Quarterly Journal of Speech*, *66*(2), 140–154.

Hynes, H. P. (2016). The legacy of Agent Orange in Vietnam. *Peace Review: A Journal of Social Justice*, *28*, 114–122.

Kelsey, S. G., & Laditka, S. B. (2009). Evaluating the roles of professional geriatric care managers in maintaining the quality of life for older Americans. *Journal of Gerontological Social Work*, *52*, 261–276.

Kiesinger, C. E. (2002). My father's shoes: The therapeutic value of narrative reframing. In A. P. Bochner & C. Ellis (Eds.), *Ethnographically speaking: Autoethnography, literature, and aesthetics* (pp. 95–114). Walnut Creek, CA: AltaMira.

Lacan, J. (2014). *Anxiety: The seminar of Jacques Lacan, book* X. J. Miller (Ed.). Cambridge, UK: Polity.

Langellier, K. M. (1989). Personal narratives: Perspectives on theory and research. *Text and Performance Quarterly*, *9*, 243–276.

Link, B. G., & Phelan, J. C. (2001). Conceptualizing stigma. *Annual Review of Sociology*, *27*, 363–385.

Lipka, M. (2015, January 9). 5 facts about Catholicism in the Philippines. *Pew Research Center*. Retrieved from http://www.pewresearch.org/fact-tank/2015/01/09/5-facts-about-catholicism-in-the-philippines/

Lockford, L. (2002). Breaking habits and cultivating home. In A. P. Bochner & C. Ellis (Eds.), *Ethnographically speaking: Autoethnography, literature, and aesthetics* (pp. 76–86). Walnut Creek, CA: AltaMira.

McArthur, J. (2013). *Rethinking knowledge within higher education: Adorno and social justice*. London, UK: Bloomsbury Academic.

McLaren, P. (1999). *Schooling as a ritual performance: Toward a political economy of educational symbols and gestures* (3rd ed.). Lanham, MD: Roman & Littlefield.

Mingé, J. M., & Sterner, J. B. (2014). The transitory radical: Making place with cancer. In R. M. Boylorn & M. P. Orbe (Eds.), *Critical autoethnography: Intesecting cultural identities in everyday life* (pp. 33–46). Walnut Creek, CA: Left Coast Press.

Mitnick, S., Leffler, C., & Hood, V. L. (2010). Family caregivers, patients and physicians: Ethical guidance and optimize relationships. *Journal of General Internal Medicine*, *25*, 255–260.

Nadeau, M. M., Balsan, M. J., & Rochien, A. B. (2016). Men's depression: Endorsed experiences and expression. *Psychology of Men & Masculinity*, *17*(4), 328–335.

Nakayama, T. K., & Halualani, R. T. (2010). (Eds.). (2010). *The handbook of critical intercultural communication*. Malden, MA: Wiley-Blackwell.

Nasu, M. (2015). *Children of the paper crane: The story of Sadako Sasaki and her struggle with A-bomb disease* (E. W. Baldwin, S. L. Leeper, & K. Yoshida, Trans.). New York, NY: Routledge. (Original work published 1991)

Parrott, R., & Kreuter, M. N. 2003. Multidisciplinary, interdicisplinary, and transdisciplinary approaches to health communication; Where do we draw the lines? In T. L. Thompson, R. Parrott & J. F. Nussbaum (Eds.), *The Routledge Handbook of Health Communication* 2nd ed. pp. 3–17. New York, NY: Routledge.

Pecchioni, L. L., & Nussbaum, J. F. (2000). The influence of autonomy and paternalism on communicative behaviors in mother–daughter relationships prior to dependency. *Health Communication*, *12*(4), 317–333.

Pelias, R. J. (1999). *Performance studies: The interpretation of aesthetic texts*. Dubuque, IA: Kendal/Hunt.

Pineau, E. L. (2002). Critical performative pedagogy: Fleshing out the politics of liberatory education. In N. Stucky & C. Wimmer (Eds.), *Teaching performance studies* (pp. 41–54). Carbondale: Southern Illinois University Press.

Reagan, L. J. (2016). 'My daughter was genetically drafted with me': US-Vietnam war veterans, disabilities and gender. *Gender & History*, *28*(3), 833–853.

Roter, D. L., & Hall, J. A. (1998). Why physician gender matters in shaping the physician–patient relationship. *Journal of Women's Health*, *7*, 1093–1097.

Roter, D. L., & Hall, J. A. (2004). Physician gender and patient-centered communication: A critical review of empirical research. *Annual Review of Public Health*, *25*, 497–519.

Roter, D. L, & Hall, J. A. (2011). How medical interaction shapes and reflects the physician-patient relationship. In T. L. Thompson, R. Parrot, & J. F. Nussbaum (Eds.), *The Routledge handbook of health communication* (pp. 55–68). New York, NY: Routledge.

Roter, D. L., Hall, J. A., & Aoki, Y. (2002). Physician gender effects in medical communication: A meta-analytic review. *Journal of the American Medical Association*, *288*, 756–764.

Roter, D. L., Lipkin Jr., M., & Korsgaard, A. (1991). Sex differences in patients' and physicians' communication during primary care medical visits. *Medical Care*, *29*, 1083–1093.

Sanchez, F., & Gaw, A. (2007). Mental health care of Filipino Americans. *Psychiatric Services*, *58*(6), 810–815.

Smith, R. A. (2011). Stigma, communication, and health. In T. L. Thompson, R. Parrott, & J. F. Nussbaum (Eds.), *The Routledge handbook of health communication* (pp. 455–468). New York, NY: Routledge.

Toyosaki, S. (2013). Pedagogical love as critical labor: Relational pedagogy of whiteness. *Qualitative Communication Research*, *2*(4), 411–433.

Toyosaki, S., & Pensoneau-Conway, S. L. (2013). Autoethnography as a praxis of social justice: Three ontological contexts. In S. Holman Jones, T. E. Adams, & C. Ellis (Eds.), *Handbook of autoethnography* (pp. 557–575). Walnut Creek, CA: Left Coast Press.

Trujillo, N. (1991). Hegemonic masculinity on the mound: Media representations of Nolan Ryan and American sports culture. *Critical Studies in Mass Communication*, *8*, 290–368.

Wakamatsu, S., Morikawa, T., & Ito, A. (2013). Air pollution trends in Japan between 1970 and 2012 and impact of urban air pollution countermeasures. *Asian Journal of Atmospheric Environment*, *7*(4), 177–190.

CHAPTER FOURTEEN

Photovoice and Photobodies: Public Pedagogies of Health

BY PHILLIP E. WAGNER

Social theorists have long speculated that the Western world is in the midst of a shift from a modern industrial culture to a postmodern culture of consumption (see Baudrillard, 1981; Derrida, 1966; Lyotard, 1984). As culture shifts, so do cultural practices. As practices shift, so do sites of social dialogue. The body—a site of longstanding cultural critique and social dialogue—is a primary site for observing this shift. Indeed, the body has become a site for consumption, where others can observe social etchings of power. And here in the West, where many of us research, teach, and toil, the borders between the body and the rest of the world are rendered even more blurred through bodily performances that are willingly (and strategically) shared publicly on social media platforms.

These public performances do not occur through the body alone; indeed, the channels by which they are possible are digital. For public health practitioners and scholars, this is exciting, as digital data is ever present. As teachers, this should also prove exciting, as the means by which our students are familiar with cultivating a sense of responsibility, identification, and understanding are *familiar,* leading to a litany of potential in the classroom. These digital means of understanding are not often welcomed with open arms, however. Cell phones, cameras, and other digital gadgets were once regarded solely as means of distraction in the classroom. Yet the ubiquity and utility of such tools now all but requires instructors to tap into the power and opportunity that lie within them. So, do they? Rarely, it seems. Though there is no specific data on instructors' use of technology in the classroom, recent results from the Student Pulse Survey (Top Hat, 2017) reveal that 94% of students desire to use their cell phones (more) in class. And of those that *did* use their phone in class for learning-specific outcomes, cited activities were using it to "check-in" or answer questions or to access a digital textbook (Top Hat, 2017).

Given what we *study* and what we *teach*, it seems that this is a prime opportunity gone to waste. How then can those who teach at the intersections of health and culture move past the trepidation they may have over inviting technologies into the classroom? And, once they do, how can they harness the power of digital performances of identity to bring about a greater understanding of intercultural/ international health communication? This chapter will present *photovoice* as both a research-oriented framework and a public pedagogy for better understanding the intersections between bodies, health, culture, and communication.

Photovoice

No doubt, the body is a visual artifact. In the modern era, there are many things that the body *does*; some physical, some social, some cultural—and nearly *all* observable thanks to the extensive self-security afforded by the technology that rests in our pockets. Though they are often taken for granted as mere pedestrian preoccupations, these modern practices of self-security—which include selfies, Instastories, and brief documentaries ala Snapchat—are spaces rife with potential for cultivating a deeper understanding of lived experience, particularly in light of international health communication. What if, in fact, these were not mere digital preoccupations, and, instead, served as the catalyst for pedagogical breakthrough in the arena of global public health?

Researchers have long tapped into the power of the visual. Though relatively underutilized, photovoice is a digital research methodology that uses photographic works to better understand lived experience. Originally developed by Wang and Burris (1997) for an investigation of health in China, photovoice is a participatory action research methodology that seeks to give "voice" to those taking the photos. As Chio and Fandt (2007) note, most often such people—which can range from those marginalized, those who have directly experienced the issue being examined in the community, or even those who have no distinct identification with this issue (e.g., students)—are not "typically represented in official decision-making (or texts)" and, therefore, to not have an opportunity to record or represent the concerns impacting their community or day-to-day lives (p. 486). For critical scholars and practitioners, this also helps us address the call to tear down the walls between the knower (or "expert") and the known (those being studied; see Chio & Fandt, 2007; Harding, 1998; Mohanty, Russo, & Torres, 1991).

Photovoice is inherently transgressive, as it democratizes research (Novak, 2010) and places value on subjective lived experience. Sitting squarely within the domain of critical approaches to consciousness-raising and understanding, photovoice provides a valuable opportunity for individuals to navigate the social, political, global, digital, and contextual conditions that lead to, facilitate, permit, or aggravate social issues. But the answer to the questions that are raised throughout this process are unapologetically individual and subjective. Whereas traditional scientific ways of knowing are often only legitimized when regarded as objective, photovoice boldly embraces subjective lived experience as the true catalyst for action-oriented advocacy and learning. As Pollock (1996) notes, "Everyone has a specific story, a particular experience of the configurations of class, race, gender, sexuality, family, country, displacement, alliance … Those stories are mediated by the forms of representation available in the culture" (p. xv). Photovoice provides a means for the representation of those stories, prioritizing them as highly relevant in the investigation of social problems.

Known also as photo interviewing (Hurworth, 2003), photofeedback (Sampson-Cordle, 2001), autodriving (Heisley & Levy, 1991), reflexive photography (Douglas, 1998), and photo novella (Wang & Burris, 1994), photovoice involves the integration of photographs in the research process (Harper, 1998). These (auto)ethnographic photo endeavors are situated in the wider spectrum of Arts-Based Research (ABR), a collective body of philosophical and theoretical perspectives on "research guided by aesthetic features" (Barone & Eisner, 2012, p. xi). Leavy (2009) argues that these visual methods "adapt the tenets of the creative arts in order to address social research questions in holistic and engaged ways in which theory and practice are intertwined" (p. 3). Yet, isn't this, too, what faculty seek to do in their courses—interweave theory and practice with the end goal of cultivating a sense of personal engagement, responsibility, and action with their students?

Photovoice offers a valuable perspective in the examination of intercultural health, not only because of the critical foundations of the field, but also because of the visual nature of many topics of interest within the domain of global health. This method is also valuable because of the ways in which it stretches the field in new directions. Novak (2010) contends that Communication Studies, as a discipline, can benefit greatly from the incorporation of photovoice and other digital methods; he asserts that the field of Communication Studies, like many other disciplines in the social sciences, has privileged the written word and disregarded visual data as "nonacademic, nonscholarly, or merely performative," ultimately begging the question, "What knowledge and ways of knowing are being sacrificed at the altar of textocentric academic communities and their journals?" (p. 294). Tracy (2007) asserts that photovoice allows for the examination of "everyday interaction" and the "context of meaning making" (p. 32)—core elements in the study of human communication.

Finally, photovoice, quite frankly, is a simplistically useful and intriguing method for capturing meaning that could not be produced by the researcher (or, in this case, the instructor) in traditional ways. In many ways, it "democratizes" the qualitative research process, and the "privileged voice of the researcher is challenged" (Novak, 2010, p. 307). In terms of pedagogy, the voice being challenged is the teachers' and the assumed universal correctness of "the text" or course materials (which often go unchecked and are assumed faultless). This photographic method allows the integration of *more* voices—not just verbal ones—and helps tear down "the (false) binary between visual and verbal communication as images and words work in tandem to tell participants' stories" (Novak, 2010, p. 308). Photovoice is an effective pedagogical platform upon which we can prioritize the *visualization* of experience, *showing* the multiple dimensionalities of lived experience that transcends the typical *telling* of those experience that emerges with a singular method, alone.

Though often regarded as a research tool, photovoice is inherently pedagogical at its function. As a research methodology, it breaks down binaries between researcher and subject, placing the burden of meaning solely into the hands of those documenting the world around them. As a pedagogical tool, it serves a similar focus by placing students in the position of developing the very knowledge that they are to be learning, making them collaborators in the learning environment. Pulling heavily on Freirean (1970) principles, photovoice equips students to not only investigate social problems but to participate in addressing them and creating change.

Photovoice sits at the crossings of scholarship and advocacy, serving as an excellent means by which to help meet increasing demands for community engagement and applied learning in the classroom. It also helps bridge the connection between scholarship and application, setting students up to be not only *thinkers*, but *doers*. And for Communication faculty, this practice upholds the deep roots of the field by ensuring that "truth" is never found in one actor or orator alone, but is instead democratized throughout the learning process (Habermas, 1984; see also Cook & Quigley, 2013). When using photovoice as pedagogy, the burden of work rests with students; the instructor's role is merely to facilitate discussion, reflection, and scaffold an understanding of the major themes that have emerged across the "data" gathered by students. Though the instructor plays a significant role, the real value of photovoice is that it empowers students to (1) identify a need, (2) document and build a critical understanding, and (3) lead towards action by addressing that need.

Photovoice as Practice

Identifying a need, documenting and building a critical understanding, and developing an action-oriented outcome are the crux of photovoice in practice. Though photovoice can take many different forms and is easily adaptable across a wide array of pedagogical styles and preferences, the process of involves several distinct steps. Massengale and colleagues (2016) further flesh out these steps: "Conceptualize the issue, define goals and objectives, take photos of scenes in the community that represent the issue, facilitate group discussion about the photos, write captions for the photos, select photos that strongly represent the issue, make a public community presentation of the photos to which decision makers are invited, and advocate for policy change to make positive change around the issues of concern" (p. 118). Below, I outline each of these steps briefly to help provide a greater understanding of the ways in which photovoice can be adopted/adapted in intercultural health courses to bring about action-oriented results.

Conceptualize the Issue

While one of photovoice's greatest strengths is the familiarity many students have with using photographic means to construct an understanding of their day-to-day lives, this process does differ significantly from the (semi) random process of snapping photos as an opportunity arises. Instructors must play a heavy role here, designing courses and facilitating content delivery in a way that invites an open-ended response. The "issue" that serves as a catalyst for students' photovoice investigations could be the culminating theme of the entire course. Or, the process could serve as a weekly investigation of relevant themes found in the course. The depth and breadth of photovoice assignments is entirely up to the wishes of the instructor; however, each photovoice encounter must first begin by prioritizing the issues at hand.

Photovoice's research orientation may prove effective for instructors when conceptualizing the issues to be explored. It is important to note that photovoice's research bend does not simply *go away* when using it as a pedagogical device; in many ways, what students produce through this activity is *data*—and legitimate qualitative data, at that; thus, thinking as a researcher can be an effective way to conceptualize the issue. This conceptualization requires a clearly defined topic (e.g., global health disparities) that invites multiple perspectives that emerge from individual accounts of lived experience. This concept should first be well-defined, and a core anchor point for learning in the course; photovoice works well when the issues it centers are as clear as possible. "Issues" is a key term here, as many photovoice projects seek to investigate, clarify, or further trouble some existing social problem. Identifying that problem/issue/topic is a key first step.

Define Goals and Objectives

Once a particular issue or problem has been identified and the larger boundaries of the project are solidified, students should work one-on-one with their instructor, within a designated small group (when the instructor has assigned topics to groups, for instance), or with the greater learning community to define specific goals and objectives for the photovoice project. Here, the researcher orientation of photovoice can again prove helpful. Establishing broad research questions can help create a common ground for students and help to tie in assignment-related concerns. Of note, the goals and objectives of the photovoice activity should not simply be the goals and objectives of the photovoice *assignment(s).*

Instructors should note that *assignment instructions* are not appropriate goals and objectives alone. The *goals* of a photovoice assignment are not to "take three images that reflect ______________." These outcomes should be thought of in a way similar to the listed learning outcomes listed in course syllabi; they reflect what is *to be learned* upon completion of this assignment—not the steps necessary to secure the desired grade. In order to be consistent with the democratic nature of photovoice work, instructors should also invite students to participate in the development of these goals and objectives, using course materials in tandem with individual and course-related goals to sculpt a list of objectives that will allow a level-playing while also promoting the value of individual investigation and identification with the topics at hand.

Still, some of these objectives can be (and might need to be) left up entirely to the instructor (e.g., how many photos must be taken). Ground rules are critical and are really subject to the pedagogical preferences and the disciplinary constraints of the course. A key distinction the instructor will need to make is the ways in which *self* and *other* factor into the photovoice project. As noted above, *everyone has a story;* those stories and their connection to greater identity variables (i.e., heritage, race/ethnicity, sexuality, ability, immigration status) all feature prominently in the discourse on intercultural health. However, there are a variety of reasons why an instructor may want to specifically make known the subject/object differential in the photovoice assignment.

Some instructors may find that students with a largely privileged background are not fully able to *find* themselves in the photovoice project. For instance, in a project on health disparities, how can a student who has had consistent access to health insurance, wellness initiatives, adequate nutrition, and a host of support for health and wellness truly understand the complexity of health disparities by featuring themselves prominently in that conversation? Here, it is up to the instructor to draw boundaries. In some settings, it may make sense for students to (forcibly) find themselves in the data; in others, it may be valuable to take an other-oriented approach. This can occur through (carefully- and appropriately-contextualized) role-play, by embodying characters within a textualized case study or fictional actor, or any other means by which the instructor makes this distinction. Still, in order to truly get at the action-oriented thrust of photovoice pedagogy, students must understand that the goal here is to further illuminate problems and highlight the complexities of lived experience within these intercultural health domains in a way that surpasses what is already known in traditional textocentric spaces.

Take Photos

Of course, the thrust of photovoice work is the visual outcome it yields. As noted at the front end of this chapter, the process of documenting the world around them is one that is quite familiar to our students. Still, it must be made explicitly clear that photovoice is not merely a scholarly selfie endeavor; it is deliberate and, at its most successful, abstract. Instructors will need to first present some sort of training to students on how/where/when photos should be taken. Again, these considerations are not assignment specifics; they have to do with the ethics of visual documentation, consent, and framing. Before students begin collecting photos, the instructor should provide training on key aspects of the study.

Access. As critical scholars and practitioners, it is important to keep in mind the lived experiences of our students. Many may not possess the financial means to have appropriate technologies (e.g., smartphones, cameras, etc.) to engage in this activity. Instructors who plan to use photovoice can help mitigate this at the beginning of the term by placing a statement on their syllabus indicating that the course requires digital engagement and/or providing an anonymous survey to students to ensure that all have available technology. If a student does *not* have access to some means to capture photos, instructors may be able to work with university services (e.g., the library, information technology, etc.) to identify technology that is available for rent or loan at little to no cost to the student. These access considerations may also apply further than just the means available to take a photo. Students may have varying forms of technology with different levels of advancement. Photovoice does not require that all students have the same technology; in fact, quality of photos and different modes of presentation can further enhance the individual and subjective nature of this exploration.

Consent. Of course, there are a variety of ethical considerations that must be made when involving the visual element of lived experience. Though these issues are not situated prominently in students' day-to-day photographic social media adventures, the sensitive nature of many photovoice explorations—in tandem with its scholarly applications—necessitates that those engaging in it prioritize consent, safety, and ethics. Students should be provided with clear instructions on how to obtain consent from those they capture in their images (e.g., a signed consent document). Further, if students are documenting themselves in any image, they, too, should provide documented consent to help ensure there are no liability issues. Of course, instructors may wish to forgo consent altogether by instructing students to avoid capturing any (identifiable) humans in their images. This requirement also helps ensure that students are engaging in the necessary depth of critical thinking and abstraction required for photovoice to be successful.

Abstraction. A successful photovoice investigation does not merely substitute images for textual answers to the questions asked. While it might be easy for a student to take an image that reflects an answer to a simple question (e.g., "What people group experiences the greatest health disparities worldwide?"), photovoice does not seek answers—it seeks action; action which, most of the time, requires that we further muddy the waters. The questions that frame the photovoice investigation should be broad enough to invite a litany of subjective lived experience (e.g., "What is one of the most significant obstacles in your local community for people seeking healthcare?"). The more abstraction loaded into the questions asked, the more that subjective lived experience can shine through. Instructors should encourage students to answer the question in a meaningful way but to avoid trying to document an answer in a way that might be clear without their explanation. Here, the abstract visual serves as a means for eliciting audience anticipation and interest—both important elements of photovoice's end goals of eliciting a community response.

Excellence. Though many students are highly familiar with the process of taking digital images, photovoice can also serve as a means for enhancing both their creative and artistic skills. Recognizing that not all instructors are proficient in photography and arts-based methods, it may be worthwhile for instructors to partner with other available resources—either on campus or in the community—to help students understand how to capture photos that are clear and interesting. Instructors must keep in mind that, as noted above, students may not all have access to the same technologies and that some photos may, by default, be of lesser quality. The extent to which the instructor can control other variables here related to photographic excellence, the more level the playing field for students.

To be fair, though, the purpose of photovoice as a pedagogical device is not photographic excellence—the purpose is engaged and personalized learning. Ultimately, instructors should ensure that all students are comfortable with the process but allow *process*—not just *outcome*—to drive students forward. To achieve comfort with the process, instructors can utilize photovoice in the moment (for face-to-face courses; e.g., a daily self-portrait) or in low-stakes settings (for online courses; e.g., integrating a required photo into a weekly discussion forum post).

Key Considerations. The beauty and success of photovoice comes from the individuality and subjectivity that it highlights. The adaptability it presents allows it to be used in nearly any course that requires critical self-reflection and identification. Even instructors who teach online can use this technique to facilitate engagement among their students. However, when coupled with the explicit instructions to pursue abstract reflections of understanding, students (especially those in online courses) may be tempted to simply copy and paste images found online. This is *not* photovoice; it is a mere photo-montage (which, in its own right, could have significant pedagogical value). Instructors should be clear that students must *take* all photos themselves and that each photo should be an intentional reflection, with the focus on the defined goals and objectives for the assignment.

Submission and Image Selection. Instructors should work with their students on a submission process that fits within the parameters of the course. Students may choose to upload all images to a shared online space, within a course learning management system, or print them out and bring them to the physical classroom. For professors who are slow to embraced technology and/or ambivalent to it, there are a variety of ways that photos can be gathered. Utilizing Instagram (with a common course hashtag used to identity student images), Snapchat (with an identified course space or centralized account), or other forms of social media may be advantageous and simple for those who already use these technologies. For others, a commonly shared online space (e.g., GoogleDrive, Dropbox, Box, etc.), may be the best option, as the modality often used in many universities for collaboration and such academic spaces may provide specific course support to faculty hoping to utilize the space for these pedagogical means. Photovoice does not specify which of these is most effective; instead, the goal should be to gather images and situate them in a way that will allow for reflection and discussion.

This reflection is first personal, and students should work within the confines of the assignment to "select" photos that are most meaningful. Often, this requires the instructor to specify how many pictures were to be taken, and how many photos should make it into the final selection for each student. Students should may work individually or within a group to identify which images and—a la discussion—which themes were most salient to their investigation. The final collection of images that is brought forward for greater discussion most likely will not (and probably should not) be *all* of the images taken. In order for true abstraction to synthesis to occur, students may need to take a few images that help frame their own understanding but are not necessarily pertinent to the final outcome.

Facilitate Group Discussion About Photos, Write Captions, and Select Photos

Photovoice is, by its very nature, simultaneously very personal and very public. Its subjective orientation requires those capturing the photo to find some form of identification with the topic at hand, yet the end goal is never personal reflection alone. As a research methodology, photovoice seeks to drive action, change policy, and create change. So, too, as a pedagogical tool, does it seek a very public outcome to a very personal (and, at times, vulnerable) process of critical reflection. Once instructors have identified the means by which a set amount of photos are brought forward as the final "data," they will need to then identify an open environment for sense-making. Again, when done properly, photovoice should lean towards the abstract; by their very nature, successful photovoice adventures require conversation surrounding those images. These conversations may take a variety of different forms, largely left up to the discretion of the instructor. But the end goal is to help build community around shared themes and make sense of divergent themes. In many ways, the group driving action (in this case, students in a course) should ensure they are all on the same page, even if not all agree on the pertinent issues emerging from the data.

Though the particulars of the discussion about these photos is open to interpretation, pedagogical uses of photovoice may also find it beneficial to borrow from the mnemonic device often used to stimulate participant discussion of images taken in formal research studies—SHOWeD:

- What do you **S**ee here?
- What is really **H**appening?
- How does this relate to **O**ur lives?
- **W**hy does this problem exist?
- What can we **D**o about it?

Instructors may first wish to have students engage in freewriting about the images selected, pulling together an organized textual framework to situate their photographic works. In courses where the photovoice endeavors are group-based, this might be something the group constructed together through collaborative writing. Regardless, the end outcome here is to provide students with a safe place to discuss their motivations for taking the photo, the feelings elicited in those photos, and the ways in which they see those photos as a form of representation of the problem or related solution. By prioritizing vulnerability over diplomacy or well-grounded rhetoric, instructors can provide their students with a space to practice critical thinking, reflection, and argument crafting.

Additionally, throughout this process, instructors should invite students to (thoughtfully) *caption* their images. To do this, students should attempt to textually represent the major themes found in their photo. The goal here is not to simply *title* the photo, but to provide a textual *jumping off point*; in essence, if the image were hanging in an art gallery, what textual representation might be situated alongside it to stimulate further conversation and thinking?

After using SHOWeD (or another method that makes sense within the confines of the course) and captioning images, instructors should then have students engage in collaborative discussion, again working to build a greater community (i.e., in the course) understanding of the major themes emerging through the data. The instructor should take great care to ensure that pertinent course outcomes are mapped onto this activity and that students emerge with a coherent understanding of the themes relevant to the data. Because these projects tend to yield dozens to hundreds of photos, the instructor will likely want to select a few images from the ones taken that reflect the major themes found across that data; this can occur before or after the captioning and sense-making process.

Make a Public Presentation to Advocate for Change

Breaking the private/public dichotomy, the final goal of photovoice is to present the images to the public—namely policy makers, key stakeholders, and relevant members of the community. This can occur in a variety of ways. For online courses, a digital archive, complete with extended textual analysis or voiceovers, can be an effective way to show the breadth and scope of an issue. In traditional brick and mortar settings, inviting key stakeholders to an exhibit of sorts can also help bridge the divide between the academy and the community and build connections between courses/departments/colleges and the communities in which they reside. Of course, the students who have taken these images should be present, engaging the community members in discussion on those themes and potential recommendations for future action. Often, the burden of this work falls upon the faculty member, who may find it advantageous to contact a sympathetic local council person, head of a government entity, or even an engaged university administrator.

As a participatory action research method, the utility and success of photovoice requires the enactment of both—*participation* and *action.* The participatory function is actualized through the collaborative group process of building towards change (i.e., students working together towards a common goal). But the full participatory potential of photovoice as pedagogy is actualized when students engage members of the community in sense-making and leading towards collaborative action. This action is key, too. The goal should not be to merely set up a pop-up gallery for enjoyment; instead, photovoice should drive action. Students and their instructors should develop a specific plan for continued engagement with those who attend the exhibit (or are brought into the loop if another method of delivery is used). Especially ambitious instructors may wish to contact the local press or their university's marketing unit to help provide increased publicity, and, thus, increased *accountability* for continued engagement and action.

Overwhelmed? Don't Be!

Anytime instructors attempt to navigate the complexities and unknowns of a new pedagogical device, it can be overwhelming. The integration of photovoice is not designed to be highly technological, complex, or cumbersome. In fact, the key value of photovoice as a pedagogical method is the simplicity and mundane regularity of this technology. Despite the cumbersome specifics above, photovoice is a highly flexible and adaptable pedagogical method. Though the specifics above delve into some strategies for combating the complexity of integration, truthfully, photovoice is quite simple. For those inclined to use it but overwhelmed, here's a simple step by step guide:

- Develop open-ended prompts surrounding complex, multidimensional social issues related to course content and themes.
- Ask students to respond to those prompts/themes through *both* image(s) and written word, crystallizing the abstract with the concrete.
- Gather, disseminate, view, and share images in a way that makes sense for the pedagogical space.
- Facilitate an open atmosphere for sharing and discussion surrounding the images, where students can navigate the complexities of the social issue/themes with others, finding both convergences and divergences.
- Share the images openly with key stakeholders and all interested parties, helping to provide an academically-grounded, data-driven, and creative understanding of the problems and issues they address in their day-to-day lives.

Why Photovoice?

As can be derived from the extensive overview above, photovoice is not a tool that should be used by instructors who are merely seeking to fulfill course learning objectives. The activity requires an extensive amount of preparation throughout all stages. The process can be exhausting and even runs the risk of failure—pictures may not fully document an idea appropriately, technological issues may abound, communities may not respond as expected; put simply, there are a litany of reasons as to why photovoice as a pedagogy might bring pause. Yet these obstacles may prove small when stacked against the numerous benefits that photovoice as a pedagogical tool brings into courses exploring issues of culture and health.

Instructors utilizing photovoice—especially those utilizing it for the first time—may be (positively) surprised at the level of energy and engagement that this pedagogy tends to elicit. Students often find the process cumbersome yet enjoyable, in part due to the familiarity of the digital documentation of everyday life. Instructors seeking to enhance creativity, critical thinking, and many of the other learning outcomes that are difficult to conceptualize may also find the process quite enjoyable as it is highly subjective and, thus, personally meaningful to each student. Photovoice allows us a rare window into our students' intimate ways of thinking, knowing, and understanding, increasing the relational connection between teacher and student, ultimately working to dismantle those titles in favor of everyone working together as participatory actors leading towards change. And, of course, though often pitted against each other, the relationship between the public and the academy can be strengthened through this process; external community partners often enjoy seeing the level of engagement that our students have in the community.

Beyond enjoyment, photovoice also instills within students a sense of personal responsibility to identify and address community needs. In many ways, students engage in advocacy work through this process, whereby they combine "individual and social actions designed to gain political commitment, policy support, and social acceptance to change community conditions" related to culture and health (Massengale, Strack, Orsini, & Herget, 2016, p. 118; see also Goodhart, 2002). This advocacy should not be regarded as merely a political endeavor alone; indeed, this advocacy reflects many of the 21st century skills most sought after in the world of work (Casner-Lotto & Benner, 2006). Photovoice gives students a chance to find their voice and use it to empower others, create change, and enhance their local community, putting principles of ethical leadership, critical thinking, diversity and inclusion, and communication into practice all along the way.

For instructors teaching at the intersections of culture and health, photovoice can help us harness the *power* of the abstract. Many of the issues we address (e.g., reproductive rights, global health disparities, etc.) are so subjective and grounded in lived experience. Many students may have never had the opportunity to experiences those disparities or to examine them beyond one-dimensional textual accounts. In many ways, subjectivity has been lambasted but for intercultural health scholars and practitioners, we know that our content is personal and *the personal is political.* Photovoice serves as a crystallization method, wherein students can find greater personal identification with key issues and themes and cultivate a well-rounded and multidimensional understanding of those themes, particularly as they related to lived experience.

As culturally-minded health practitioners and instructors, we regard these skills as some of those most critical to the health profession. When carefully designed, photovoice can prove to be an effective pedagogical tool to help enhance students' learning and identification with concepts that may otherwise prove to be abstract and impersonal. Rather than decrying modern digital tools as mere distractions, instructors can use these tools to further blur the lines and borders of the body—between the self and other and between the body of knowledge and the general public.

References

Barone, T., & Eisner, E. W. (2012). *Arts based research.* Thousand Oaks, CA: Sage.

Baudrillard, J. (1981). *Simulacra and simulation.* Translated by S. F. Glaser. Ann Arbor: University of Michigan Press.

Casner-Lotto, J., & Benner, M. W. (2006). Are they really ready to work? Employers' perspectives on the basic knowledge and applied skills of new entrants to the 21st century U.S. workforce. Retrieved from http://www.p21.org/storage/documents/FINAL_REPORT_PDF09-29-06.pdf

Chio, V. C. M., & Fandt, P. M. (2007). Photovoice in the diversity classroom: Engagement, voice, and the "eye/I" of the camera. *Journal of Management Education, 31*, 484–504.

Cook, K., & Quigley, C. F. (2013). Connecting to our community: Utilizing photovoice as a pedagogical tool to connect college students to science. *International Journal of Environmental & Science Education, 8*(2), 339–357.

Derrida, J. (1966). Structure, sign, and play in the discourse of the human sciences. In A. Bass (trans.), *Writing and difference* (pp. 278–282). Chicago, IL: University of Chicago Press.

Douglas, K. B. (1998). Impressions: African American first-year students' perceptions of a predominately White university. *Journal of Negro Education, 67*, 416–431.

Friere, P. (1970). *Pedagogy of the oppressed.* New York, NY: Continuum.

Goodhart, F. W. (2002). Teaching advocacy to public health students: The New Jersey experience. *Health Promotion Practice, 3*, 341–346.

Habermas, J. (1984). *The theory of communicative action: Reason and the rationalization of society* (Vol. 1). Boston, MA: Beacon Press.

Harding, S. G. (1998). *Is science multicultural? Postcolonialisms, feminism, and epistemologies.* Bloomington: Indiana University Press.

Harper, D. (1998). An argument for visual sociology. In J. Prosser (Ed.), *Image based research: A sourcebook for qualitative researchers* (pp. 24–42) New York, NY: Routledge.

Heisley, D., & Levy, S. (1991). Autodriving: A photoelicitation technique. *Journal of Consumer Research, 18*, 157–172.

Hurworth, R. (2003). Photo-interviewing for research. *Social Research Update—Sociology at Surrey, 40*, 1–4.

Leavy, P. (2009). *Method meets art: Arts-based research practice.* New York, NY: Guilford.

Lyotard, J.-F. (1984). *The postmodern condition: A report on knowledge.* Minneapolis: University of Minnesota Press.

Massengale, K. E. C., Strack, R. W., Orsini, M. M., & Herget, J. (2016). Photovoice as pedagogy for authentic learning: Empowering undergraduate students to increase community awareness about issues related to the impact of low income on health. *Pedagogy in Health Promotion, 2*, 117–126.

Mohanty, C. T., Russo, A., & Torres, L. (1991). *Third world women and the politics of feminism.* Bloomington: Indiana University Press.

Novak, D. R. (2010). Democratizing qualitative research: Photovoice and the study of human communication. *Communication Methods and Measurements, 4*, 291–310.

Pollock, G. (1996). *Generations and geographies in the visual arts: Feminist readings.* New York, NY: Routledge.

Sampson-Cordle, A. V. (2001). *Exploring the relationship between a small in Northeast Georgia and its community: An image-based study using participant produced photographs* (Unpublished doctoral dissertation). University of Athens, Georgia.

Top Hat. (2017). Cellphones in school are essential to learning, say students. Retrieved from https://tophat.com/blog/cellphones-in-school-student-survey/

Tracy, K. (2007). The role (or not) for numbers and statistics in qualitative research: An introduction. *Communication Methods and Measures, 1*, 31–35.

Wang, C. C., & Burris, A. (1994). Empowerment through photo novella: Portraits of participation. *Health Education Quarterly, 21*, 171–186.

Wang, C. C., & Burris, A. (1997). Photovoice: Concept, methodology, and use of participatory needs assessment. *Health Education and Behavior, 24*, 369–387.

CHAPTER FIFTEEN

When Cultural Identity Impacts Health Decisions: Using *Grey's Anatomy* to Teach Communication Theory of Identity and Agency-Identity Model

BY KALLIA O. WRIGHT

Introduction

While populations are becoming more diverse, there are still undergraduate students, particularly those in predominantly white institutions (PWI), with limited interaction with persons of cultural backgrounds different from their own. Students who are preparing to work in health services need to be trained in theoretically-sound practices that factor in the impact of culture in health decision-making. A pedagogical concern for health communication teachers is determining which instructional strategies can most effectively help students sensitively navigate a culturally-impacted healthcare terrain. Often, students learn through observation. This chapter proposes a pedagogical activity that can be used in health communication classes to demonstrate the intersection of health and cultural identity. This pedagogical activity has four objectives: (1) students will understand the main principles of the Communication Theory of Identity (CTI) (Hecht, Warren, Jung, & Krieger, 2005) and the Agency-Identity Model (Villagran, Fox, & O'Hair, 2007); (2) students will be able to articulate the similarities between the concepts, and each one's unique perspective; (3) students will identify principles as they view clips from an episode of the television series, *Grey's Anatomy* (Rhimes & Tinker, 2005); and, (4) students will apply those concepts to the scenes and beyond to real-life scenarios.

The chapter begins by outlining the current social environment that demands that students be educated about the intertwined relationship between health and culture. The section that follows is a brief literature review on theoretical perspectives that have been applied to *Grey's Anatomy*, noting the lack of storylines that feature diverse cultural perspectives or approaches to health. The chapter then describes the suggested pedagogical design that could be adopted by health communication instructors. In that section, instructors receive an overview of the CTI and the Agency-Identity Model and suggestions on how to debrief the episode in class.

I have shown this episode in both my health communication and my intercultural communication courses that I teach at a PWI. For many of the students, this is their first time learning of the Hmong culture featured in the episode and the role of the "shaman" in Asian cultures. I have observed that as the students view the hospital scene which depicts a clash of two perspectives or cultural borders on health and healing—biomedical versus religious/supernatural—many experience discomfort. They struggle to reconcile the familiar biomedical model which they find credible, with this other model of healing which honors "weird," and unfamiliar cultural practices. They struggle openly with this embodiment of health and culture. The in-class discussions that follow are tentative as the students attempt to confront their engrained frame of reference about health. This chapter aims to guide instructors through these reflections.

Current Social Environment Demands

Particularly in North America, students live in a society characterized by increasing social, cultural, and economic diversity. By 2020, approximately half of the nation's children will be categorized as people of color (Colby & Ortman, 2015). Ultimately, the overall population will follow suit so that by 2044 over half of the US population will have people of color as its majority. Additionally, the Census report projects that by 2060, about 19% of the US population will be foreign-born; this will be an increase from 14% in 2014. Furthermore, data from the 2013 American Community Survey showed that about 60 million persons speak a language other than English in their home—an increase of almost 2 million from 2010 (Ryan, 2013). This means that one in five US residents speaks a foreign language at home. These developments signal an influx of cultural backgrounds that are uniquely dissimilar from the current dominant culture. Not only do these cultures introduce different languages, but also perspectives and approaches to health and healing that are divergent from established western biomedical practices. Particularly for students who wish to work in health services, committing to understanding, respecting, and learning how to negotiate with persons from cultures that are unlike their own is essential to building relationships and ethically operating in this field. A path to achieving this success is by being an effective and culturally competent communicator.

Significantly, the US government has recognized the importance of nurturing cultural competency and ensuring that employees in the field are trained in these skills. Government reports and research have revealed the existence of the health disparities experienced by minorities in the US and the need for more training in cultural competence. For instance, the 1985 Heckler Report found that sensitivity to culture is lacking in healthcare for minorities and that health professionals needed more education about the cultural beliefs, concerns, and attitudes of minority patients (Heckler, 1985). From that report emerged the Office of Minority Health in the US Department of Health and Human Services which aims to eliminate health disparities throughout the country. The Office provides educational opportunities for health service organizations interested in improving how they respond to the diverse cultural beliefs and practices of their patients (Office of Minority Health, 2018). Taking the lead from that governmental agency, one educational institution asserts that culturally competent communication focuses on being "open to learning about the family values, societal norms, and healthcare beliefs of minority groups" (Georgetown University Health Policy Institute, 2004, para 1) and verbally and nonverbally engaging with minority groups in a sensitive manner that takes these values, norms and beliefs into consideration. Importantly, research has found that practitioners without an understanding of cultural differences will likely do more harm, than help in medical treatment (Dutta & de Souza, 2008). Dutta-Bergman (2005) goes on to encourage an embracing of "multiple realities" where the health knowledge of those on the margin is considered just as valid as those rich in biomedical knowledge.

The practice of culturally competent communication has far-reaching effects. The practitioner must commit to sensitively and openly communicating with the patient about cultural perspectives that may impact the patient's health. Additionally, the practitioner must be self-aware about personal and professional biases and background experiences that may prevent a collaborative relationship with the patient from forming. Finally, the practitioner also must commit to working on creating a space that will ensure that open collaborations take place (Fuller, 2003). Fuller (2003) explains that sensitive communication must involve knowledge or an inquisitiveness when they interact with persons from other cultures. Sensitivity also accepts a self-awareness that a practitioner does not know everything about all cultures. Additionally, part of that knowledge is recognizing that a patient operates within a cultural web. At any given moment, one aspect of that patient's culture may be more significant than another and only through communication can the practitioner determine which aspect for example, religious or socioeconomic, must be considered in the approach to health and healing. Galanti (2014) recommends that practitioners interacting with patients from other cultures should ask three questions: "What do you think is wrong?" "What do you think caused your problem?" "How do you cope with your condition?" There are mutual benefits to be experienced when the practitioner is engaged in a reflective approach—one that is introspective, but also one that is interested in patients and how the patients define the illness and its impact on their lives. That is the start to culturally competent communication or collaboration in the healthcare setting. If a real-life scenario cannot be experienced, then the use of popular media is the best glimpse into this world. As such this chapter focuses on the popular television series, *Grey's Anatomy*, as one option to demonstrate how practitioners can practice cultural sensitivity and accommodation in the health care context. The episode also shows how a fictional scenario can be used to teach theories that can ground the behavior of students when they are in the real-world setting.

Theoretical Perspectives Applied to *Grey's Anatomy*

Over the years, research on popular culture has demonstrated that this form of media succeeds at not only entertaining, but also educating, whether correctly or incorrectly, its audiences. More specific to *Grey's Anatomy*, several studies, using theoretical lenses as their foundation, have examined the potential impact this show can have on audiences (Hetsroni, 2014; Quick, 2009a). Researchers of the series have found that the scenes are instructive for both medical students and patients who may be watching the show to determine how to interact with each other (Mickel, McGuire, & Gross-Gray, 2013). For instance, an application of the communication accommodation theory revealed that in the show medical practitioners both accommodated and did not accommodate the needs of patients (Mickel et al., 2013). The study concluded that practitioners need to know that viewers of the show may enter a healthcare context with unrealistic expectations of how to be treated as patients. Also, the study noted that the show can build expectations of the quality of communication expected from practitioners. Researchers have also found that there is a cultivation effect present among viewers of the show. Quick (2009a) found that not only did audience members view doctors as courageous, but that this perception led to a positive patient satisfaction. Also, this perception cultivated certain predispositions toward interactions with doctors. Hetsroni (2014) also found that loyal viewers often overestimated the number of illness diagnoses that occur in the society. Additionally, the study revealed that these audiences had a dramatic perception of the development and treatment of illnesses. Studies have also focused on specific storylines in the series for example, organ donation (Morgan, Movius, & Cody, 2009; Quick, 2009b) and the BRCA1 breast cancer gene mutation (Hether, Huang, Beck, Murphy, & Valente, 2008). The studies found that there was an impact on the knowledge, attitudes, and behaviors of the audiences, with audiences becoming more likely to talk about a health situation or engage in behavior to either support prevention or to educate others (application of the social learning theory). Connected to these findings is the fact that audiences are more inclined to adopt behaviors if they are emotionally involved and if they perceive that the narrative is consistent with everyday life (Morgan et al., 2009). Additionally, the more consistent the narrative, the more positive the perception of medical practitioners (Cho, Wilson, & Choi, 2011). However, while the show has been positively received as a potential teaching tool, there are critiques, with the most common one the lack of or inconsistent portrayal of cultural diversity in the storylines. Hetsroni (2009) found that there was a lack of Hispanic representation in the medical drama. While there was a celebrated portrayal of a Black character struggling with a mental disability (rare occurrence), it was noted that the show portrayed this female doctor's disability as a liability. This was a "bad" disability which author argued would have been portrayed more positively if the character had been a white male (Orem, 2017). Cramer (2016) noted that the show neutralized race by making absent any references to the impact of race at the personal or social levels whether on the lives of the practitioners or the patients. Finally, if the show is representative of practices in the medical field, researchers have found that there is still need for improvement in cultural sensitivity. Ye and Ward (2010) noted that there was still a heavy bias toward the use of the biomedical approach, rather than a bio-cultural or a socio-cultural approach. Donaldson (2008) argued that the mechanical approach toward patients was not effective in interactions with patients. Instead, the researcher argued for practitioners both in the show and in real life to encourage patients to tell their illness narratives. All in all, the show is influential in the portrayal of illnesses, medical practitioners, and in teaching and impacting behavior. With this in mind, this chapter now focuses on how to capitalize on that influence to help students understand how health and culture can intersect and how they can navigate that situation sensitively, effectively and ethically.

Suggested Pedagogical Design

In this section, I describe the suggested pedagogical design for health communication teachers which is as follows: (a) a description of the CTI and the Agency-Identity Model (emphasizing the intrapersonal/personal, interpersonal/relational, and sociocultural/communal self-concepts); (b) a synopsis of how these theories have grounded and been applied to research conducted by health communication scholars; (c) a description of the episode's content which would be viewed by students in a live class session; (d) and finally, debriefing suggestions that will help students first identify the principles of the theory and model in the scenes, then problematize the messages, and examine the interaction between the patient, doctors, and family members.

Communication Theory of Identity

Identity is communicative. In this section, I detail the main characteristics of the CTI and how it posits that identity is intertwined with communication. According to Hecht et al. (2005), "identity is formed, maintained, and modified in a communicative process and this reflects communication" (p. 262). The authors go on to assert that "identity ... is acted out and exchanged through communication" (p. 262). In earlier work, Hecht (1993) noted that identity is formed through social interaction when people internalize and associate symbolic meanings with the self. Additionally, individuals place themselves into social and cultural categories because of social interaction. Importantly, there will be specific categorizations that call for certain expectations and expressions of identity. All this happens even as society ascribes and communicates categorizations to us. The theory acknowledges the individual (Carbaugh, 1989) and the social loci of identity (Burke & Reitzes, 1981) and presents four layers of identity: personal, enacted, relational, and communal. Hecht et al. (2005) noted that all four are intertwined and always operate in concert with the others even when contradictions exist.

Each layer has particular characterizations. The personal layer refers to the individual's self-concept or how the person defines him/herself generally or in specific contexts. The enacted layer is the performance of that self or personal identity. Through social behavior and/or symbols, the individual communicates or expresses that self. In the relational layer, the individual's identity is based on how others view the individual, especially their social categorizations. The individual's identity is shaped in part by the interaction with other relational partners for example, one's family. Additionally, the individual identifies herself and the meaning of that identity through the relationship with others for example, I am a daughter. Also, one's role is a hierarchically ordered social role. In this communal layer, people with similar characteristics, histories, and experiences forge a sense of belonging with each other.

Agency-Identity Model

Related to the CTI is the Agency-Identity model premised by Villagran et al. (2007) (See Table 1). The Agency-Identity Model was discussed against the background of cancer diagnosis and care. However, the main principles of the model are applicable to other illness contexts, particularly those also impacted by culture. The model posits that all illness has the potential to damage the physical body, but also the self and the social self. The authors note that among the responses to illness is assertive action in the decision-making process regarding treatment. They note that the agency an individual exercises takes place at the intrapersonal, interpersonal, and sociocultural levels. Stohl and Cheney (2001), define agency in communication as seeing an individual become the "originator of action, a source of messages" (p. 239). This person will advocate for him/herself whenever illness or perceptions of an illness act as a barrier to one's agency. Like the personal layer in the CTI, the intrapersonal aspect of identity is one's personal assertion of the physical and cognitive self (Villagran et al., 2007). Here, the patient takes control of the physical and emotional self and can confidently and objectively become involved in the decisions about treatment. As the patient becomes more assertive, the more the identity is strengthened and the more likely relationships with others will be maintained. The model also identifies the interpersonal aspects of identity.

Table 1: Comparing communication theory of identity and agency-identity model

Communication Theory of Identity		Agency-Identity Model
• Personal Layer	⟷	Intrapersonal Aspect (agency)
• Relational Layer	⟷	Interpersonal Aspect (agency)
• Communal Layer	⟷	Sociocultural Aspect (agency)
• Enacted Layer	⟷	(Agency Enacted throughout)

Similar to the relational aspect of CTI, this aspect focuses on significant relationships for example, family. According to the model, once a patient begins to take more control over the process, alienation from important primary relationships lessens. This interpersonal identity invites family members into the decision-making process so that they become co-partners in the health care. Additionally, by disclosing information, seeking support and involving primary relationships in the decision-making process, the relationship between members is strengthened. Finally, the model highlights the sociocultural aspects of identity which is akin to the social layer of the CTI. The sociocultural identity highlights the cultural values, beliefs and practices and symbolic interactions that emerge from the environment or cultural context of which the individual is a part. When the patient begins to maintain cultural roles by which she defines herself, then she experiences more agency in the sociocultural identity. The patient also enacts agency through the communication process as she redefines the cause of the illness or the treatment through the lens of culture. Agency exists when the patient refuses to be passive and resists skepticisms and aversions to her perspective on health which is embedded in her culture.

Examples of Research Focused on Identity and Health

Over the years, health communication scholars have realized the far-reaching effects of illness on a patient's identity. Research has found that illness can cause a patient to re-define oneself (Arrington, 2003; Charmaz, 1987; Harwood & Sparks, 2003; Montali, Frigerio, Riva, & Invernizzi, 2011). Research has looked at how patients have enacted their identity during illness (Nuttbrock, 1986) and how illness can change individuals' social categorizations and ultimately, their social network (Darrow, Speyer, Marcus, Ter Maat, & Krome, 1998; Kundrat & Nussbaum, 2003). More specifically, there has been research that has examined how patients communicate their identity when culture and health collide (Fadiman, 1997; Goode, 1993; Mendenhall, Fernandez, Adler, & Jacobs, 2012). The research also highlights dialectic tensions that exist as persons attempt to enact both the personal and social identities while struggling against the meanings attached to their illness. For instance, men with mental illness, such as schizophrenia, have used exercise to combat cultural perceptions of the illness while struggling to live up to social perceptions of masculinity and strength and acknowledging the truth of their illness (Carless & Douglas, 2008). Cancer patients, such as mothers, grapple to maintain that identity even as the illness forces them to move from the social role of being the family member in charge of everyone's health to being dependent on others (Mathieson & Stam, 1995). Also, African-American women with cancer wrestle with the social construction of the "strong black woman" while living with the disease (Madlock Gatison, 2016).

Episode Description

In October 2005, the television series, *Grey's Anatomy* aired an episode titled, "Bring the Pain" (Season 2, episode 5) (Rhimes & Tinker, 2005). In this episode doctors, Meredith Grey and Derek Shepherd meet a female patient (Anna) from the Hmong culture. In their first scene together, Anna is dressed in a hospital gown laying on the bed. She is being examined by Dr. Shepherd. She describes her illness experience which involve back pain and numbness in her legs. At the end of the examination, Anna's parents rush into the room. Her father is wearing a black business suit and her mother is in a light blue long jacket over a white top and a long black skirt. Her father asks, "Anna, why didn't you call us before coming down here?" The doctors report to both Anna and her parents that there is a tumor in her spinal canal. They note that she has a 95% chance of recovering fully, but they must operate immediately because of the aggressive nature of the tumor.[1] Anna looks to her father:

Anna:	Father?
Mr. Chue:	No (shakes his head). No surgery
Dr. Shepherd:	Mr. Shu, without surgery, Anna will be paralyzed probably within the next 24 hours.
Mr. Chue:	There will be no surgery today, we're taking her home.
Dr. Grey:	Anna needs the surgery
Mr. Chue:	She can have it at another time.
Dr. Shepherd:	No, Mr. Chue
Mr. Chue (interrupts and says firmly):	We are taking our daughter home.
Dr. Shepherd (looks to Anna):	Anna, you're over 18. You don't need your father's consent.
Anna (looks to her father and responds):	I'm Hmong and my father is the elder (she looks at the doctors). He says I go home, I go home.

The scene ends with both doctors walking fast up a stairwell in the hospital. Dr. Shepherd, in exasperation, orders Dr. Grey to do some research so that they will know more about the Hmong culture. In the second scene, only Dr. Grey and Anna are interacting. In their dialogue, Anna challenges Dr. Grey's perceptions of her as a patient and Dr. Grey learns more about how the Hmong culture views health and healing.

Anna:	Why do the lights keep flickering?
Dr. Grey:	Something about a backup generator. This pump will provide you with the morphine drip. It should stop your pain.
Anna:	I told you. I don't need it. I'm going home.
Dr. Grey:	You realize you will have to sign an AMA [against medical advice] form saying you're leaving against medical advice.
Anna (closes her eyes in pain):	Fine.
Dr. Grey:	I know this is new and confusing. I called a social worker and she's willing to come down and talk to you.
Anna (interrupts and looks directly at her):	Spare me the white girl cultural divide love. I grew up down the street from here. I play in a band. I went to UW [University of Washington]. I get it. My father doesn't. He says no, it's no.
Dr. Grey:	We're talking about your ability to ever walk again.
Anna:	That's what you're talking about. I'm talking about my family. Have you ever even heard of the Hmong people? Our religion has got rules that are way old and way set in stone and way spiritual and you don't mess with them. You don't anger the ancestors. Even if you pierce your tongue and play in a band.
Dr. Grey:	What are the rules, exactly?

In the next scene in this story line, Dr. Grey tells Dr. Shepherd that he needs to be the one to talk with Anna's father. She notes that, "I would do it myself, but I guess having testicles is a requirement." Dr. Grey reveals, from her conversation with Anna, that Anna's father believes that his daughter is missing one of her souls and that according to Hmong culture, only a shaman can restore that soul. The soul must be restored prior to surgery. The next scene presents Dr. Shepherd walking outside with an umbrella to protect himself from the rain. He approaches Anna's father who is standing with an umbrella and smoking a cigar. Dr. Shepherd begins a process of negotiation with this primary caregiver and decisionmaker.

Mr. Chue:	Anna needs to have her souls intact before she has surgery. She needs a shaman.
Dr. Shepherd:	Well, you could have told me that.
Mr. Chue:	Why, so you could call me a fool?
Dr. Shepherd:	I respect that you have traditions that I can't understand. But you're standing beside me in a

	$3000 suit, so I also know that you respect the fact that I'm telling you Anna needs the surgery in the next 24 hours if she's going to continue to walk. She can't leave this hospital.
Mr. Chue:	She can't undergo surgery without her soul. She'll die.
Dr. Shepherd:	Alright, then. We're just gonna have to get a shaman ... today ... in the hospital.
Mr. Chue:	Shamans aren't listed in the yellow pages. Our shaman is 500 miles from here. You're an arrogant man.
Dr. Shepherd:	No. I'm just a guy with access to a helicopter.
Mr. Chue (hands Dr. Shepherd a cigar):	Finding her soul won't be easy.
Dr. Shepherd (smiles and walks away):	It never is.

The story ends with the shaman arriving at Anna's hospital room. He begins the ritual. Prior to the ritual the doctors had stopped the morphine drip to honor Anna's request not to be medicated while the shaman tries to find her soul. She noted that medication would make it more difficult for her soul to be found. There is a moment in the ritual when she nods to Dr. Grey, who has been watching, as an indication that her soul has been restored.

The narrative is an intriguing one as it introduces most of the students to a culture of which they were not aware. Additionally, it draws them into a reflective process as they must examine their personal reactions to the patient and her family's insistence on resisting medical advice. Also, the story presents one possible option of how to go about negotiating between two seemingly dissimilar cultural values regarding health. After students have viewed the scene, the next process is to help them process the information and as this chapter suggests, through the lenses of the CTI and the Agency-Identity Model. The section that follows presents a list of suggestions, albeit, not an exhaustive list.

Debriefing Process

The CTI and the Agency-Identity Model are frameworks which may be taught in a Communication Theory, a Health Communication, or an Intercultural Communication course. The use of the storyline is one way to introduce the concepts or to help make the premises in each framework clearer. The following suggestions are presented with the assumption that the students have not yet been introduced to the two frameworks.

Opening Questions

Whether as a larger class or in pairs or small groups ask students:

i. For their initial impressions of the storyline.
ii. How they would have responded when the father first refused to have his daughter undergo surgery.
iii. How they would have solved the problem if they had no access to a helicopter.
iv. To describe the intertwined relationship between culture, health, and identity in the storyline. The students need to think of how culture impacted identity and how that identity impacted the health decision-making. They could also think of how decision-making impacted cultural identity for example, did it change it, reinforce it?

Identifying the Principles of the CTI and Agency Identity Model

In this next section, the instructor may present questions which begin to have the students move from a superficial description into engaging in critical thinking and preparing them for deeper analysis. As students respond, the professor may write the responses on the board or an electronic screen. Keeping the information or responses in front of the students will help them retain the ideas and aid in the discussion process. Therefore, whether as a larger class or in pairs or small groups ask students:

i. To describe how Anna identifies herself. Instruct them not to include any reference to the Hmong cultural group. With this question, the students begin to identify the personal layer or the intrapersonal aspect of identity. Ask students why she chose to present those characteristics as exemplary of who she was. How would knowing those personal characteristics help a medical practitioner in her efforts to treat her patient?
ii. To describe how Anna identifies herself in relation to her relationships, more specifically, her relationship with her family. With this question, the students begin to identify the social layer or the interpersonal aspect of identity. Ask students to explain how this identity affected the decision-making regarding her health.
iii. To describe how Anna identifies herself in relation to her culture, the Hmong people. With this question, the students begin to identify the communal layer or the sociocultural aspect of identity. Ask students to explain how this identity affected how she engaged with the treatment

process. Note that it may also be beneficial to begin this analysis section by starting with this question that focuses on the larger picture. The impact of the Hmong culture in the narrative may be more evident to the students. Moving from the broader concept to the smaller (personal) may help students see the differences between the layers of identity.

iv. To describe how Anna enacted her agency at the personal (e.g. how does she assert herself and become part of the decision-making process?), social (how does she incorporate her family members and make them co-partners in the interaction?) and sociocultural levels (what symbolic interactions or cultural practices does she invoke in her interactions with the practitioners) in that storyline. Ask them to identify what she said to family members and the practitioners for each level.

Problematizing Identity

In the following section, the instructor continues to guide the students through the process of identifying how culture, health and identity may be intertwined. Another path to achieving this is by problematizing the process. In this phase, the instructor may don a "devil's advocate" stance to have students think creatively about their responses and the responses portrayed in the televised story. Therefore, ask students:

i. To describe the problems that these identities introduced into the interaction.
ii. To explain the tensions that exist between or among the identities. How was one identity positively or negatively impacting the other?
iii. To describe Anna's response if the medical practitioner had insisted that she forget about her Hmong culture (sociocultural/communal identity) or her family (relational/interpersonal identity) in this context. What impact would that have had on the patient? For instance, the instructor could ask the students what if the practitioner had told her that she was in the United States now and that she needed to follow this country's rules and not those of her culture?
iv. State what harm could have been done to the patient had the medical practitioner ignored the cultural rules.

Reflecting on the Doctor-Patient-Family Interaction

In this final phase, the students reflect on the interaction between the patient, doctors and family members more positively. Galanti (2014) recommended that the practitioner use a reflective approach when engaging with patients from other cultures. In this section:

i. Tell students of Galanti's (2014) three suggested questions: What do you think is wrong? What do you think caused your problem? And How do you cope with your condition? Ask how those questions could have changed the interaction.
ii. Remind students that cultural sensitivity involves self-awareness on the part of the medical practitioner, an inquisitiveness about other cultures, and a commitment to meet a goal to create a space where open negotiations about health and healing can take place (Fuller, 2003). Ask students to describe how the medical practitioners in the narrative attempted to achieve these three goals. One aspect to note is that Dr. Grey recognized that she was not be the best option to speak with Anna's father. She relinquished her own gendered identity before the patriarchal cultural norms of the Hmong culture. Ask students whether they thought this was an ethical approach for practitioners? Would it be right for one individual in the communication process to surrender their own personal and sociocultural identity so that another's thrives?
iii. Ask students for suggestions for other ways to address the situation.

At the end of this question and answer process, the instructor may begin teaching the principles of the CTI and the Agency-Identity Model. In particular, the instructor can note how illness can instigate discussions of cultural identity because illness can either change, add to, or reinforce cultural behavior and perceptions.

Suggestions for Applications of Alternative Intercultural Communication Theories

While this chapter has focused on how instructors may introduce the frameworks of the CTI and Agency-Identity Model, it must be noted that the clip is versatile and other frameworks can be applied to facilitate the learning process. One of the first that could be applied is the Intersectional Theory (Bauer, 2014) which reminds us that no human being is simply one characteristic or one identity. Instead, the theory emphasizes that humans operate within a larger social context. Our personal identities will always interact or collide with larger sociocultural identities. A person cannot be the sum of all the identities. Neither is it possible to rank order the identities and determine which is more important at a particular time and this is because all identities are intricately intertwined. Additionally, the intersectional theory forces us to avoid subscribing to generalizations for example, as Dr. Grey did when she stated to Anna, "I know this must be new and confusing for you." She assumed that the patient had little formal education about or exposure to the biomedical world. An instructor can either teach the intersectional theory using the clip or can use the clip to demonstrate how identities are intersectional in nature. Finally, intersectional theory emphasizes that practitioners must get to know their patients so that they determine how overlapping identities can define or guide approaches to health and healing.

A second framework that could be applied is the Communication Accommodation theory. This theory posits that when interacting, individuals will either adapt their communication style so that is similar to the one used by the conversational partner (converge) or an individual will communicate so differently from another that it could result in a distancing effect between the communication partners (diverge) (Giles, Mulac, Bradac, & Johnson, 1987). This intercultural communication theory demonstrates the push and pull involved in the communication process as individuals seek to attain understanding particularly when they are from different backgrounds. In this storyline Dr. Shepherd begins his description of the illness using convergence. However, he diverges when the father insists on no surgery. Dr. Shepherd's divergence is seen as he turns to Anna and reminds her that she is an adult. Divergence is also evident in the exchange between Dr. Grey and Anna. Dr. Grey notes that, "We're talking about your ability to ever walk again." Anna counters by stating, "That's what you're talking about. I'm talking about my family." Anna observes that they each were making significant or meaningful two different ideas. However, converging efforts are also present. At the end of that exchange, Dr. Grey converges through a simple question, "What are the rules, exactly?" In this one question she draws closer to Anna's communication and begins to operate from her perspective. Dr. Grey also converges when she tells Dr. Shepherd that a male doctor needs to negotiate with Mr. Chue, rather than a female doctor (herself). Finally, Dr. Shepherd engages in convergence when he approaches Mr. Chue in the rain and determines a compromise—getting the shaman to the hospital. Essentially, there are many ways to engage the students and help them both learn and retain communication concepts that can be applied to real-world settings.

Conclusion

All in all, this narrative of the Hmong culture is one that is a valuable pedagogical tool within the classroom. Visual popular culture captures the interest of students. Narrative is a powerful tool for maintaining that interest. Finally, when the information is relevant and consistent with a broader body of knowledge (communication), the information will more likely be retained for a longer period. Importantly, for a number of students in PWI's, this may be the closest interaction with another culture that they may receive prior to working in the field. By illustrating, modeling, challenging, and applying concepts, they draw closer to becoming sensitive communicators and being the kind of practitioners that persons from other cultures enjoy engaging with. The author acknowledges that this pedagogical activity focuses on educating the cultural mainstream and notes that there is a risk of further marginalizing a culture and reinforcing the sense of difference between cultures. Rather than avoid the activity, instructors are encouraged to engage their students in dialogue about the power dynamics in intercultural conversation, how persons can remain marginalized even while being accommodated, and finally, how they can help reduce that sense of difference in real-life settings. In summary, the chapter has sought to ensure that students will understand the main principles of the CTI (Hecht et al., 2005) and the Agency-Identity Model (Villagran et al., 2007); that students will be able to articulate the similarities between the concepts, and unique perspectives presented by each; that students will identify principles as they view clips from an episode of the television series, *Grey's Anatomy*; and, finally, that students will apply those concepts to the clip and beyond to real-life scenarios. The suggested questions are aimed at interrogating the students and helping them engage in a more structured and meaningful analysis of a popular culture media. Rather than stopping at the question, "What did you think?" this chapter reminds instructors that intercultural experience is much more nuanced, and the experiences can be pulled out through thoughtful planning. Additionally, the exercise reminds students not to dismiss the cultural experiences of patients and their families. Instead, practitioners need to be reminded to slow down and engage wholly with clients who may be from backgrounds different from their own. Finally, the exercise reminds students that culture is a complex web. No one experience is solely impacted by one cultural characteristic. Instead, effort must be made to determine how culture can impact health decisions and what is most appropriate or sensitive route that can be taken to ensuring that patient and practitioner's needs are met and are mutually beneficial.

Note

1. See (https://www.imdb.com/title/tt0592905/ for more information).

References

Arrington, M. I. (2003). "I don't want to be an artificial man": Narrative reconstruction of sexuality among prostate cancer survivors. *Sexuality & Culture*, *7*(2), 30–58.

Bauer, G. R. (2014). Incorporating intersectionality theory into population health research methodology: Challenges and the potential to advance health equity. *Social Science & Medicine*, *110*, 10–17. doi: 10.1016/j.socscimed.2014.03.22

Burke, P. J., & Reitzes, D. C. (1981). The link between identity and role performance. *Social Psychology Quarterly*, *44*, 83–92.

Carbaugh, D. (1989). *Talking American: Cultural discourses on Dunahue*. Norwood, NJ: Ablex.

Carless, D., & Douglas, K. (2008). Narrative, identity and mental health: How men with serious mental illness re-story their lives through sport and exercise. *Psychology of Sport and Exercise*, *9*(5), 576–594. https://doi.org/10.1016/j.psychsport.2007.08.002

Charmaz, K. (1987). Struggling for a self: Identity levels of the chronically ill. In J. Roth & P. Conrad (Eds.), *Research in the sociology of health care* (pp. 283–321). Greenwich, CT: JAI Press.

Cho, H., Wilson, K., & Choi, J. (2011). Perceived realism of television medical dramas and perceptions about physicians. *Journal of Media Psychology: Theories, Methods, and Applications*, *23*(3), 141–148. doi: 10.1027/1864-1105/a000047

Colby, S. L., & Ortman, J. M. (2015). *Projections of the size and composition of the U.S. population: 2014 to 2060. Population estimates and projections*. United States Census Bureau. Retrieved from https://www.census.gov/content/dam/Census/library/publications/2015/demo/p25-1143.pdf

Cramer, L. M. (2016). The whitening of Grey's Anatomy. *Communication Studies*, *67*(4), 474–487. doi: 10.1080/10510974.2016.1205640

Darrow, S. L., Speyer, J., Marcus, A. C., Ter Maat, J., & Krome, D. (1998). Coping with cancer: The impact of the cancer information service on patients and significant others. *Journal of Health Communication*, *3*, 86–96.

Donaldson, E. J. (2008). Transforming how doctors are trained: Dissonance and harmony in medical humanities. *Interdisciplinary Humanities*, *25*(1), 26–32.

Dutta, M. J., & de Souza, R. (2008). The past, present, and future of health development campaigns: Reflexivity and the critical-cultural approach. *Health Communication*, *23*, 326–339.

Dutta-Bergman, M. J. (2005). Theory and practices in health communication campaigns: A critical interrogation. *Health Communication*, *18*, 103–122.

Fadiman, A. (1997). *The spirit catches you and you fall down: A Hmong child, her American doctors, and the collision of two cultures*. New York: Farrar, Straus and Giroux.

Fuller, J. (2003). Intercultural health care as reflective negotiated practice. *Western Journal of Nursing Research*, *7*, 781.

Galanti, G.-A. (2014). *Caring for patients from different cultures* (5th ed.). Philadelphia: University of Pennsylvania Press.

Georgetown University Health Policy Institute. (2004). Cultural competence in healthcare: Is it important for people with chronic conditions? Retrieved from https://hpi.georgetown.edu/agingsociety/pubhtml/cultural/cultural.html

Giles, H., Mulac, H., Bradac, J., & Johnson, P. (1987). SAT expanded and renamed CAT. In M. L. McLaughlin (Ed.), *Speech accommodation theory: The first decade and beyond* (pp. 13–48). Newbury Park, CA: Sage.

Goode, E. E. (1993, February 15). The cultures of illness. *US World News & World Report, 114*, 74–76.

Harwood, J., & Sparks, L. (2003). Social identity and health: An intergroup communication approach to cancer. *Health Communication, 15*, 145–159.

Hecht, M. L. (1993). A research odyssey: Towards the development of a communication theory of identity. *Communication Monographs, 60*, 76–82.

Hecht, M. L., Warren, J. R., Jung, E., & Krieger, J. L. (2005). The communication theory of identity: Development, theoretical perspective, and future directions. In W. B. Gudykunst (Ed.), *Theorizing about intercultural communication* (pp. 257–278). Thousand Oaks, CA: Sage.

Heckler, M. M. (1985). *Report of the Secretary's task force on Black and Minority health.* U.S. Department of Health and Human Services. Retrieved from https://ia800501.us.archive.org/32/items/reportofsecretar00usde/reportofsecretar00usde.pdf

Hether, H. J., Huang, G. C., Beck, V., Murphy, S. T., & Valente, T. W. (2008). Entertainment-education in a media-saturated environment: Examining the impact of single and multiple exposures to breast cancer storylines on two popular medical dramas. *Journal of Health Communication, 13*(8), 808–823. doi: 10.1080/10810730802487471

Hetsroni, A. (2014). Ceiling effect in cultivation: General TV viewing, genre-specific viewing, and estimates of health concerns. *Journal of Media Psychology: Theories, Methods, and Applications, 26*(1), 10–18. doi: 10.1027/1864-1105/a000099

Hetsroni, A. (2009). If you must be hospitalized, television is not the place: Diagnosis, survival rates and demographic characteristics of patients in TV hospital dramas. *Communication Research Reports, 26*(4), 311–322. doi: 10.1080/08824090903293585

Kundrat, A. L., & Nussbaum, J. F. (2003). The impact of invisible illness on identity and contextual age. *Health Communication, 15*, 331–347.

Madlock Gatison, A. D. (2016). *Health communication and breast cancer among black women: Culture, identity, spirituality, & strength.* Lanham, MD: Lexington Books.

Mathieson, C. M., & Stam, H. J. (1995). Renegotiating identity: Cancer narratives. *Sociology of Health and Illness, 17*(3), 283–306. https://doi.org/10.1111/1467-9566.ep10933316

Mendenhall, E., Fernandez, A., Adler, N., & Jacobs, E. (2012). *Susto, coraje,* and abuse: Depression and beliefs about diabetes. *Culture, Medicine & Psychiatry, 36*(3), 480–492. doi: 10.1007/s11013-012-9267-x

Mickel, J. T., McGuire, S., & Gross-Gray, S. (2013). Grey's Anatomy and communication accommodation: Exploring aspects of nonverbal interactions portrayed in media. *Interpersona*, *7*(1), 138–149. doi: 10.5964/ijpr.v7i1.95

Montali, L., Frigerio, A., Riva, P., & Invernizzi, P. (2011). 'It's as if PBC didn't exist': The illness experience of women affected by primary biliary cirrhosis. *Psychology & Health*, *26*(11), 1429–1445. doi: 10.1080/08870446.2011.565876

Morgan, S. E., Movius, L., & Cody, M. J. (2009). The power of narratives: The effect of entertainment television organ donation storylines on the attitudes, knowledge, and behaviors of donors and nondonors. *Journal of Communication*, *59*(1), 135–151. doi: 10.1111/j.1460-2466.2008.01408.x

Nuttbrock, L. (1986). The management of illness among physically impaired older people: An interactionist interpretation. *Social Psychology Quarterly*, *2*, 180.

Office of Minority Health. (2018). *Cultural competency: NCLAS standards*. Retrieved from https://minorityhealth.hhs.gov/omh/browse.aspx?lvl=2&lvlid=53

Orem, S. (2017). (Un)necessary procedures: Black women, disability, and work in Grey's Anatomy. *African American Review*, *50*(2), 169. doi: 10.1353/afa.2017.0020

Quick, B. L. (2009a). The effects of viewing Grey's Anatomy on perceptions of doctors and patient satisfaction. *Journal of Broadcasting & Electronic Media*, *53*(1), 38–55. doi: 10.1080/08838150802643563

Quick, B. L. (2009b). Coverage of the organ donation process on Grey's Anatomy: The story of Denny Duquette. *Clinical Transplantation*, *23*(6), 788–793. doi: 10.1111/j.1399-0012.2008.00937.x

Rhimes, S. (Writer), & Tinker, M. (Director). (2005, October 23). Bring the pain. [Television series episode] In T. A. Casper, R. Corn, M. Schmir, G. G. Stanton, & H. Werksman (Producer), *Grey's Anatomy*. Hollywood: American Broadcasting Company.

Ryan, C. (2013). *Language use in the United States: 2011. American community survey reports*. United States Census Bureau. Retrieved from https://www.census.gov/prod/2013pubs/acs-22.pdf

Stohl, C., & Cheney, G. (2001). Participatory processes/paradoxical practices: Communication and the dilemmas of organizational democracy. *Management Communication Quarterly*, *14*, 349–407.

Villagran, M. M., Fox, L. J., & O'Hair, D. H. (2007). Patient communication processes: An agency-identity model for cancer care. In H. D. O'Hair, G. L. Kreps, & L. Sparks (Eds.), *The handbook of communication and cancer care* (pp. 127–144). Cresskill, NJ: Hampton Press, Inc.

Ye, Y., & Ward, K. E. (2010). The depiction of illness and related matters in two top-ranked primetime network medical dramas in the United States: A content analysis. *Journal of Health Communication*, *15*(5), 555–570. doi: 10.1080/10810730.2010.492564

CHAPTER SIXTEEN

Intercultural Health Communication Studies: Looking Forward

BY SATOSHI TOYOSAKI AND ANDREW R. SPIELDENNER

A few years ago, we met at a National Communication Association convention. Our life and professional paths crossed. Since then, we have been good colleagues and friends. I (Satoshi) specialized in critical intercultural communication studies. I was just embarking a new research project; I was interested in global peace pedagogy in and about Japan, paying attention to the atomic bomb survivors' narratives. I wanted to contemplate on a peace pedagogy that would connect atomic bomb survivor narratives and today's US-American students' intersectional identities. I wanted to work toward a peace pedagogy that would bridge intercultural, intergenerational, and interlinguistic gaps. Thinking about such a peace pedagogy might give me some hints about understanding various global conflicts, post-conflict healing, and peace-building. As I met with survivors and planed a study-abroad program to Japan, something hit me hard. I was conceiving of my research agenda as critical intercultural communication studies and pedagogy. Or at least, I thought I could approach it from those perspectives. I was wrong.

I had an opportunity to work with an atomic bomb survivor from Hiroshima a few years ago. I interpreted his lived experiences into English when he spoke in public settings in the United States. It was a precious professional and personal experience to me as a Japanese person and as a critical intercultural communication researcher/pedagogue. His story included Little Boy (the uranium atomic bomb dropped in Hiroshima), US-Japan histories, Japan's schooling back then, the day on which the bomb hit Hiroshima, his family, his friends, his recovery from injury and radiation sickness, and his hope and peace messages for future generations. I was reminded how international politics implicated people—their lives, their bodies, their health, their families, their classmates, and their friends. As a communication scholar, I was just starting to think of and questioning the boundary between intercultural communication and health communication. That was when I met Andy. I was drawn to his research, activism, public service, and his vision of being a university professor.

When I (Andrew) first met Satoshi, I wanted to know more. We had gone on different journeys—our lives vary wildly in experience and nationality—and ended up in the same space. At this academic conference, we stood out amidst our overwhelmingly White colleagues. Over the years, we have found common ground in trying to describe community processes within the narrow definitions of communication sub-disciplines. How is community trauma transmitted? How do people share and build resilience in the midst of structural and historical violence?

My own work has centered on HIV and its attendant contexts (in the US, this is mostly around sexuality, race, poverty, criminalization and substance use). When I was a teenager, I started in HIV because my boyfriend at the time got me a job. That boyfriend had HIV already and he taught me a lot about following my passions (especially comic books) and the joys of travel. Vince is Chamorro and learned his sexuality in New York City in the 1980s: a time and place where the lines between homosexual and heterosexual were far more blurred, especially in some venues (Delany, 1999). He also supported my experience that the categories of race and sexuality in the United States were not so strict, that there are liminal spaces for people like us; we remain friends to this day.

Since then, I have been involved in the HIV community in a variety of ways. Professionally, I have worked at a large health department as well as several community-based organizations. As I entered academia, I maintained my connection to HIV through national advocacy groups such as the US People living with HIV Caucus. Currently I am the North American Non-Governmental Organization representative to UNAIDS, the United Nations joint program on HIV. I have seen how multilateral and international concerns about HIV are not reflected accurately in the US context, where health departments and federal agencies are developing "End the Epidemic" plans. This distortion between the historicizing of HIV in the US and the still-present epidemic going on in the Global South has made me rethink my own approach.

As a health communication researcher and health advocate, I recognize that the US creates its own echo chamber: we read and write in English, we publish in the journals that are largely US-based, we convene largely with each other to discuss conditions in this country and imagine these are universal. Health communication needs to be able to engage voices and lives beyond our own borders. There is a need in health for frameworks that include international concerns and intercultural methods and theories.

So we met. Since then, we have been working together on this book project whose goal is to bridge health communication and international/intercultural communication studies particularly through interpretive and critical methodologies (Miller, 2002). We have been wanting to do interdisciplinary labor to bring Health Communication and Intercultural Communication together. Our labor is predicated upon our belief: Our disciplinary demarcations are artificial. This recognition is important especially for the field of communication studies because communication knows no boundaries. We believe the importance of interdisciplinary approaches in order to study and teach communication in a more holistic manner.

Such interdisciplinary approaches help us recognize how the field of communication studies has historically been implicated by racial and heterosexual structures (Yep, 2003, 2010) and other—isms (e.g., sexism, ableism, classism, etc.). Hannawa, Kreps, Paek, Schulz, Smith, and Street (2014) observe that "it is often challenging to publish a paper in top health communication journals with data collected outside of the United States" (p. 960). Toyosaki (2016), for example, writes that whiteness has crafty ability to hinge upon other oppressive systems, such as educational institutions and global knowledge economy (Toyosaki, 2018). These observations all point at that our research and education are not culturally neutral and invite us to be reflexive of how we research, learn, and teach communication. It is beneficial to develop more complicated and interdisciplinary approaches to study messy realities of health and cultures while recognizing that we productively fail to capture the holistic picture ever. Our epistemological labor toward complicated analyses of health and cultures is worth exploring in order to capture messy intersections of health and cultures.

Health communication and intercultural communication can benefit from each other. Such interdisciplinary initiative has already been taking place (Hannawa et al., 2014). Intercultural communication studies offer theoretical and methodological frameworks through which health politics can be interrogated in culturally complex manners. Intercultural communication studies benefits from studying health politics in order to meaningfully complicate cultural analysis and critique. This book celebrates that such labor has been taking place in both fields and continues to bring health communication and intercultural communication together particularly through a variety of interpretive and critical methodological approaches (Miller, 2002).

It has been such a privilege and honor to work with these exciting authors featured in this collection. As scholars who are interested in the critical intersection between health communication and international/intercultural communication studies, we have learned so much from these authors and their research projects. Working on this collection reminds us that it is essential that we continue to explore the interdisciplinary intersection. We are so vividly reminded that both health and cultures are unstable and messy concepts. We try to conceptually anchor and/or isolate them through our research methodologies (e.g., variables, communities, etc.); however, such anchoring and isolating might not reflect how people "experience" health and cultures simultaneously. Health and cultures are historically, communally, socially, economically, capitalistically, politically, and ideologically constructed and situated within global and domestic discourses and people's lives. Dutta (2008) explains that the biomedical model is indeed a cultural and institutionalized product that reinforces a particular kind of health, such as the Western view, and that permeates through the world via today's various globalizing effects (e.g., information and capital movements, etc.). Exploring how people experience the intersections of health and cultures ought to be messier than any singular methodological isolation and operationalization can accomplish.

Both health communication studies and intercultural communication studies use post-positivistic approaches (Miller, 2002) in order to isolate, define, and operationalize what it is that is being studied. For example, one particular health condition (e.g., cancer, HIV, depression, etc.) or one national/cultural identity (e.g., Japanese, African American, etc.) can function as a nominalist variable for analysis, which helps situate replicability in research, identify behavioral trends, and maximize predictability. Such methodological isolation, definition, and operationalization also function as a set of criteria for identifying research subject pools. These disciplines do this kind of work very well, and this approach is effective for what it is supposed to do.

Is this enough? Generally speaking, much of health communication scholarship aims at operationalizing and generalizing research findings. What becomes overlooked and neglected in the historical sweep of quantitative health communication research is how "health" moves through and among people, relationships, communities, societies, cultures, and worlds. Intercultural communication studies, globally speaking, follows the social scientific rubrics in generating research while it has been diversifying its methodological approaches. We need methodological approaches that help us capture messy realities that blur health and cultures and how we experience them simultaneously. Such a call has already been made for health communication studies (see Parrott & Kreuter, 2003; Hannawa, García-Jiménez, Candrian, Rossmann, & Schulz, 2015). Hannawa et al. (2014) indicate the future directions of the field of health communication. They write that "health communication researchers need to expand their international and interdisciplinary horizons" and that "health communication researchers need to collaborate intensively ... to expand their own interdisciplinary and intellectual networks" (p. 960). We are in agreement with these authors.

Intercultural communication scholars have been explicitly addressing this question, proposing dialectic approaches to intercultural communication research (Martin & Nakayama, 1999). Martin and Nakayama discuss four prominent paradigms utilized in the field of culture and communication; they are the functionalist, interpretive, critical humanist, and critical structuralist paradigms. The functionalist approach generally describes and predict human behaviors and sees culture as "a variable, defined a priori by group membership" (p. 4). Interpretivist researchers try to understand "the world as it is" (p. 5) and communication behaviors in contexts, rather than predicting them (p. 6). "Culture ... is generally seen as socially constructed and emergent" (p. 6). Critical humanist researchers understand human communication to be "dominated by ideological superstructures and material conditions that drive a wedge between them and a more liberated consciousness" (p. 8). Their research goal is to change social injustice created by ideological superstructures and material conditions. They see culture as "a site of struggle" for meanings (Fiske cited in Martin & Nakayama, 1999). The critical structuralist paradigm similarly promotes change as the critical humanist paradigm does. It sees culture as "societal structures." "This approach emphasizes the significance of the structures and material conditions that guide and constrain the possibilities of cultural contact, intercultural communication, and cultural change" (p. 9).

Martin and Nakayama (1999) labor toward a dialectic approach. "A dialectic approach accepts that human nature is ... both creative and deterministic; that research goal can be to predict, describe, and change; that the relationship between culture and communication is ... both reciprocal and contested" (p. 13). Thus, the dialectic approach to culture and communication helps us render more holistic and comprehensive understanding of cultures/communication within communication/cultures. It situates "the possibility of engaging multiple, but distinct, research paradigms [and] the possibility to see the world in multiple ways and to become better prepared to engage in intercultural interaction" (p. 13). Thus, the dialectic approach helps us get at the dynamic terrains of cultures and communication with paradigmatic and methodological agility, flexibility, and complexity.

Thinking of intercultural health communication studies, we believe that Martin and Nakayama's (1999) dialectic approach can function as an effective model. The dialectic approach to intercultural health communication studies is more comprehensive and productively messy in sprit of trying to get at people's lived experiences of health and cultures. The functionalist approach operationalizes health and cultures as variables. The interpretive approach understands health and cultures as socially constructed and co-emerging. The critical humanist approach emphasizes health and cultures as sites of struggle for competing meanings. Finally, the critical structuralist researchers see health and cultures as societal structures that hinge up each other to (re)produce materialistic realities. The dialectic approach, separately yet collectively, engages in research that predict, understand, and change human communicative practices at the intersections of health and cultures.

This book, in particular, engages the intersections among health and cultures from interpretive and critical perspectives, acknowledging that the fields have been effectively engaging the functionalist research (Cross, Davis, & O'Neil, 2017). Considering such approaches, we identify several major discussion points that intercultural health communication scholars can continue engaging. First, we need to host rigorous discussions in order to see how health communication theories and intercultural communication theories can inform and develop each other further. Interdisciplinary theory-building is advantageous for intercultural health communication.

Second, we need to attend to "theory" and "context" carefully in developing intercultural health communication studies further. We understand the importance of complex, particular, and nuanced contexts where health and cultures co-construct each other. How do we understand "context" in relation to research methodologies and theory-building? Oftentimes, in research "context" is filtered out through reductionist data analyses. How do we treat "context" methodologically in relation to theory-building in intercultural health communication studies? In situating the dialectic approach to intercultural health communication studies, we need to discuss a role of theory as we focus on the significance of politically complex, situationally particular, and ephemerally nuanced contexts where communication takes place. How do we research intercultural health communication in "moving contexts and factors such as histo[ies], structures, and economics" (Halualani & Nakayama, 2010, p. 10)? Halualani and Nakayama further complicate a relationship between theory and context. They explain Grossberg's point: "Critical work recognizes that there is no theory in advance and no social process of culture without some theoretical sense-making; it travels through a trajectory of theory from and toward context" (p. 9). The from-and-toward relationship of theory and context blurs the distinction between them and challenges us to (re)examine how we deploy and develop theories in our research. It may be productive to pause to (re) evaluate the important relationship between theory and context for intercultural health communication studies.

Third, intercultural health communication studies needs to engage more community-based ethnographic research. Such an approach productively complicates the notion and foregrounds the importance of "context." It also helps us reflexively challenge taken-for-granted assumptions (Davies, 1999) about health and cultures that we "acquire" often from our own cultural assumptions and educational training (Conle, 2004; Pathak, 2013) and that we embody—consciously or not—in our research, such as biomedicalism (Dutta, 2008), whiteness (Yep, 2010), ableism, heteronormativity (Yep, 2003), classism, masculinity, and so on. The concept of "community" is also important as some communities organize around specific health issues, as in the case of HIV (Spieldenner et al., 2019). Other times, the health issue impacts a particular community in a specific way, as in the case of police violence and the African American community. As a community, members are able to advocate for social justice and equity, as well as challenge social norms about illness. These communities develop their own borders and cultural practices that can be understood and navigated through intracultural communication. The communal borders are always redefined, reaffirmed, challenged, and changing as no community is simply homogenous, static, and isolated. Communities are internally shifting, externally overlapping, and constantly changing. Thus, examining the intersections among health and cultures requires complex and nuanced intercultural analysis. Community-based and ethnographic research in intercultural health communication studies is productive in getting "at" the localized complexities, nuance, and particularities (Spieldenner, 2017).

Fourth, it may be productive for intercultural health communication scholars to engage complex studies of intersectional identity/ies among various health situations and cultures. Identity research oftentimes relies on consensual theorization (Toyosaki, 2012). Consensual theorization is built on an assumption that "a common language serves to promote consensus by communicating shared meanings" (Fiske, 1991, p. 332). Theorizing identity management, for example, Imahori and Cupack (2005) focus on the communal, such as "shared systems of symbols and meanings as well as norms/rules for conduct" (p. 197). Communities are organized but are not homogenous. While the consensual approach renders productive analyses and findings, it may overlook the conflictual nature of intersectional identities present at a particular community; symbols and meanings are socially constructed and contested, and norms and rules for conduct are oftentimes reproductive of power, contended, and reconstituted (Spieldenner, 2016; Spieldenner et al., 2019). While the consensual approach is productive in one way, it may fall short in another way, which by the way is a nature of any methodological approach. Thus, our intention here is not to critique it but diversify our approaches especially when we engage the intersections among health situations and cultures.

For example, thick intersectionalities (Yep, 2010) and intersectional reflexivity (Jones, 2010) may function as methodological approaches to get at people's complex lived intercultural health experiences. Yep (2010) write;

> Thick intersectionalities call for an exploration of the complex particularities of individuals' lives and identities associated with their race, class, gender, sexuality, and national locations by understanding their history and personhood in concrete time and space, and the interplay between individual subjectivity, personal agency, systemic arrangements, and structural forces. (p. 173)

Thick intersectionalities is a significant research approach to explore how we live and experience the intersections among health situations and cultures. Rather than just listing identity markers (Jones & Calafell, 2012), intersectional analysis gets at the simultaneity of multiple identities at work while some aspects of intersectional identities may be emphasized, salient, and played up, and other aspects subdued, played down, and ignored. Thus, this invites our reflexive and ongoing efforts to make our intersectional analyses thicker. Jones (2010) explains;

> Engaging in intersectional reflexivity requires one to acknowledge one's intersecting identities, both marginalized and privileged, and then employ self-reflexivity, which moves one beyond self-reflection to the often uncomfortable level of self-implication. (p. 122)

Employing thick intersectionalities (Yep, 2010), we can interrogate contextually rich intersections of health situations and cultures, attending our intersecting identities at work. This thick intersectional approach helps us embody the from-and-toward relationship of theory and context in research and get "at" people's everyday lived-and-living intercultural health experiences.

Finally, it is productive that intercultural health communication scholars wrestle with how we situate "praxis" in our research. Schrag (1997) explains that praxis-oriented self is "defined by its communicative practices, oriented toward an understanding of itself in its discourse, its action, its being with others, and its experience of transcendence" (p. 9). In praxis-oriented research and pedagogy, we make our presence matter as narrative, self-reflexive, social, and cultural constructs for one another. Praxis-oriented research assists us pay attention to the "living" context and time. Schrag emphasizes the importance of the "living"; "the self is implicated in its discourse as a who that … understands itself as a self that has already spoken, is not speaking, and has the power yet to speak, suspended across the temporal dimensions of past, present, and future" (p. 17). Thus, the space and time of the "living" is the connective tissue of the past and future where possibility of human agency lies. In the "living," theory and context collide; we are to navigate the from-and-toward relationship of theory and context in observing, examining, analyzing, theorizing, critiquing, hoping, acting, and transforming.

Schrag (2003) further explains that "I" and "you" are coemergents within a network of intersubjectivities. "Every subject is a piece of the continent of other subjects" (p. 125). Our identities are necessarily dialogical, relational, and communal (Baxter & Montgomery, 1996). A praxis-oriented approach to intercultural health communication studies labors toward building networks of (inter)subjective narratives to catch how health situations and cultures intersect in the world in which we coexist. McKerrow (1993) warns our attempt to make a master text of social analysis; he, instead, endorses that "the goal is to pull together those fragments whose intersection in real lives has meaning for social actors ... As such, the invented text functions to enable historicized subjects to alter the conditions of their lived experiences" (p. 62). The act of "pulling together" to build the networks of praxis-oriented research labors toward social justice. Warren (2011) writes, "For me, social justice is about seeing the world in all its loss and imagining ways of healing" (p. 30). We as social beings are all implicated as subjects of social injustice either simultaneously as victims, doers, perpetuators, spectators, and/or accomplices. Social injustice works its way throughout various human activities, ranging from societal structures to our everyday ephemeral actions. Praxis-oriented intercultural health communication research pulls together narratives of the "living" to construct networks of the narratives to catch the world of social injustice and conceives of the "living" as the site of possibility for social justice.

Intercultural health communication studies cannot afford any paradigmatic battle on our research approaches. In front of us, we have a messy world to catch together. Human communicative practices of intersectional health-and-culture politics are drastically morphing and just too messy in various moving contexts whose borders are blurred and refuse to be demarcated. We need all available means to get at small pieces of the intersectional politics through our research, put them in dialogue, and pull them together if we want to catch it.

References

Baxter, L. A., & Montgomery, B. M. (1996). *Relating: Dialogue and dialectics.* New York, NY: The Guilford Press.

Conle, C. (2004). Texts, tensions, subtexts, and implied agendas: My quest for cultural pluralism in a decade of writing. *Curriculum Inquiry, 34*, 139–167.

Cross, R., Davis, S., & O'Neil, I. (2017). *Health communication: Theoretical and critical perspectives.* Cambridge, UK and Malden, MA: Polity Press.

Davies, C. A. (1999). *Reflexive ethnography: A guide to researching selves and others*. London, UK: Routledge.

Delany, S. R. (1999). *Times square red, times square blue*. New York, NY: New York University Press.

Dutta, M. J. (2008). *Communicating health: A culture-centered approach*. Cambridge, UK: Polity Press.

Fiske, J. (1991). Writing ethnographies: Contribution to a dialogue. *Quarterly Journal of Speech, 77*, 330–335.

Halualani, R. T., & Nakayama, T. K. (2010). Critical intercultural communication studies: At a crossroads. In T. K. Nakayama & R. T. Halualani (Eds.), *The handbook of critical intercultural communication* (pp. 1–16). Malden, MA: Wiley-Blackwell.

Hannawa, A. F., García-Jiménez, L., Candrian, C., Rossmann, C., & Schulz, P. J. (2015). Identifying the field of health communication. *Journal of Health Communication*, *20*(5), 521–530.

Hannawa, A. F., Kreps, G. L., Paek, H., Schulz, P. J., Smith, S., & Street, R. L. (2014). Emerging issues and future directions of the field of health communication. *Health Communication, 29*, 955–961.

Imahori, T. T., & Cupach, W. R. (2005). Identity management theory: Facework in intercultural relationships. In W. B. Gudykunst (Ed.), *Theorizing about intercultural communication* (pp. 195–210). Thousand Oaks, CA: Sage.

Jones, R. G., Jr. (2010). Putting privilege into practice through "intersectional reflexivity:" Ruminations, interventions, and possibilities. *Reflections: Narratives of Professional Helping, 16*(1), 122–125.

Jones, R. G., Jr., & Calafell, B. M. (2012). Contesting neoliberalism through critical pedagogy, intersectional reflexivity, and personal narrative: Queer tales of academia. *Journal of Homosexuality, 59*(7), 957–981.

Martin, J. N., & Nakayama, T. K. (1999). Thinking dialectically about culture and communication. *Communication Theory, 9*(1), 1–25.

McKerrow, R. E. (1993). Critical rhetoric and the possibility of subject. In I. Angus & L. Langsdorf (Eds.), *The critical turn: Rhetoric and philosophy in postmodern discourse* (pp. 51–67). Carbondale: Southern Illinois University Press.

Miller, K. (2002). *Communication theories: Perspectives, process, and contexts*. Boston, MA: McGraw Hill.

Parrott, R., & Kreuter, M. W. (2003). Multidisciplinary, interdisciplinary, and transdisciplinary approaches to health communication: Where do we draw the lines? In T. L. Thompson, R. Parrott, & J. F. Nussbaum (Eds.), *The Routledge handbook of health communication* (2nd ed., pp. 3–17). New York, NY: Routledge.

Pathak, A. (2013). Musings on postcolonial autoethnography. In S. Homan Jones, T. Adams, & C. Ellis (Eds.), *Handbook of autoethnography* (pp. 595–608). Walnut Creek, CA: Left Coast Press.

Schrag, C. O. (1997). *The self after postmodernity*. New Haven, CT: Yale University Press.

Schrag, C. O. (2003). *Communicative praxis and the space of subjectivity*. West Lafayette, IN: Purdue University Press.

Spieldenner, A. R. (2016). PrEP whores and HIV prevention: The queer communication of HIV Pre-Exposure Prophylaxis (PrEP). *Journal of Homosexuality*, *63*(12), 1685–1697.

Spieldenner, A. R. (2017). Infectious sex?: An autoethnographic exploration of HIV prevention. *QED: A Journal in LGBTQ Worldmaking*, *4*(1), 121–129.

Spieldenner, A. R., Sprague, L., Hampton, A., Smith-Davis, M., Peavy, D., Bagchi, A., … Brewer, R. (2019). From consumer to community-based researcher: Lessons from the PLHIV Stigma Index. In P. Kellett (Ed.), *Narrating patienthood: Engaging diverse voices on health, communication, and the patient experience* (pp. 151–166). New York, NY: Lexington Press.

Toyosaki, S. (2012). Praxis-oriented autoethnography: Performing critical selfhood. In N. Bardhan & M. P. Orbe (Eds.), *Identity research and communication: Intercultural reflections and future directions* (pp. 239–251). Lanham, MD: Lexington Books.

Toyosaki, S. (2016). Praxis-oriented whiteness research. *Journal of Multicultural Discourses*, *11*(3), 243–261.

Toyosaki, S. (2018). Toward de/postcolonial autoethnography: Critical relationality with the academic second persona. *Cultural Studies ↔ Critical Methodologies*, *18*(1), 32–42.

Warren, J. T. (2011). Social justice and critical/performative communicative pedagogy: A storied account of research, teaching, love, identity, desire, and loss. *International Review of Qualitative Research*, *4*, 21–33.

Yep, G. A. (2003). The violence of heteronormativity in communication studies: Notes on injury, healing, and queer world-making. *Journal of Homosexuality*, *45*(2–4), 11–59.

Yep, G. A. (2010). Toward the de-subjugation of racially marked knowledges in communication. *Southern Communication Journal*, *75*(2), 171–175.

About the Contributors

Nora Abdul-Aziz (Pre-Medicine student, University of Toledo) is Syrian-French-American pre-med undergraduate student who aims to specialize in surgery and improve the quality of care for underserved populations. Having witnessed the collective trauma in the Syrian diaspora and the emotional toll it has taken on her community, after obtaining her medical degree she aspires to engage in medical humanitarian action in the Middle East and North Africa with organizations such as *Médecins Sans Frontières.*

Ambar Basu (Ph.D., Purdue University) is a Professor in the Department of Communication at the University of South Florida. His research explores how intercultural communication provides a framework to understand meaning making on health, illness, and living in marginalized contexts. Philosophies of critical intercultural communication guide his scholarship. With particular emphasis on theorizing culture as a site of globalization and social change, Dr. Basu documents and analyzes intercultural health narratives that emerge from dialogue between the researcher and research participants. His research interest is in locating communication across cultures within geopolitical discourses of power, subordination, resistance, and agency.

Yea-Wen Chen (Ph.D., University of New Mexico) is an Associate Professor in the School of Communication at San Diego State University. Her research examines how communication—including silence—about cultural identities impacts diversity, inclusion, and social justice across contexts such as pedagogy, intercultural relating, and nonprofit organizing. She is currently serving as a Professor of Equity in Education leading and facilitating seminars on implicit biases and microaggressions on her campus.

Spring Cooper (Ph.D., Pennsylvania State University) is a social researcher with academic qualifications in public health, health promotion, and sexuality. Her academic background is in BioBehavioral Health, an interdisciplinary approach to health and prevention. Her Ph.D. focused on the sexual health education implications of menstrual attitudes and knowledge among women of varying socio-economic status in the United States. Since graduating Dr Cooper traveled to Australia, to undertake a Postdoctoral Fellowship with The University of Sydney at The Children's Hospital at Westmead Clinical School. She then taught for three years in the Masters of HIV, STIs, and Sexual Health at The University of Sydney. She joined CUNY SPH in 2015. Her current research interests are in adolescent sexual health, adolescent online and offline social networks, health promotion, health communication, and prevention of disease through behavior change and vaccination.

Patrick J. Dillon (Ph.D., University of South Florida) is an Assistant Professor in the School of Communication Studies at Kent State University at Stark. His scholarship explores health inequality in contemporary society. He uses qualitative research methods to examine how the day-to-day health experiences of marginalized populations are impacted by macro-level social forces, such as health policy, economic inequality, and racism. He focuses, in particular, on advancing health communication scholarship in three areas: (1) end-of-life, (2) HIV/AIDS, and (3) substance abuse.

Mohan J. Dutta (Ph.D., University of Minnesota) is Dean's Chair Professor of Communication and the Director of the Center for Culture-Centered Approach to Research and Evaluation, developing culturally-centered, community-based projects of social change that articulate health as a human right. His research examines the role of advocacy and activism in marginalizing structures, the relationship between poverty and health, political economy of global health policies, the mobilization of cultural tropes for the justification of neo-colonial health development projects, and how participatory culture-centered processes and strategies of radical democracy serve as axes of global social change.

Shinsuke Eguchi (Ph.D., Howard University) is Associate Professor in the Department of Communication and Journalism at the University of New Mexico.

Their research interests focus on global and transcultural studies, queer of color critique, intersectionality and racialized gender politics, Asian/Pacific/American studies, and performance studies. Their recent work has appeared for publication in *China Media Research*, *Critical Studies in Media Communication*, *Cultural Studies↔Critical Methodologies, Departures in Critical Qualitative Research*, and *Journal of Homosexuality*. They are also the co-editor of *Queer Intercultural Communication: The Intersectional Politics of Belonging in and across Differences* released from Rowman & Littlefield (Lanham, MD).

Tina M. Harris (Ph.D., University of Kentucky) is the Manship-Maynard Endowed Chair of Race, Media, and Cultural Literacy in the Manship School of Mass Communication at Louisiana State University. Her primary research interest is interracial communication. Her specific foci are critical communication pedagogy, race and identity, diversity and media representations, racial social justice, mentoring, and racial reconciliation, among others. She is a well-published and very active senior scholar with many accolades and awards for her longstanding continued contributions to the communication discipline.

Leandra H. Hernández (Ph.D., Texas A&M University), Assistant Professor of Communication Studies, enjoys teaching health communication, gender studies, and media studies courses. She utilizes Chicana feminist and qualitative approaches to explore Latina/o cultural health experiences, Latina/o journalism and media representations, and Latina/o cultural identities in reproductive justice and gendered violence contexts. She is the co-author of "Challenging Reproductive Control and Gendered Violence in the Americas: Intersectionality, Power, and Struggles for Rights," recipient of the 2018 NCA FWSD Studies Division Bonnie Ritter Award. She is also the co-editor of *This Bridge We Call Communication: Anzalduan Approaches to Theory, Method, and Praxis* and *Military Spouses with Graduate Degrees: Interdisciplinary Approaches to Thriving amidst Uncertainty*. She is the co-editor of the Lexington Press book series Lexington Studies in Health Communication and the Peter Lang Cultural Media Studies book series. Furthermore, as the Chair of the NCA La Raza Caucus and Latina/o Communication Studies Division, she works to foster the study of Latina/o Communication Studies for students and scholars alike.

Satveer Kaur-Gill (Ph.D., National University of Singapore) is an Instructor with the Chua Thian Poh Community Leadership Center (CTPCLC) at the National University of Singapore. Satveer's current research interests are in critical health communication, specifically looking at health experiences and inequalities among migrant domestic workers and low-income communities in Singapore. Her doctoral dissertation focused on heart health disparities among low-income

Malay community members. Satveer has published on the disenfranchisement of migrant domestic workers, media portrayals of migrant workers, and health information-seeking behaviors.

Nivethitha Ketheeswaran is a Ph.D. student in the Department of Communication at the University of South Florida. She has a M.A. in Communication from the University of South Florida. Her M.A. research focused on the intersections of race, policy, reproductive health, and communication. As a Ph.D. student Nivethitha continues to study health communication as well marginalization and resistance within organizations.

Lara Lengel (Ph.D., Ohio University) began her research program on intercultural and transnational communication as a Fulbright Research Scholar in Tunisia (1993–1994). Her refereed articles appear in, among others, *Journal of Health Communication*, *Journal of International and Intercultural Communication*, *International and Intercultural Communication Annual*, *French Journal for Media Research*, *Journal of Communication Inquiry*, *Feminist Media Studies*, *International Journal of Women's Studies*, *Text and Performance Quarterly*, and *Studies in Symbolic Interaction.*

Annette Madlock Gatison (Ph.D., Howard University) is an independent scholar and university professor. Gatison completed her doctoral work in Communication and Culture at Howard University. She is an award-winning author with over 40 publications and over 45 national and international professional presentations and workshops. Dr. Gatison's notable publications include: *Health Communication and Breast Cancer Among Black Women: Culture, Identity, Spirituality and Strength*, Lexington Books; and *Communicating Women's Health: Social and Cultural Norms that Influence Health Decisions*, Routledge.

P. Christopher Palmedo (Ph.D. and MBA, Portland State University) is an associate professor at the City of New York Graduate School of Public Health and Health Policy. Chris Palmedo teaches courses in health communications, social marketing, and health advocacy, and conducts an online certificate program in social marketing for health. His research focuses on junk food marketing to urban youth and on college student access to mental health and health insurance. He recently co-authored a college textbook which covers personal health in a public health context.

Sarah Parsloe (Ph.D., Ohio University) focuses on how individuals communicate to construct empowering health and disability identities in the face of uncertainty, doubt, stigma, and ableism. She considers how biosocial communities organize for collective and connective action. Her research has been featured in *Health*

Communication, The Journal of Applied Communication Research, Departures in Critical Qualitative Research, and *Information, Communication, & Society*. Her forthcoming book, *Falling in Love with the Process: Cultivating Resilience in Health Crises*, explores stroke survivorship and advocacy.

Gloria N. Pindi (Ph.D., Southern Illinois University Carbondale) is an Assistant Professor in the Department of Communication at California State University San Marcos. Her research lies in the area of critical intercultural communication, Black feminisms, and performance of the self in transnational context. Her scholarship focuses on African immigrants' process of identity negotiation in diasporic context with a critical approach to diversity and social justice.

Tomeka M. Robinson (Ph.D., Texas A & M University) is an Associate Professor of Rhetoric and Public Advocacy and is the Director Forensics at Hofstra University. Dr. Robinson's primary research and teaching foci are in Health, Organizational, and Intercultural Communication. She also regularly conducts research in forensic pedagogy. Additionally, Dr. Robinson serves at the Immediate Past President of Pi Kappa Delta National Forensics Honorary Association, on the Executive Boards of the Interstate Oratorical Association and the Southern and Northern Atlantic Forensic Union, and is a member of the Equity, Diversity, and Inclusion Committee of the National Forensics Association.

Shaunak Sastry (Ph.D., Purdue University) is an Associate Professor in the Department of Communication at the University of Cincinnati and Affiliate Faculty, Center for Culture-centered Research and Evaluation (CARE) at Massey University, New Zealand. His research and teaching interests are in the areas of health and culture, globalization and health, and community-partnered research. Some of his current projects explore structural and cultural politics of infectious and "emerging" diseases in the global South. Another line of research involves community-based interventions addressing racial and socioeconomic disparities in health outcomes in the United States. His work has been published in leading international peer-reviewed journals like *Health Communication, Communication Theory, Journal of Health Communication, Culture, Health & Sexuality, Frontiers in Communication, and Journal of International* and *Intercultural Communication*, in addition to several book chapters and more than 30 paper presentations at national and international conferences. He sits on the editorial boards of the journals *Health Communication* and *Frontiers in Communication*.

Katie D. Scott holds a BAC from the University of Tennessee and is a graduate student at the University of Georgia. Katie's research interests center on women's health communication, especially qualitative inquiry into communication about chronic pelvic and genital pain. She has also contributed to publications addressing issues of communication and race. Outside of the academy, Katie works as an advocate for residents at a domestic violence shelter.

Patrick Seick (M.A., Eastern Michigan University) is a doctoral candidate in the Department of Communication Studies at Southern Illinois University, Carbondale where his research interests include intercultural communication, critical communication pedagogy, disability studies, performances of disability, and popular culture representations of disability. Seick also serves as the Director of Forensics and as an instructor of communication studies at Eastern Michigan University.

Adam Smidi (Doctoral student, Bowling Green State University) is an advocate for and leader within the Muslim American community, involved in initiatives that focus on reversing the hateful rhetoric that has become associated with Islam. He has published and presented work in the areas of organizational and intercultural communication, the contested terrain of religious freedom for Muslims in the U.S., and how interfaith community-building can reduce religious and cultural marginalization.

Andrew R. Spieldenner (Ph.D, Howard University) is Associate Professor of Health Communication at California State University-San Marcos. He coordinates the US implementation of the Stigma Index for the Global Network of People with HIV/AIDS/North America, and serves as Vice-Chair of the US People Living with HIV Caucus. He currently represents Civil Society as North American Delegate to UNAIDS, the UN Joint Programme on HIV.

Shelby Swafford (M.A., Southern Illinois University, Carbondale) is a PhD student in Performance Studies and Women, Gender, and Sexuality Studies at Southern Illinois University, Carbondale. Her research interests broadly include feminist performance praxis, automethodologies, and reproductive justice. Specifically, her scholarship focuses on embodiments of reproductive health and storied health experiences.

Satoshi Toyosaki (Ph.D., Southern Illinois University, Carbondale) is an associate professor and the director of International Studies in the Department of Languages, Cultures, and International Trade at Southern Illinois University. He conducts interdisciplinary research on intercultural issues by employing qualitative, interpretive, and critical methodologies. In his recent research, he employs ethnographic methods and studies human health politics and intercultural/-linguistic/-generational peace pedagogy. He values, theorizes, and practices autoethnography as a pedagogical and dialogical mode for intercultural understanding.

Jillian A. Tullis (Ph.D., University of South Florida) is Associate Professor in the Department of Communication Studies at the University of San Diego. Her professional interests focus on health communication, specifically communication about dying and death. Tullis uses qualitative methods to study hospice team communication, tumor boards, quality of life, and a "good death." Her research has appeared in *Health Communication*, *Qualitative Research in Medicine & Healthcare*, *Journal of Medicine and the Person*, *Behavioral Sciences*, and *Departures in Critical Qualitative Research*.

Darren J. Valenta (M.A., West Chester University of Pennsylvania) is a doctoral candidate in the Department of Communication Studies at Southern Illinois University Carbondale. His research interests include stand-up comedy, anxiety, mental illness stigma, performance studies, critical communication pedagogy, and autoethnography.

Lindy Wagner (M.S., Kansas State University) is a doctoral student in the Communication Studies program at Southern Illinois University Carbondale where her focus of study is Intercultural Communication. Her research interests include colorism, dialogue, intercultural training, identity, and higher education institutions.

Phillip E. Wagner (Ph.D., University of Kansas) is a Clinical Assistant Professor of Communication in the Mason School of Business at the College of William and Mary, after having served as faculty member of Communication Studies and Regional Assistant Vice Chancellor of Academic Affairs at the University of South Florida Sarasota-Manatee. His research uses arts-based methods to interrogate issues of the body and identity. Phil's work has been featured in *Communication Quarterly*, the *Journal of Applied Communication Research*, *Women and Language*, and on the TED stage.

Kallia O. Wright (Ph.D., Ohio University) is a teacher-scholar. She has taught a variety of courses, including intercultural communication and health communication. She has been involved in several experiential-learning initiatives that focus on intercultural interactions. She has also received awards for teaching excellence. Originally from Jamaica, she is a qualitative researcher who examines narratives about chronic illness experiences and the impact of culture on those experiences. She has published work in the *Health Communication* journal, communication encyclopedias, and chapters of edited books.

Index

A

B

C

D

E

H

I

J

N

Q

R

S

Y

Health Communication

Gary L. Kreps, Series Editor

This series examines the powerful influences of human and mediated communication in delivering care and promoting health.

Books analyze the ways that strategic communication humanizes and increases access to quality care as well as examining the use of communication to encourage pro-active health promotion. The books describe strategies for addressing major health issues, such as reducing health disparities, minimizing health risks, responding to health crises, encouraging early detection and care, facilitating informed health decisionmaking, promoting coordination within and across health teams, overcoming health literacy challenges, designing responsive health information technologies, and delivering sensitive end-of-life care.

All books in the series are grounded in broad evidence-based scholarship and are vivid, compelling, and accessible to broad audiences of scholars, students, professionals, and laypersons.

For additional information about this series or for the submission of manuscripts, please contact:

Gary L. Kreps
University Distinguished Professor and Chair, Department of Communication
Director, Center for Health and Risk Communication
George Mason University Science & Technology 2, Suite 230, MS 3D6
Fairfax, VA 22030-4444
gkreps@gmu.edu

www.ingramcontent.com/pod-product-compliance
Ingram Content Group UK Ltd.
Pitfield, Milton Keynes, MK11 3LW, UK
UKHW021836100926
8556IPUK00004B/366

9 781433 156526